PEDIATRIC ONCOLOGY

Alberto Pappo (Ed.)

Pediatric Bone and Soft Tissue Sarcomas

With 65 Figures and 26 Tables

Springer

Alberto Pappo, MD
Department of Pediatrics
The Hospital for Sick Children
555 University Avenue
Toronto, ON M5G 1X8, Canada

Library of Congress
Control Number 2005925686

Springer Berlin Heidelberg New York
ISBN 978-3-540-40843-7
Springer Berlin Heidelberg New York
ISSN 1613-5318

Springer is a part of Springer Science+Business Media

springeronline.com

Medical Editor: Dr. Julia Heidelmann, Heidelberg, Germany
Desk Editor: Meike Stoeck, Heidelberg, Germany
Cover design: Erich Kirchner, Heidelberg, Germany
Layout: Bernd Wieland, Heidelberg, Germany
Production: Pro Edit GmbH, Heidelberg, Germany
Reproduction and typesetting: AM-productions GmbH, Wiesloch, Germany

21/3151 – 5 4 3 2 1 0
Printed on acid-free paper

Dedication

To my children Jonathan and Danielle,
who define the essence of my daily life.

To Jack, my brother and trusted friend.

To my patients and their families,
from whom I learn the meaning of compassion,
courage and caring.

Preface

The purpose of this book is to integrate the most recent advances in the diagnosis and treatment of pediatric bone and soft tissue sarcomas. The book is divided into two major sections, the first of which presents salient concepts in epidemiology, the impact of novel tools in imaging and molecular biology, and the underlying principles for continued drug development. In the second section, the book embarks on an up-to-date survey of the diagnosis and treatment of each specific disease, with particular emphasis on the need for an integrative, multidisciplinary approach to diagnosis and treatment.

I am indebted to my colleagues and collaborators who have contributed their ideas, time, and knowledge to this project. I am also grateful for the contributions and support of my colleagues and friends at The University of Texas Southwestern Medical School, St. Jude Children's Research Hospital, and the Hospital for Sick Children in Toronto. In particular, I would like to thank Drs. George Buchanan, Charles Pratt, William Crist, David Parham, Jim Anderson, and Larry Kun for their friendship, mentorship, and wisdom. Their teachings will continue to be an endless source of passion and inspiration. It is my wish that this book will provide answers, guidance and hope to medical professionals, children, and their families.

Alberto Pappo, MD

Contents

4 Local Control Issues in Pediatric Bone and Soft Tissue Sarcomas

John C. Breneman, David Rodeberg, Ruth F. Lavigne, Ken Brown, Eugene S. Wiener

5 Drug Discovery in Pediatric Bone and Soft Tissue Sarcomas Using In Vivo Models

Jennifer K. Peterson, Peter J. Houghton

6 Pediatric Rhabdomyosarcoma: Biology and Results of the North American Intergroup Rhabdomyosarcoma Trials

Alberto Pappo, Fred G. Barr, Suzanne L. Wolden

7 Non-Rhabdomyosarcoma Soft Tissue Sarcomas

Sheri L. Spunt, Suzanne L. Wolden, Deborah E. Schofield, Stephen X. Skapek

8 Fibrous and Fibrohistiocytic Tumors

Diane Nam, Benjamin A. Alman

Contributors

Benjamin A. Alman, MD
Division of Orthopaedic Surgery
and Program in Developmental Biology
Hospital for Sick Children, University of Toronto
555 University Avenue
Toronto, ON M5G 1X8, Canada

Fred G. Barr, MD
Department of Pathology and Medicine
The Children's Hospital of Philadelphia
34th Street and Civic Center Boulevard
Philadelphia, PA 19104-4399, USA

John C. Breneman, MD
Department of Radiation Oncology
University of Cincinnati, Barrett Cancer Center
234 Goodman Street, Cincinnati, OH 45219, USA

Ken Brown, MD
Department of Orthopedics
Vancouver Children's Hospital
4480 Oak Street, Room A207
Vancouver, British Columbia V6H 3V4, Canada

Thomas D. Henry, MD
Department of Radiological Sciences
Division of Diagnostic Imaging
St. Jude Children's Research Hospital
332 N. Lauderdale St.
Memphis, TN 38105-2794, USA

Fredric A. Hoffer, MD
Department of Radiological Sciences
Division of Diagnostic Imaging
St. Jude Children's Research Hospital
332 N. Lauderdale St.
Memphis, TN 38105-2794, USA

Peter J. Houghton, PhD
Department of Molecular Pharmacology
St. Jude Children's Research Hospital
332 N. Lauderdale Street
Memphis, TN 38105-2794, USA

Joseph Khoury, MD
Department of Pathology
St. Jude Children's Research Hospital
332 N. Lauderdale Street
Memphis, TN 38105-2794, USA

Matthew Krasin, MD
Radiological Sciences
St. Jude Children's Research Hospital
332 N. Lauderdale Street
Memphis, TN 38105-2794, USA

Ruth F. Lavigne, MD
Radiation Oncology, Barrett Cancer Center
234 Goodman Street, Cincinnati, OH 45219, USA

Mary E. McCarville, MD
Department of Radiological Sciences
Division of Diagnostic Imaging
St. Jude Children's Research Hospital
332 N. Lauderdale St.
Memphis, TN 38105-2794, USA

Paul A. Meyers, MD
Department of Pediatrics
Memorial Sloan Kettering Cancer Center
1275 York Ave., New York, NY 10021, USA

Rajaram Nagarajan, MD
Department of Pediatrics, Division of Epidemiology
University of Minnesota, 420 Delaware Street
SE, MMC 715, Minneapolis, MN 55455, USA

Diane Nam, MD
Resident in Orthopaedic Surgery
Hospital for Sick Children, University of Toronto
555 University Avenue
Toronto, ON M5G 1X8, Canada

Fariba Navid, MD
Department of Hematology/Oncology
St. Jude Children's Research Hospital
332 N. Lauderdale Street
Memphis, TN 38105-2794, USA

Alberto Pappo, MD
Department of Pediatrics
The Hospital for Sick Children
555 University Avenue
Toronto, ON M5G 1X8, Canada

Jennifer K. Peterson, PharmD
Department of Molecular Pharmacology
St. Jude Children's Research Hospital
332 N. Lauderdale Street
Memphis, TN 38105-2794, USA

David Rodeberg, MD
Pediatric Surgery, Mayo Clinic
200 1st Street, SW, Rochester, MN 55905, USA

Carlos Rodriguez-Galindo, MD
Department of Hematology/Oncology
St. Jude Children's Research Hospital
332 N. Lauderdale Street
Memphis, TN 38105-2794, USA

Julie A. Ross, PhD
Department of Pediatrics, Division of Epidemiology
University of Minnesota, 420 Delaware Street
SE, MMC 715, Minneapolis, MN 55455, USA

Deborah Schofield, MD
Department of Pathology
Children's Hospital of Los Angeles
4650 Sunset Boulevard, Los Angeles, CA 90027, USA

Stephen X. Skapek, MD
Department of Hematology/Oncology
St. Jude Children's Research Hospital
332 N. Lauderdale Street
Memphis, TN 38105-2794, USA

Logan Spector, PhD
Department of Pediatrics, Division of Epidemiology
University of Minnesota, 420 Delaware Street
SE, MMC 715, Minneapolis, MN 55455, USA

Sheri L. Spunt, MD
Department of Hematology/Oncology
St. Jude Children's Research Hospital
332 N. Lauderdale Street
Memphis, TN 38105-2794, USA

Timothy Triche, MD
Department of Pathology
Children's Hospital of Los Angeles
4650 Sunset Boulevard, Los Angeles, CA 90027, USA

Eugene S. Wiener, MD
Children's Hospital of Pittsburgh
3705 Fifth Avenue, Pittsburgh, PA 15213, USA

Suzanne L. Wolden, MD
Department of Radiation Oncology
Memorial Sloan Kettering Cancer Center
1275 York Avenue, New York, NY 10021-6094, USA

Epidemiology of Bone and Soft Tissue Sarcomas

Logan G. Spector, Julie A. Ross,
Rajaram Nagarajan

Contents

1.1 Descriptive Epidemiology of Bone Tumors

Osteosarcoma (OS) and Ewing's sarcoma (ES) together form the large majority of bone cancers in persons less than 20 years old. The contrast between the patterns of incidence of these two malignancies is interesting, particularly with respect to race and tumor location. Thus, perhaps more so than for other childhood cancers, the descriptive epidemiology has guided etiologic investigations of OS and ES.

1.2 Worldwide Statistics

Bone sarcomas are rare worldwide, with combined rates mostly between 2 and 8 cases per 1,000,000 children aged 0–14 years (Parkin et al. 1998). Figure 1.1 shows the incidence rates for OS and ES in 50 populations worldwide. Whereas the rates of OS are similar between nations, a severalfold difference in incidence of ES is apparent when comparing white Europeans and Americans to Asians, Africans, and black Americans. However, the two cancers are similar in that incidence peaks during adolescence in most nations.

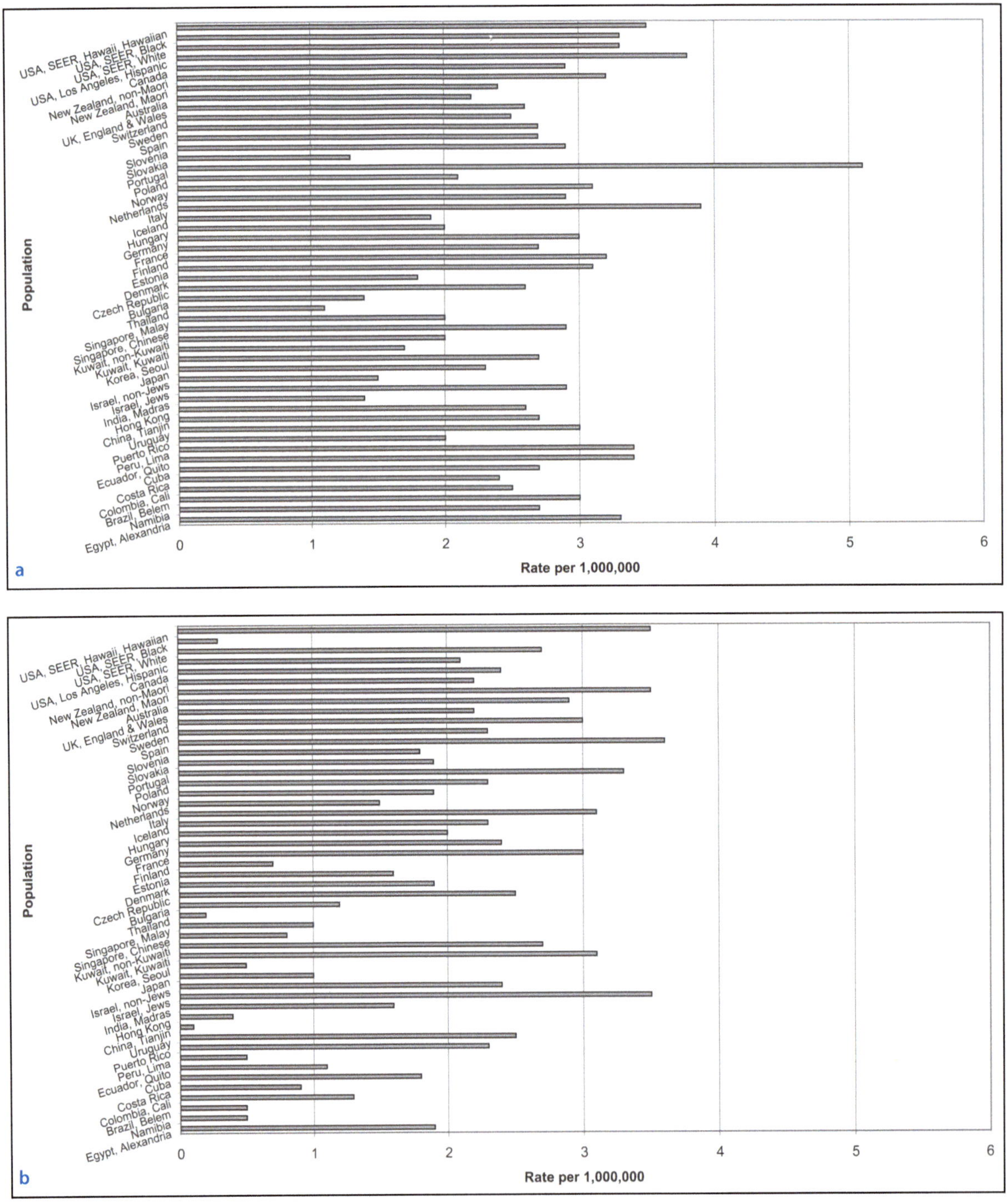

Figure 1.1

a Worldwide rates of osteosarcoma, ages 0–14 years. **b** Worldwide rates of Ewing's sarcoma, ages 0–14 years

1.3 North American Statistics

An estimated 650–700 bone cancers are diagnosed each year in the United States in children 0–19 years of age, 53% of which are OS and 35% ES (Ries et al. 1999; Ries et al. 2004). In Canada 57% and 38% of the 357 cases diagnosed in children 0–19 years of age in 1996–2000 were OS and ES, respectively (McLaughlin et al. 2004). Chondrosarcomas account for about half of the remaining bone tumors. Together the bone sarcomas accounted for 5.5% of malignancies in persons younger than 20 years in North America (McLaughlin et al. 2004; Ries et al. 2004).

The overall rates for OS are 4.6 and 4.5 cases per million children ages 0–19 years in the United States (Ries et al. 2004) and Canada (McLaughlin et al. 2004), respectively. The corresponding rates for ES are 3.0 and 2.9 cases per million children. Overall rates, however, do not convey the substantial variation in incidence of the bone sarcomas by age (Fig. 1.2). Both OS and ES are very rare in early childhood but have a markedly peaked incidence in adolescence (Ries et al. 2004). It should also be noted that incidence among young adults (20–24 years) is also substantial but lower than at the peak during adolescence (Wu et al. 2003). Neither the rate of OS nor of ES has changed significantly between 1987 and 2001 in the United States (Ries et al. 2004).

The rate of the bone sarcomas is somewhat higher in males than in females (ratio 1.2:1) (Ries et al. 1999). Figure 1.3 shows the sex-specific incidence rates in SEER by single year of age. Interestingly, the peak incidence in females comes 2 years earlier, at age 13, than does that of males.

Osteosarcoma occurs at roughly the same rate among blacks and whites, with the ratio being 1.15 (Gurney et al. 1995). Ewing's sarcoma, by contrast, has a substantially higher rate of occurrence in white than in black children. The rate of ES in the former group is 11 times that of the latter (Gurney et al. 1995).

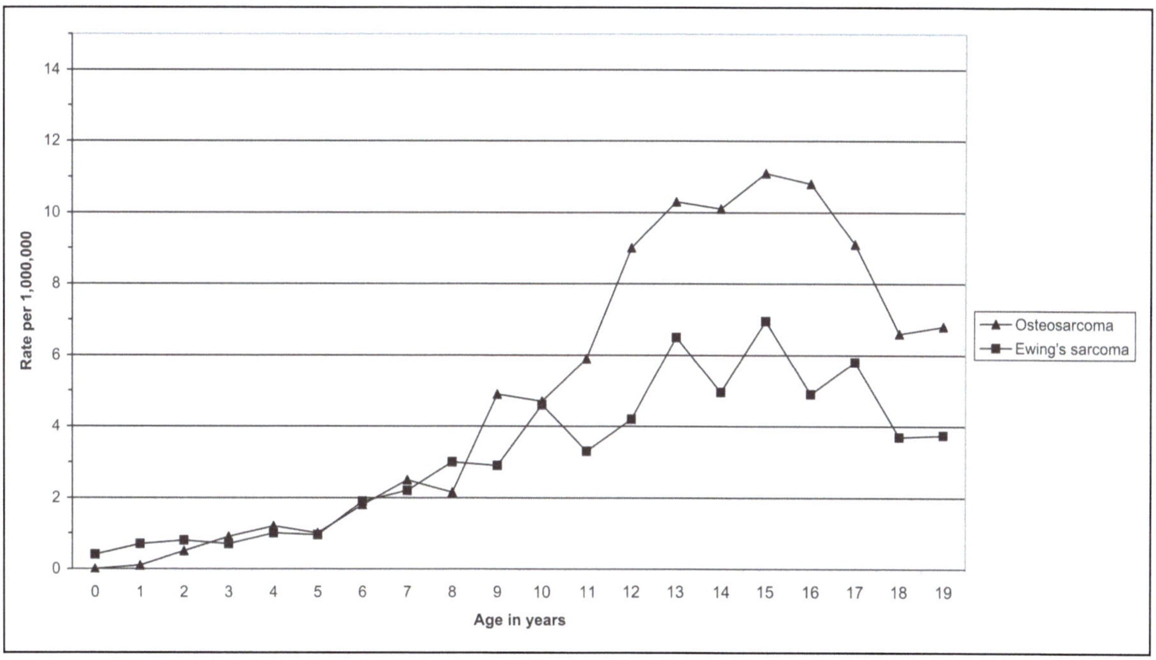

Figure 1.2

Incidence rates of osteosarcoma and Ewing's sarcoma by single year of age, SEER, 1976–1984 and 1986–1994, combined

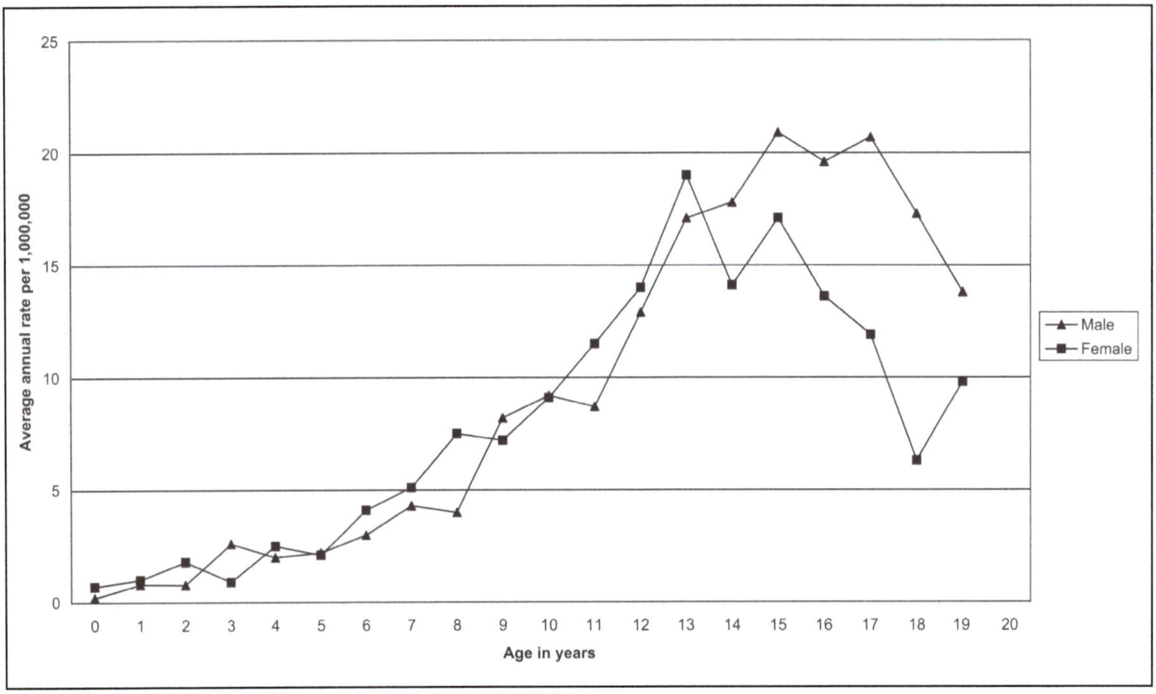

Figure 1.3

Bone cancer incidence rates by sex, SEER, 1976–1984 and 1986–1994

Tumor location is also strikingly different between the two main bone sarcomas. Nearly 80 % of OS cases occur in the long bones of the lower limbs and only about 5 % in the central axis. However, 45 % of ES cases occur in the central axis and 30 % in the lower limbs (Ries et al. 1999). Less than 20 % of OS (Kager et al. 2003; Kaste et al. 1999) and ES (Paulussen et al. 1998) present with metastatic disease at diagnosis.

These facts suggest that OS and ES have distinct etiologies. It was noted some time ago that the age-incidence curve of bone tumors closely follows the childhood growth curve (Fraumeni 1967) and, moreover, the incidence of bone tumors peaks earlier in females, which coincides with their reported earlier growth spurts (Staheli 2003). These data indicate that bone growth and development play a role in the occurrence of bone sarcomas and OS in particular, since OS, but not ES, appears frequently in the distal femur and proximal tibia (Price 1958), which are sites that contribute the most to the lengthening of the leg during the adolescent growth spurt (Staheli 2003). Meanwhile, the gross racial disparity in the occurrence of ES and its more proportional distribution among the bones of the body imply a genetic predisposition.

1.4 Mortality and Survivorship

Mortality due to malignant bone tumors is higher than that for childhood cancers overall. In 1985–2000 in SEER the 5-year survival rate was 65.4 % for bone cancers among children aged 0–19 years compared to 76.1 % for all childhood cancers combined (Ries et al. 2004). However, the survival rate for childhood bone cancers in the most recent decades shows a substantial improvement over the previously reported rate of

42% for the 1975–1984 period (Ries et al. 1999). Survival is only slightly higher for OS than for ES, with respective rates of 64.3% and 61.5%. Survival of females is noticeably better than that for males for both bone sarcomas. Among females 68% with OS and 67% with ES survive 5 years compared with about 62% and 58% of males (Ries et al. 2004).

As more pediatric bone tumor patients are surviving their bone cancer, there will be more survivors who have been exposed to the high doses of chemotherapy and suffered the effects of surgery (limb-sparing or amputation) or radiation. The effects of chemotherapy range from potential cardiotoxicity to development of secondary malignancies and are described elsewhere (Bhatia et al. 2003). Unique to bone tumor survivors are issues relating to the methods of surgical removal of the tumor. Since the vast majority of bone tumor lesions occur in the extremities, amputation had been the standard of care. Over time limb sparing surgery techniques (e.g., endoprosthesis, allografts and composites) came to the forefront on the belief these techniques would provide improved function and quality of life over amputation. This has been borne out in the upper extremity lesions (Aboulafia and Malawer 1993; Cheng and Gebhardt 1991), but substantial differences have not been found in the lower extremity (Nagarajan et al. 2002). Overall it appears that bone tumor survivors do well over time; however, prospective follow-up of these survivors is needed to further assess the impact of the diagnosis and treatment, especially since surgical techniques and materials are continually evolving.

1.5 Etiology of Bone Sarcomas

Etiologic studies of bone sarcomas are few, but intriguing. Most studies have distinguished between OS and ES, though some have lumped them together. More recently ES and primitive neuroectodermal tumors (PNETs) have been grouped together in studies as the Ewing sarcoma family of tumors (ESFT), based on the observation that both malignancies display t(11;22) chromosomal rearrangements (Arvand and Denny 2001).

As with most childhood cancers only a few risk factors are firmly established which account for a minority of cases. However, some putative risk factors have been associated with ES with surprising consistency for such a small literature. Furthermore, though a link between OS and bone development is not consistently seen in analytic studies it is strongly implied by the descriptive epidemiology. Many other exposures have been the subject of exploratory study.

Risk of OS is decidedly raised in children with Li-Fraumeni (Li et al. 1988), hereditary retinoblastoma (Hansen et al. 1985; Wong et al. 1997), and Rothmund-Thomson syndromes (Leonard et al. 1996). Germline mutations of p53, Rb, and RECQL4, respectively, underlie these syndromes. Somatic mutations of the former two genes are commonly found in sporadic OS (Miller et al. 1996) while those in the latter are not (Nishijo et al. 2004). Given the rarity of these genetic syndromes they account for only a small percentage of OS cases. The dramatic racial difference in ES incidence (Ries et al. 1999) suggests a genetic predisposition for the disease. However, the data offer little support for a raised risk of ES or other cancers among family members of cases (Buckley et al. 1996; Hartley et al. 1991; Li and Hemminki 2002; Novakovic et al. 1994).

Previous treatment for cancer is a known risk factor for bone sarcomas. Radiation and alkylating agents both increase risk independently in a dose-dependent manner (Hawkins et al. 1996; Tucker et al. 1987). However, absolute risk of secondary bone sarcoma is still low, with only about 1% of childhood cancer survivors developing it within 20 years of primary diagnosis in one cohort (Hawkins et al. 1996).

Height is one aspect of development that has frequently been examined in the bone sarcomas. An early impetus for this line of research was the observation that OS in dogs is more common in large breeds than in small ones (Tjalma 1966). In humans, Fraumeni found that cases of OS, and to a lesser degree ES, were significantly taller at diagnosis than were children with other cancers (Fraumeni 1967). The finding that OS cases are taller than controls has been corroborated in two studies (Gelberg et al. 1997; Ruza et al. 2003) but not others (Buckley et al. 1998; Operskalski et al. 1987). Height was not a significant risk factor for ES in two studies (Buckley et al. 1998; Holly et al. 1992). Lastly, Cotterill et al. compared the heights of United Kingdom OS and ES case series to national reference data (Cotterill et al. 2004). They found that OS patients were significantly taller, adjusted for age and sex, than the general UK population ($p = 0.001$); this association was especially pronounced for tumors located in the femur ($p = 0.0001$). While ES patients were not significantly taller than the reference population overall, those diagnosed at ages less than 15 years were ($p = 0.004$).

One reason for the inconsistency of these findings may be the complexity of growth. The absolute height at diagnosis may not be as relevant as the rate at which it was attained. Meanwhile, anthropometric studies do not indicate that taller children necessarily grow faster than do smaller ones (Gasser et al. 1985a, 1985b; Largo et al. 1978; Tanner et al. 1976). In light of this, some investigators have attempted to quantify cases' and controls' rate of growth (Buckley et al. 1998; Gelberg et al. 1997; Operskalski et al. 1987). Another method has been to examine birth weight and length (Buckley et al. 1998; Gelberg et al. 1997; Hartley et al. 1988; Operskalski et al. 1987), which may be proxies for the rate of growth in later life (Sorensen et al. 1999). Neither approach has revealed a consistent pattern with OS or ES.

The age at puberty, as measured by the appearance of secondary sexual characteristics, has also been of interest. Two studies of OS did not find significant associations with these variables (Buckley et al. 1998; Gelberg et al. 1997). One study of ES found a significant inverse trend in risk of the disease with the age at first shave (Valery et al. 2003), while another found little association with pubertal factors (Buckley et al. 1998). Earlier age at puberty implies an earlier onset of the adolescent growth spurt, which has itself been investigated in relation to the bone sarcomas to little effect (Buckley et al. 1998; Gelberg et al. 1997).

However, one study in Rottweiler doges suggested that endogenous hormone exposure itself may influence risk of OS apart from growth (Cooley et al. 2002). In this study the investigators found that the risk of OS rose significantly with an earlier age of gonadectomy among both male (p for trend $= 0.008$) and female (p for trend $= 0.006$) dogs, independent of size.

Parental occupational exposures have been frequent topics of study in bone sarcoma etiology. In general this line of research has generated only isolated reports of associations with OS (Buckley et al. 1998; Gelberg et al. 1997; Hartley et al. 1988; Hum et al. 1998; Operskalski et al. 1987) or ES (Buckley et al. 1998; Hartley et al. 1988; Holly et al. 1992; Hum et al. 1998; Valery et al. 2002). However, parental agricultural work has been significantly associated with ES, or nearly so, in three studies (Holly et al. 1992; Hum et al. 1998; Winn et al. 1992). In a fourth study parental occupation in agriculture was significantly associated with ESFT at ages less than 20 years, though not overall (Valery et al. 2002). Farm work implies exposure to a number of possible risk factors, including zoonoses and pesticides. Pesticides have been investigated in two studies (Holly et al. 1992; Valery et al. 2002), one of which found a significant positive association with ES (Holly et al. 1992).

Intriguingly, an association of ES with hernia has been suggested by four studies. Holly et al. first reported that risk of ES was increased in children with hernias diagnosed by age 3 years ($p = 0.11$) (Holly et al. 1992) and Winn et al. reported a significant association with any type of hernia without reference to age (OR = 5.7; 95% CI: 1.7–19.3) (Winn et al. 1992). Two later studies found significant associations specifically with inguinal hernias (Cope et al. 2000; Valery et al. 2003). A fifth study appears not to have found an association of ES with hernia (Buckley et al. 1998). Hernias, and the surgery to correct them, are memorable events, so these findings are unlikely to be due to recall bias. The etiology of hernias is itself obscure, but some seem to have their origin during gestation (Clarnette and Hutson 1996; Greer et al. 2003). Thus the apparent association with hernia may signal that in utero exposures play a role in the development of ES.

Several case-control studies have examined exposures to fluoride and radium, mainly in drinking water, in relation to bone sarcomas. Both substances are deposited in the bones and the latter is, of course, radioactive. Three studies found no association of OS with fluoride (Gelberg et al. 1995; McGuire et al. 1991;

Moss et al. 1995). Of the three studies that have examined radium in drinking water, one found no association while the others tentatively suggested a weak positive association (Finkelstein 1994; Finkelstein and Kreiger 1996; Moss et al. 1995).

Some evidence hints that infections have a role in bone sarcoma etiology, though few epidemiological studies have directly addressed the topic. Simian virus 40 (SV40), JC, and BK viruses comprise the polyomavirus family. The T antigen expressed by polyomaviruses interferes with the function of the p53 and Rb tumor suppressor genes (Barbanti-Brodano et al. 1998; Fanning 1998) and defects in these genes increase the risk of OS. SV40 has been show to induce OS in hamsters (Diamandopoulos 1973) and has been detected in OS tissue (Carbone et al. 1996; Mendoza et al. 1998; Yamamoto et al. 2000). However, studies that have followed children who received early batches of poliovirus vaccine that were contaminated with SV40 have not generally supported an increased risk of OS (Carroll-Pankhurst et al. 2001; Engels et al. 2003; Fisher et al. 1999; Olin and Giesecke 1998; Strickler et al. 1998). Case-control studies of the bone sarcomas have not indicated an association with childhood (Hartley et al. 1988; Holly et al. 1992) or maternal infections (Hartley et al. 1988). Also, little evidence supports the temporal (Glass and Fraumeni 1970; Moss et al. 1995; Ross et al. 1999) or spatial (Glass and Fraumeni 1970; Silcocks and Murrells 1987) clustering of bone sarcoma diagnoses, which can be indicative of an infectious etiology.

Lastly, a number of exploratory analyses of other factors have not demonstrated any noteworthy associations with bone sarcomas. These include parental smoking (Hartley et al. 1988; Holly et al. 1992; Valery et al. 2003; Winn et al. 1992), medications taken by mother or child (Hartley et al. 1988; Holly et al. 1992; Valery et al. 2003; Winn et al. 1992), and in utero or postnatal diagnostic X-rays (Hartley et al. 1988; Holly et al. 1992; Operskalski et al. 1987; Valery et al. 2003; Winn et al. 1992). An association with bone fracture, particularly at the tumor site, was suggested by one study (Operskalski et al. 1987) but not in subsequent studies (Buckley et al. 1998; Holly et al. 1992).

1.6 Bone Sarcomas: Future Directions

As with much of cancer epidemiology, molecular methods will become increasingly important in the study of bone sarcoma etiology. Growth and development are under substantial genetic control (Sharma 1983; Silventoinen et al. 2003) and genes that regulate these processes would be a natural starting point for future investigations. At least one study has already followed this line of research. Ruza et al. compared the frequency of polymorphisms in the vitamin D receptor, estrogen receptor, and collagen Iα1 genes in a small, hospital-based series of Spanish bone sarcoma cases (72 OS, 53 ES) to that of controls with mostly null results (Ruza et al. 2003). The striking racial disparity in ES may also be exploited using admixture analysis to identify chromosomal regions involved in disease susceptibility (Smith et al. 2004). Research into the etiology of the bone sarcomas continues to hold promise.

1.7 Epidemiology of Soft Tissue Sarcomas

The soft tissue sarcomas (STS) comprise a diverse group of malignancies. Rhabdomyosarcoma (RMS) is the largest diagnostic group and is itself divided into embryonal and alveolar types. Non-RMS diagnoses include fibrosarcoma, malignant fibrous histiocytoma, leiomyosarcoma, liposarcoma, and synovial sarcoma, among others. Most of these malignancies constitute less than 5% of STS at ages 0–19 years and none constitutes more than 10%. Kaposi's sarcoma (KS) makes up an appreciable percentage of STS in adulthood but, being AIDS-related, is rare in childhood in North America (Ries et al. 1999).

Internationally the incidence of STS among children ages 0–14 years varies moderately from a low of about 3 cases per million in Asian nations to 12 cases per million in North America. However, exceptionally high rates of KS are seen in Uganda and Zimbabwe likely due to the AIDS epidemic (Parkin et al. 1998).

About 850–900 STS are diagnosed each year in the United States in children 0–19 years of age (Ries et al. 1999). About 48% of these cases are RMS and 23% FS

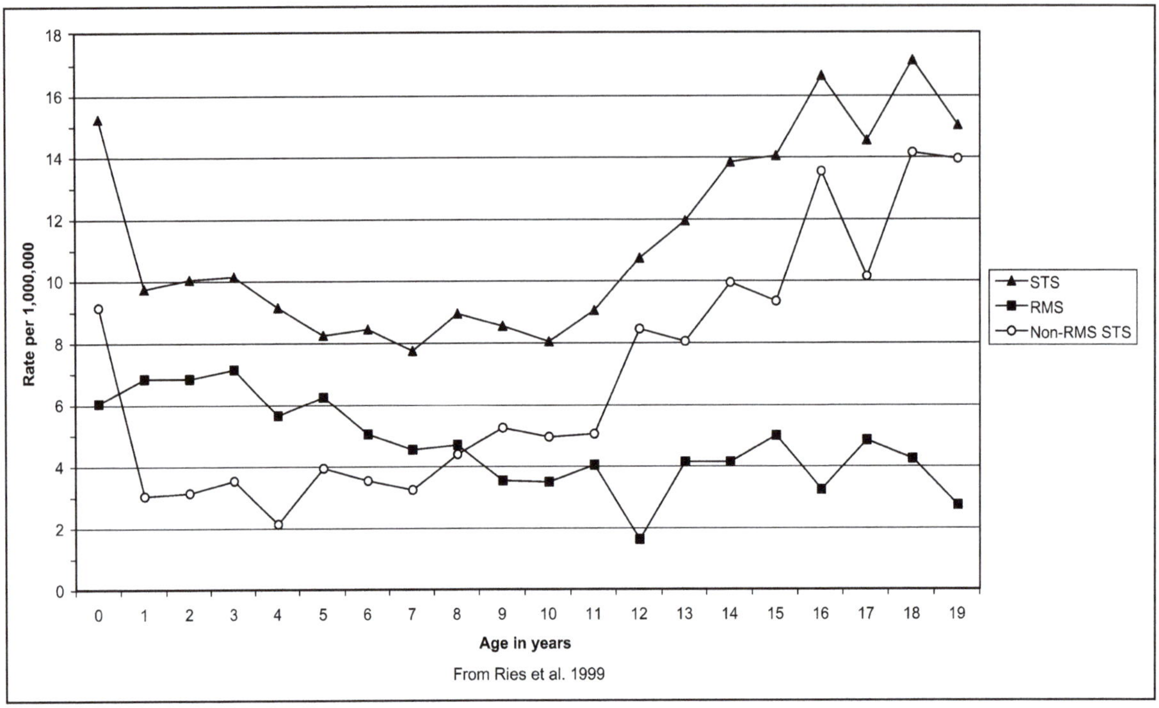

Figure 1.4

Incidence rates of soft tissue sarcoma (STS), rhabdomyosarcomas (RMS), and non-RMS soft tissue sarcomas by single year of age, SEER, 1976–1984 and 1986–1994, combined

(Ries et al. 2004). In Canada between 1996 and 2000 there were 397 cases of STS, 158 of which were RMS and 61 FS, diagnosed at ages 0–19 years (McLaughlin et al. 2004). STS comprised 6–7% of malignancies in persons younger than 20 years in North America (McLaughlin et al. 2004; Ries et al. 2004).

The rates of STS and RMS are 11.5 and 4.5 cases per million children ages 0–19 years, respectively, in the United States (Ries et al. 2004) and 10 and 4 cases per million, respectively, in Canada (McLaughlin et al. 2004). Figure 1.4 depicts the incidence of overall, RMS, and non-RMS soft tissue sarcomas by age. Incidence of RMS is highest in infancy and is lower and level at later ages. The proportion of RMS that is embryonal declines from 70% among children ages 0–5 years to 50% among children ages 15–19 years old (Ries et al. 1999). In the pediatric population non-RMS soft tissue sarcomas have their highest incidence in adolescence (Ries et al. 1999), though the rate is even higher among young adults aged 20–24 years (Wu et al. 2003). Incidence of STS is slightly higher among blacks compared to whites (ratio = 1.2) and among males compared to females (ratio = 1.15) (Ries et al. 1999). In the United States the rate of STS increased significantly ($p < 0.05$) by about 1% per year between 1975 and 2001 (Ries et al. 2004). The 5-year survival rate was 71.4% for STS and 64.9% for RMS among children aged 0–19 years in SEER in 1985–2000 (Ries et al. 2004).

Due to its rarity and diagnostic diversity very little is known about the etiology of STS in childhood. Li-Fraumeni syndrome (Li et al. 1988; Malkin et al. 1990) and neurofibromatosis (Hartley et al. 1988), involving germline mutations of the p53 and NF1 genes, respectively, are both known to increase the risk of STS. Beckwith-Wiedemann (Koufos et al. 1985) and Costello (Gripp et al. 2002) birth syndromes have been linked to STS in general and RMS in particular. Birth defects have also been so linked, though with less consistency (Hartley et al. 1994; Ruymann et al. 1988; Yang et al. 1995). Previous treatment for childhood cancer with radio- or chemotherapy has also been found to raise the risk of secondary STS (Menu-Branthomme et al. 2004). Only a small proportion of STS cases are explained by these factors.

Very few case-control studies of childhood STS (Hartley et al. 1988; Magnani et al. 1989) or RMS (Ghali et al. 1992; Grufferman et al. 1982, 1991, 1993) have been conducted, most of which included 100 or fewer cases (Ghali et al. 1992; Grufferman et al. 1982; Hartley et al. 1988; Magnani et al. 1989). There were over 300 cases of RMS and as many controls in the largest study, by Grufferman et al., which found significant positive associations of the disease with in utero X-rays and parental use of recreational drugs (Grufferman et al. 1991, 1993). Three much smaller studies found positive associations of STS or RMS with advanced maternal age (Grufferman et al. 1982; Magnani et al. 1989), maternal toxemia during pregnancy (Hartley et al. 1988), and fewer previous pregnancies among mothers (Hartley et al. 1988). Other positive associations were found with in utero exposure to radiation (Magnani et al. 1989), paternal cigarette smoking (Grufferman et al. 1982), and lower socioeconomic status (Grufferman et al. 1982). Lastly, Ghali et al. found a positive trend in the risk of RMS in children with the number of previous stillbirths in their mothers ($p = 0.0004$) (Ghali et al. 1992). Another study of relatives of STS cases suggested that fetal loss may be a function of predisposing familial cancer syndromes (Hartley et al. 1994).

Acknowledgements. This work was supported by the Children's Cancer Research Fund.

References

Aboulafia AJ, Malawer MM (1993) Surgical management of pelvic and extremity osteosarcoma. Cancer 71 (10 Suppl): 3358–3366

Arvand A, Denny CT (2001) Biology of EWS/ETS fusions in Ewing's family tumors. Oncogene 20(40):5747–5754

Barbanti-Brodano G et al. (1998) BK and JC human polyomaviruses and simian virus 40: natural history of infection in humans, experimental oncogenicity, and association with human tumors. Adv Virus Res 50:69–99

Bhatia S, Landier W, Robison L (2003) Late effects of childhood cancer therapy. In: DeVita V, Hellman S, Rosenberg S (eds) Progress in oncology. Jone and Barlett Publications, Sudbury, MA. pp 171–201

Buckley JD et al. (1996) Concordance for childhood cancer in twins. Med Pediatr Oncol 26(4):223–229

Buckley JD et al. (1998) Epidemiology of osteosarcoma and Ewing's sarcoma in childhood: a study of 305 cases by the Children's Cancer Group. Cancer 83(7):1440–1448

Carbone M et al. (1996) SV40-like sequences in human bone tumors. Oncogene 13(3):527–535

Carroll-Pankhurst C et al. (2001) Thirty-five year mortality following receipt of SV40-contaminated polio vaccine during the neonatal period. Br J Cancer 85(9):1295–1297

Cheng EY, Gebhardt MC (1991) Allograft reconstructions of the shoulder after bone tumor resections. Orthop Clin North Am 22(1):37–48

Clarnette TD, Hutson JM (1996) The genitofemoral nerve may link testicular inguinoscrotal descent with congenital inguinal hernia. Aust N Z J Surg 66(9):612–617

Cooley DM et al. (2002) Endogenous gonadal hormone exposure and bone sarcoma risk. Cancer Epidemiol Biomarkers Prev 11(11):1434–1440

Cope JU et al. (2000) Inguinal hernia in patients with Ewing sarcoma: a clue to etiology. Med Pediatr Oncol 34(3): 195–199

Cotterill SJ et al. (2004) Stature of young people with malignant bone tumors. Pediatr Blood Cancer 42(1):59–63

Diamandopoulos GT (1973) Induction of lymphocytic leukemia, lymphosarcoma, reticulum cell sarcoma, and osteogenic sarcoma in the Syrian golden hamster by oncogenic DNA simian virus 40. J Natl Cancer Inst 50(5):1347–1365

Engels EA et al. (2003) Cancer incidence in Denmark following exposure to poliovirus vaccine contaminated with simian virus 40. J Natl Cancer Inst 95(7):532–539

Fanning E (1998) Introduction to simian virus 40: getting by with more than a little help from its host cell. Dev Biol Stand 94:3–8

Finkelstein MM (1994) Radium in drinking water and the risk of death from bone cancer among Ontario youths. CMAJ 151(5):565–571

Finkelstein MM, Kreiger N (1996) Radium in drinking water and risk of bone cancer in Ontario youths: a second study and combined analysis. Occup Environ Med 53(5):305–311

Fisher SG, Weber L, Carbone M (1999) Cancer risk associated with simian virus 40 contaminated polio vaccine. Anticancer Res 19(3B):2173–2180

Fraumeni JF Jr (1967) Stature and malignant tumors of bone in childhood and adolescence. Cancer 20(6):967–973

Gasser T et al. (1985a) An analysis of the mid-growth and adolescent spurts of height based on acceleration. Ann Hum Biol 12(2):129–148

Gasser T et al. (1985b) Human height growth: correlational and multivariate structure of velocity and acceleration. Ann Hum Biol 12(6):501–515

Gelberg KH et al. (1995) Fluoride exposure and childhood osteosarcoma: a case-control study. Am J Public Health 85(12):1678–1683

Gelberg KH et al. (1997) Growth and development and other risk factors for osteosarcoma in children and young adults. Int J Epidemiol 26(2):272–278

Ghali MH et al. (1992) Association between childhood rhabdomyosarcoma and maternal history of stillbirths. Int J Cancer 50(3):365–368

Glass AG, Fraumeni JF Jr (1970) Epidemiology of bone cancer in children. J Natl Cancer Inst 44(1):187–199

Greer JJ, Babiuk RP, Thebaud B (2003) Etiology of congenital diaphragmatic hernia: the retinoid hypothesis. Pediatr Res 53(5):726–730

Gripp KW et al. (2002) Five additional Costello syndrome patients with rhabdomyosarcoma: proposal for a tumor screening protocol. Am J Med Genet 108(1):80–87

Grufferman S et al. (1982) Environmental factors in the etiology of rhabdomyosarcoma in childhood. J Natl Cancer Inst 68(1):107–113

Grufferman S, Gula MJ, Olshan AF, Falletta JM, Pendergrass TW, Buckley J, Maurer HM (1991) In utero x-ray exposure and risk of childhood rhabdomyosarcoma. Paediatr Perinat Epidemiol 5:A6

Grufferman S et al. (1993) Parents' use of cocaine and marijuana and increased risk of rhabdomyosarcoma in their children. Cancer Causes Control 4(3):217–224

Gurney JG et al. (1995) Incidence of cancer in children in the United States. Sex-, race-, and 1-year age-specific rates by histologic type. Cancer 75(8):2186–2195

Hansen MF et al. (1985) Osteosarcoma and retinoblastoma: a shared chromosomal mechanism revealing recessive predisposition. Proc Natl Acad Sci USA 82(18):6216–6220

Hartley AL et al. (1988a) Neurofibromatosis in children with soft tissue sarcoma. Pediatr Hematol Oncol 5(1):7–16

Hartley AL et al. (1988b) The Inter-Regional Epidemiological Study of Childhood Cancer (IRESCC): case control study of children with bone and soft tissue sarcomas. Br J Cancer 58(6):838–842

Hartley AL et al. (1991) Cancer incidence in the families of children with Ewing's tumor. J Natl Cancer Inst 83(13):955–956

Hartley AL et al. (1994a) Foetal loss and infant deaths in families of children with soft-tissue sarcoma. Int J Cancer 56(5):646–649

Hartley AL et al. (1994b) Malformations in children with soft tissue sarcoma and in their parents and siblings. Paediatr Perinat Epidemiol 8(4):423–432

Hawkins MM et al. (1996) Radiotherapy, alkylating agents, and risk of bone cancer after childhood cancer. J Natl Cancer Inst 88(5):270–278

Holly EA et al. (1992) Ewing's bone sarcoma, paternal occupational exposure, and other factors. Am J Epidemiol 135(2):122–129

Hum L, Kreiger N, Finkelstein MM (1998) The relationship between parental occupation and bone cancer risk in offspring. Int J Epidemiol 27(5):766–771

Kager L et al. (2003) Primary metastatic osteosarcoma: presentation and outcome of patients treated on neoadjuvant Cooperative Osteosarcoma Study Group protocols. J Clin Oncol 21(10):2011–2018

Kaste SC et al. (1999) Metastases detected at the time of diagnosis of primary pediatric extremity osteosarcoma at diagnosis: imaging features. Cancer 86(8):1602–1608

Koufos A et al. (1985) Loss of heterozygosity in three embryonal tumours suggests a common pathogenetic mechanism. Nature 316(6026):330–334

Largo RH et al. (1978) Analysis of the adolescent growth spurt using smoothing spline functions. Ann Hum Biol 5(5):421–434

Leonard A et al. (1996) Osteogenic sarcoma in the Rothmund-Thomson syndrome. Med Pediatr Oncol 26(4):249–253

Li FP et al. (1988) A cancer family syndrome in twenty-four kindreds. Cancer Res 48(18):5358–5362

Li X, Hemminki K (2002) Parental cancer as a risk factor for bone cancer: a nation-wide study from Sweden. J Clin Epidemiol 55(2):111–114

Magnani C et al. (1989) Risk factors for soft tissue sarcomas in childhood: a case-control study. Tumori 75(4):396–400

Malkin D et al. (1990) Germ line p53 mutations in a familial syndrome of breast cancer, sarcomas, and other neoplasms. Science 250(4985):1233–1238

McGuire SM et al. (1991) Is there a link between fluoridated water and osteosarcoma? J Am Dental Assoc 122(4):38–45

McLaughlin J et al. (2004) Canadian Cancer Statistics 2004. National Cancer Institute of Canada, Toronto

Mendoza SM, Konishi T, Miller CW (1998) Integration of SV40 in human osteosarcoma DNA. Oncogene 17(9):2457–2462

Menu-Branthomme A et al. (2004) Radiation dose, chemotherapy and risk of soft tissue sarcoma after solid tumours during childhood. Int J Cancer 110(1):87–93

Miller CW et al. (1996) Alterations of the p53, Rb and MDM2 genes in osteosarcoma. J Cancer Res Clin Oncol 122(9):559–565

Moss ME et al. (1995) Osteosarcoma, seasonality, and environmental factors in Wisconsin, 1979–1989. Arch Environ Health 50(3):235–241

Nagarajan R et al. (2002) Limb salvage and amputation in survivors of pediatric lower-extremity bone tumors: what are the long-term implications? J Clin Oncol 20(22):4493–4501

Nishijo K et al. (2004) Mutation analysis of the RECQL4 gene in sporadic osteosarcomas. Int J Cancer 111(3):367–372

Novakovic B et al. (1994) Increased risk of neuroectodermal tumors and stomach cancer in relatives of patients with Ewing's sarcoma family of tumors. J Natl Cancer Inst 86(22):1702–1706

Olin P, Giesecke J (1998) Potential exposure to SV40 in polio vaccines used in Sweden during 1957: no impact on cancer incidence rates 1960 to 1993. Dev Biol Stand 94:227–233

Operskalski EA et al. (1987) A case-control study of osteosarcoma in young persons. Am J Epidemiol 126(1):118–126

Parkin DM et al. (1998) International Incidence of Childhood Cancer, vol II. International Agency for Research on Cancer. Carey, NC

Paulussen M et al. (1998) Ewing's tumors with primary lung metastases: survival analysis of 114 (European Intergroup) Cooperative Ewing's Sarcoma Studies patients. J Clin Oncol 16(9):3044–3052

Price CH (1958) Primary bone-forming tumours and their relationship to skeletal growth. J Bone Joint Surg Br 40B(3): 574–593

Ries LA et al. (1999) Cancer Incidence and Survival among Children and Adolescents: United States SEER Program 1975–1995. National Cancer Institute, SEER Program: Bethesda, MD

Ries LAG et al. (2004) SEER Cancer Statistics Review, 1975–2001. National Cancer Institute, Bethesda, MD

Ross JA et al. (1999) Seasonal variations in the diagnosis of childhood cancer in the United States. Br J Cancer 81(3):549–553

Ruymann FB et al. (1988) Congenital anomalies associated with rhabdomyosarcoma: an autopsy study of 115 cases. A report from the Intergroup Rhabdomyosarcoma Study Committee (representing the Children's Cancer Study Group, the Pediatric Oncology Group, the United Kingdom Children's Cancer Study Group, and the Pediatric Intergroup Statistical Center). Med Pediatr Oncol 16(1):33–39

Ruza E et al. (2003) Analysis of polymorphisms of the vitamin D receptor, estrogen receptor, and collagen Ialpha1 genes and their relationship with height in children with bone cancer. J Pediatr Hematol Oncol 25(10):780–786

Sharma JC (1983) The genetic contribution to pubertal growth and development studied by longitudinal growth data on twins. Ann Hum Biol 10(2):163–171

Silcocks PB, Murrells T (1987) Space-time clustering and bone tumours: application of Knox's method to data from a population-based cancer registry. Int J Cancer 40(6):769–771

Silventoinen K et al. (2003) Heritability of adult body height: a comparative study of twin cohorts in eight countries. Twin Res 6(5):399–408

Smith MW et al. (2004) A high-density admixture map for disease gene discovery in African Americans. Am J Hum Genet 74(5):1001–1013

Sorensen HT et al. (1999) Birth weight and length as predictors for adult height. Am J Epidemiol 149(8):726–729

Staheli L (2003) Pediatric orthopedics, 3rd edn. Lippincott Williams & Wilkins, Philadelphia

Strickler HD et al. (1998) Contamination of poliovirus vaccines with simian virus 40 (1955–1963) and subsequent cancer rates. JAMA 279(4):292–295

Tanner JM et al. (1976) The adolescent growth spurt of boys and girls of the Harpenden growth study. Ann Hum Biol 3(2):109–126

Tjalma RA (1966) Canine bone sarcoma: estimation of relative risk as a function of body size. J Natl Cancer Inst 36(6):1137–1150

Tucker MA et al. (1987) Bone sarcomas linked to radiotherapy and chemotherapy in children. N Engl J Med 317(10): 588–593

Valery PC et al. (2002) Farm exposures, parental occupation, and risk of Ewing's sarcoma in Australia: a national case-control study. Cancer Causes Control 13(3):263–270

Valery PC et al. (2003) A national case-control study of Ewing's sarcoma family of tumours in Australia. Int J Cancer 105(6):825–830

Winn DM et al. (1992) A case-control study of the etiology of Ewing's sarcoma. Cancer Epidemiol Biomarkers Prevent 1(7):525–532

Wong FL et al. (1997) Cancer incidence after retinoblastoma. Radiation dose and sarcoma risk. JAMA 278(15):1262–1267

Wu XC et al. (2003) Cancer incidence in adolescents and young adults in the United States, 1992–1997. J Adolesc Health 32(6):405–415

Yamamoto H et al. (2000) High incidence of SV40-like sequences detection in tumour and peripheral blood cells of Japanese osteosarcoma patients. Br J Cancer 82(10): 1677–1681

Yang P et al. (1995) Association of childhood rhabdomyosarcoma with neurofibromatosis type I and birth defects. Genet Epidemiol 12(5):467–474

Pathologic and Molecular Techniques Used in the Diagnosis and Treatment Planning of Sarcomas

Timothy Triche, Deborah Schofield

Contents

2.1 Introduction

The purpose of this chapter is to describe briefly the histopathologic and genetic tools currently available to establish a specific cancer diagnosis, to predict prognosis and response to therapy and, ultimately, to identify potential novel therapeutic targets. The diagnosis of cancer has traditionally been rendered based upon the morphologic characteristics of an individual tumor interpreted within a given clinical setting. Over the years, the evaluable morphologic features have expanded from light microscopic appearance by routine hematoxylin and eosin (H&E) staining to include special and immunohistochemical stains and ultrastructural features. While these phenotypic attributes have allowed the pathologist to classify the majority of tumors, the classification is relatively subjective in some cases, maybe a "diagnosis of exclusion" in others, and does not allow reliable prediction of biologic behavior in most.

As the repertoire of techniques and tools traditionally used by the pathologist has expanded, so have those utilized by the research community. These latter advancements, such as karyotyping, PCR, FISH, DNA sequencing, and microarrays (of tissue or DNA probes), frequently result in observations about specific tumors at the genetic level that provide potentially invaluable, ancillary, diagnostic information. Concomitant development of methods that allow reliable and reproducible assessment of these additional tumor characteristics has resulted in the current global approach to cancer diagnosis – one based upon the integration of molecular genetic, histologic and clinical features. The approach is fluid in two respects – first of all, the types of information used depend upon the differential diagnosis of the tumor

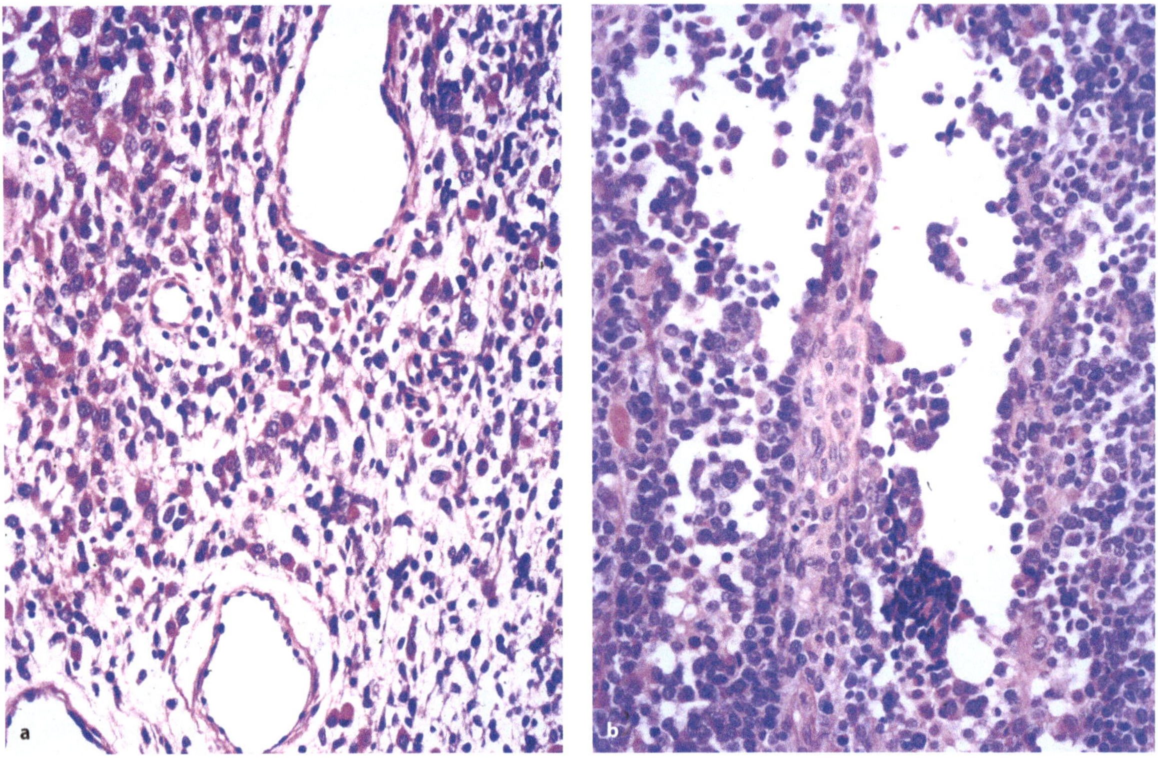

Figure 2.1

Histologic appearance of embryonal (a) vs. alveolar (b) rhabdomyosarcoma

itself and, secondly, as new information is generated and proven to be clinically useful, it is incorporated into the diagnostic process. Moreover, as the ability to refine our diagnostic capabilities increases, it carries with it the wonderful benefit of providing prognostic and therapeutic information as well, facilitating the ultimate goal of individualized tumor therapy (Brandt 2002; Cordon-Cardo 2001; Hicks et al. 2004; Millar et al. 2004).

2.2 Standard Histopathology

2.2.1 Light Microscopy

The foundation and initial step in cancer diagnosis remains the formalin fixation, routine processing to paraffin and examination of an H&E stained section of tumor tissue on a glass slide (Triche et al. 2005). In most cases, the process is an overnight procedure with generation of slides usually occurring the day following a surgical procedure or biopsy. However, if tumors are large, an additional day of formalin fixation may be needed prior to processing, and in the case of some bone-forming tumors the specimen may need to be decalcified prior to processing – a procedure that may take days or even weeks, depending upon the extent of ossification.

Interpretation of H&E stained section(s) of tumor is the "art" of surgical pathology and is based upon pattern recognition. Figure 2.1 shows the dramatic difference in appearance of a typical embryonal rhabdomyosarcoma (panel a) versus a typical alveolar rhabdomyosarcoma (panel b). Depending upon the light microscopic appearance and clinical setting

Figure 2.2

MyoD in rhabdomyosarcoma

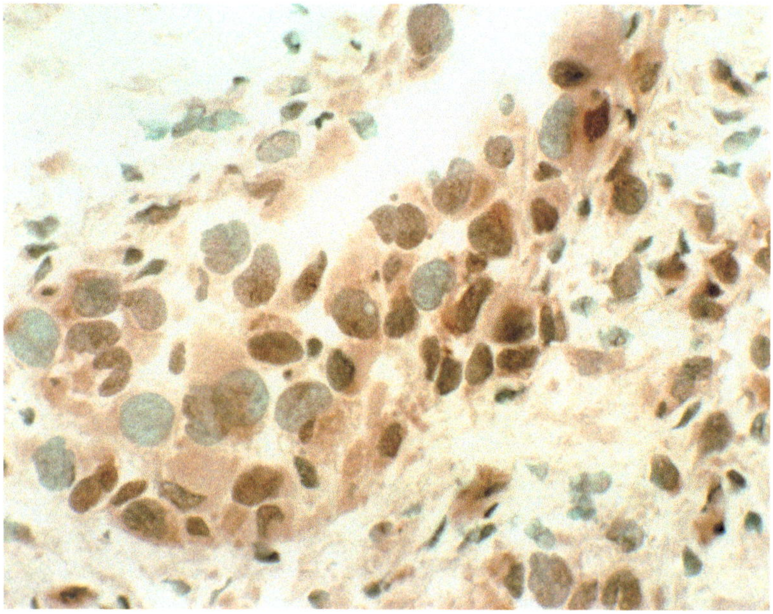

in which the tumor occurs, either a definitive diagnosis is rendered (i.e., most Wilms' tumors) or, more commonly, a working differential diagnosis is established (i.e., small round blue cell tumors, sarcomas). In the latter case, the differential diagnosis dictates the type and extent of additional and ancillary testing that will be subsequently performed (Carr et al. 2004).

2.2.2 Immunohistochemistry

One of the first steps taken to assist in the diagnostic categorization of a tumor is immunohistochemical staining (Chan 2000; Coindre 2003; Jaffer et al. 2004; Suster 2000). Antibodies developed in response to specific antigens are applied to a section of tumor prepared from the paraffin-embedded (or occasionally frozen) tissue. An avidin-biotin-based detection system results in chromogenic staining at cellular sites of antibody binding within the tumor. The technique allows assessment of a variety of cell- and tumor-specific characteristics such as differentiation or proliferative activity. This is often helpful in establishing tumor lineage, as in the differential diagnosis of undifferentiated tumors (Devoe et al. 2000; Llombart-Bosch et al. 1996; Papadimitriou et al. 2004). In other cases, it can both determine lineage and degree of differentiation (Cui et al. 1999; Dias et al. 1990). Figure 2.2 illustrates immunohistochemical detection of a myogenic transcription factor, MyoD, in tumor cell nuclei in a rhabdomyosarcoma. Note that this result documents *commitment* to a diagnostic cell lineage (e.g., rhabdomyogenesis), as opposed to actual *execution* of this lineage. As such, it is diagnostic, whether the tumor cells have actually undergone myogenesis or not. However, the number of antibodies available is limited and results must be interpreted in light of the sensitivity and specificity of any given antibody.

In addition to its role in tumor diagnosis, immunohistochemistry is also occasionally used to assist in the tailoring of tumor-specific therapy. An example of this is the expression of c-kit in gastrointestinal stromal tumors and the use of Gleevec (Went et al. 2004). The caveat to this approach to therapy is that overexpression of genes does not necessarily correlate with mutation or gene copy number (amplification) and it remains unclear as to which of these biologic misadventures may play the key role in an individual tumor or tumor type. As our understand-

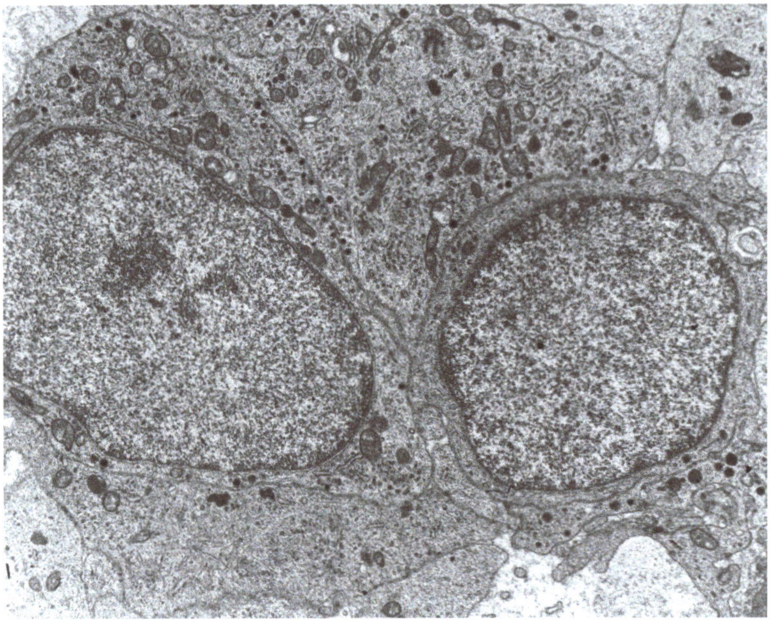

Figure 2.3

EM of dense core granules in neuroblastoma

ing of tumor biology expands, and the number of sensitive and specific antibodies produced increases, so, inevitably, will the use of immunohistochemistry. The procedure itself is simple, rapid (results are usually available within a few hours), cheap and reproducible when performed under standard clinical laboratory guidelines.

2.2.3 Electron Microscopy

Examination of tumors at the ultrastructural level prior to the introduction of immunohistochemistry was widely employed in tumor diagnosis, but has largely been supplemented by that technique in routine surgical pathology. Nonetheless, immunohistochemistry occasionally produces conflicting evidence of tumor lineage or phenotype, or none at all. In this situation, judicious use of diagnostic EM may add vital information regarding tumor lineage and differentiation that may establish a diagnosis that otherwise may be impossible by light microscopy and immunohistochemistry alone (Cui et al. 1999; Dias et al. 1990; Dickman 1987; Erlandson et al. 1988; Ghadially 1985; Lombardi et al. 1988; Mawad et al. 1994; van Haelst 1986). While only a few ultrastructural features (such as neurosecretory granules, as seen in Fig. 2.3) are diagnostic of a specific tumor type (such as neuroblastoma), a combination of features frequently support a diagnosis of one tumor type vs. another or rule out one of the tumor types in the differential diagnosis. Even basic features such as cell-cell junctions or keratin filament bundles will rule in or out an epithelial malignancy, while lack thereof would be more consistent with hematopoietic malignancy, such as lymphoma (Triche et al. 2005). Other distinguishing features often include the presence or absence of cell-associated basal lamina, pinocytotic vesicles, neurosecretory granules, various types of intercellular junctions, and various types of cytoplasmic intermediate filaments (Peydro-Olaya et al. 2003).

2.3 Cytogenetics

2.3.1 Classical Cytogenetic Analysis

The ability to karyotype tumor cells heralded a transition in the practice of traditional histopathologic tumor diagnosis (Fletcher 2004; Knuutila 2004; Sandberg et al. 1994). Karyotypic abnormalities are fre-

Figure 2.4
Ewing's t(11;22) translocation

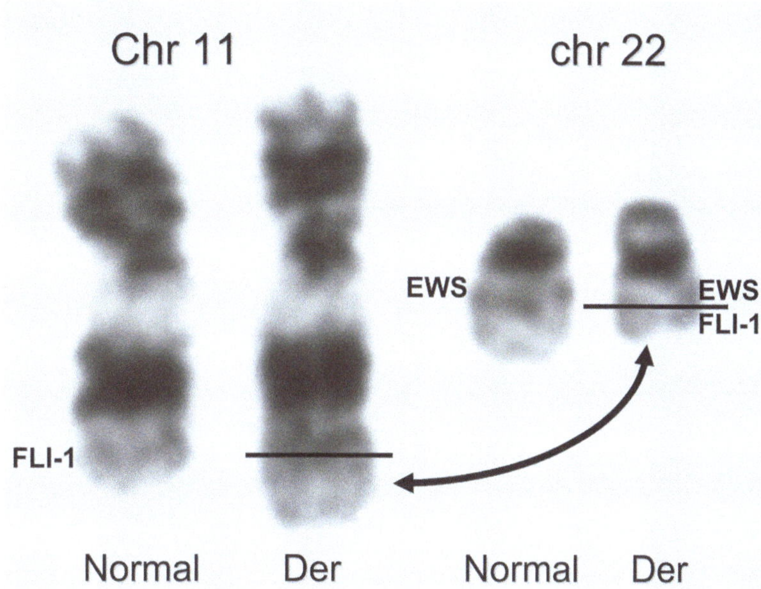

quently encountered in neoplasms and are routinely classified as either numerical or structural – numerical abnormalities being the simple gain or loss of an entire chromosome and structural abnormalities involving "movements" of pieces of chromosomes. The latter include translocations, deletions, inversions, duplications and the formation of either ring or marker chromosomes (Fletcher et al. 2001). In addition, tumor types frequently tend to be characterized by either relatively simple or relatively complex karyotypes. Ewing's sarcoma, for example, usually has a near normal karyotype with only a single or few structural and/or numerical abnormalities that tend to be consistently present within the Ewing's group of tumors. Osteogenic sarcoma, on the other hand, tends to be genetically unstable and a typical karyotype usually contains a number of different, albeit related, clones with many structural and numerical abnormalities. These genetic abnormalities are usually random in that there is great variation between individual tumors.

In contrast to tumors with complex karyotypes, those with simple karyotypes often have characteristic, nonrandom cytogenetic aberrations that are specific to certain tumor types (such as the t(11;22) in Ewing's family tumors) seen in Fig. 2.4, serving as an invaluable diagnostic adjunct (Hattinger et al. 2002; Ladanyi 1995). In addition, as karyotyping became refined (high resolution chromosomal banding), more detailed and accurate localization of these recurring genetic abnormalities facilitated identification of the specific genes involved, thus providing the foundation for the next wave of diagnostic, biologic and therapeutic advances (Liehr et al. 2002, 2004). Many of the directed techniques such as fluorescence-in-situ hybridization and PCR are based upon information derived from these types of previous karyotypic analyses.

Karyotyping is performed on fresh, unfixed tumor tissue that is minced or disaggregated with proteases into tiny fragments/single cell suspensions. The fragments/cells are placed into tissue culture media supplemented with fetal calf serum and antibiotics and allowed to proliferate. Once the cells reach a critical phase of growth (days to weeks, depending upon the tumor type), a drug (such as colchicine) is added to the media for a period of time (usually overnight) and the cells are arrested in the metaphase stage of the cell cycle. The time at which the cell suspension is harvested for analysis is critical as overgrowth of non-neoplastic elements within the tumor (such as fibroblasts or endothelial cells) may occur over time, resulting in a "falsely normal" karyotype. Hypotonic solution is added to swell the cells and separate the chromosomes and the cell suspension is then fixed in a mixture of methanol and acetic acid. The fixed cell suspension is dropped onto glass microscope slides for subsequent Giemsa staining and analysis. Much of the karyotyping process today is automated.

2.3.2 In-Situ Hybridization

In-situ hybridization, ISH, is a technique that is based upon the hybridization of a labeled nucleic acid probe to either a chromosomal metaphase spread, single cell suspension plated on a glass slide or a tissue section. If the detection system used to detect the labeled probe is fluorescently tagged, then the procedure is called fluorescence-in-situ hybridization, or FISH (Liehr et al. 2004). The technique allows localization of the probe to a specific region of a chromosome (if the target is a metaphase spread), nucleus, cell or tissue. The majority of probes are sequences of DNA, usually hundreds to thousands of bases in length, that, upon denaturation of the target DNA of interest (separation of the two nucleic acid strands, usually by heat ± variation in salt concentration), anneal with the homologous sequence as the conditions are reversed. The technique takes from hours to overnight and its usefulness is dependent upon previous knowledge of the genetic abnormality in question.

In the field of cancer diagnosis and therapy, ISH is primarily used to detect three different types of genetic abnormalities – DNA amplification, DNA deletions and chromosomal translocations. In most cases, ISH is performed on either cell suspensions or tissue sections. In the case of DNA amplification detection, such as MYC-N in neuroblastomas (Fig. 2.5), the probe is hybridized to the target of choice and amplification is manifest as either increased numbers of individual signals (if the amplification is in the form of double minutes) or as one large signal (if the amplification is in the form of homogeneous staining regions) (Mathew et al. 2001).

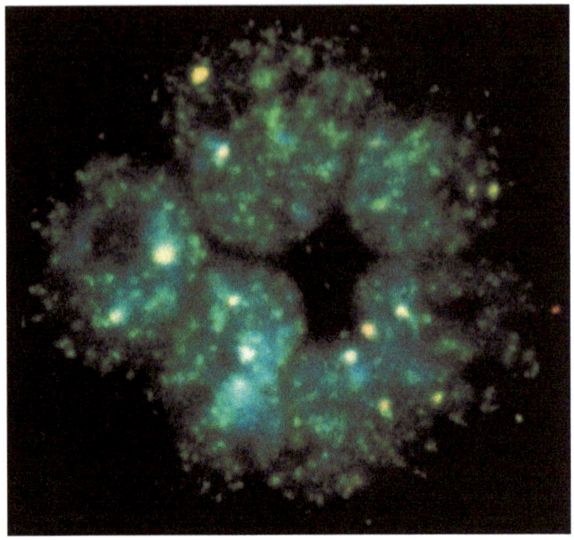

Figure 2.5
MYCN amplification in neuroblastoma

In the case of DNA deletions, two different probes are used, each labeled with a different fluorochrome (such as Cy3 and Cy5) – one probe detects the target gene/chromosomal region of interest and the second probe, hybridizing with the centromeric region of the chromosome on which the gene of interest is located, detects chromosome copy number. A deletion is present when the number of centromeric signals is greater than the number of target probe signals.

There are two FISH approaches to the detection of chromosomal translocations, both, as in the case of deletion detection, using two differentially labeled probes (Monforte-Munoz et al. 1999). In the first approach, one of the probes detects one of the translocation partner genes and spans the translocation breakpoint. The second probe is a centromeric probe that documents corresponding chromosome copy number. When a translocation is present, one copy of the probe of interest, detecting the chromosome involved in the translocation, is split, resulting in two smaller signals. The second copy of the probe of interest, detecting the normal allele, remains intact and larger in size. In the second approach to translocation testing, one of the two probes hybridizes with each of

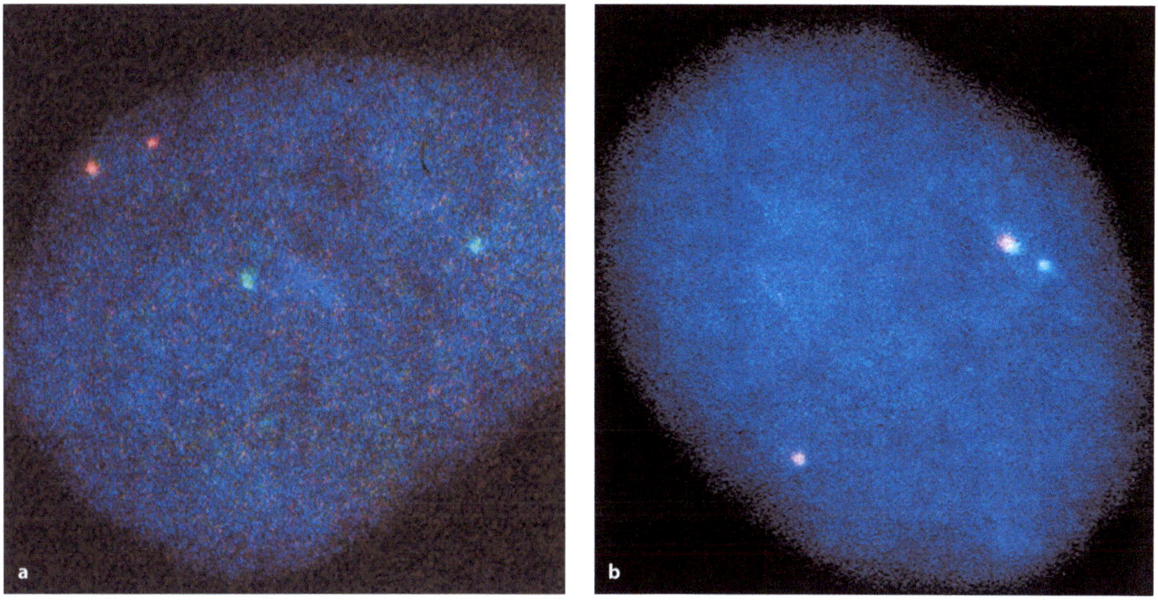

Figure 2.6 a, b

FISH of Ewing's family tumor with chromosome 11 and 22 probes

the two translocation partners – the probes hybridize with the portion of each gene that makes up the chimeric fusion gene. When a translocation is not present, the four signals are randomly scattered throughout the cell. When a translocation is present, there are three signals rather than four – two signals, one detecting each of the two translocation partners, are consistently adjacent to each other/fused, resulting in a single larger signal of "mixed" color (i.e., one red and one green appears yellow). In addition, the remaining probe for each of the two unaffected alleles not involved in the translocation is also present. This is illustrated in Fig. 2.6 in a case of Ewing's sarcoma. In the first panel (a), four signals are readily observed in a normal cell. In the second panel, the nucleus of a Ewing's tumor cell shows three signals, two smaller (e.g., untranslocated alleles) and one larger (e.g., the fused chromosome 11 and 22 chimeric gene characteristic of this tumor).

2.3.3 Spectral Karyotyping

Spectral karyotyping, or SKY, is technicolor karyotyping, combining the techniques of standard karyotyping and in-situ hybridization (Bayani and Squire 2002a; Tonon et al. 2000). It is particularly useful when karyotyping tumors that have complex karyotypes or marker chromosomes in which the origin of chromosomal material is not clear by standard Giemsa banding (Bayani and Squire 2001, 2002b). In SKY, a cocktail of short sequences of single-stranded DNA probes that hybridize along the length of each chromosome is prepared. The probes for each of the 22 autosomes and two sex chromosomes are then tagged with a different color label such that each chromosome fluoresces a unique color (Pandita et al. 1999; Zhang et al. 2000). The cocktail of probes is then applied to metaphase spreads prepared from cultures of fresh tumor material, painting the chromosomes a rainbow of colors. Analysis of the metaphase by computers allows identification of translocations, insertions and other structural abnormalities, including the origin of marker chromosomes.

2.3.4 Comparative Genomic Hybridization

Primarily used as a research tool, comparative genomic hybridization, or CGH, is a technique that is used to obtain information about unknown areas of deletion or amplification within a given tumor (Bayani et al. 1995; Bridge et al. 2000; Hughes et al. 2004; Weber-Hall et al. 1996). To perform the analysis, equal amounts of DNA are extracted from both normal and tumor cells – fresh/frozen tissue is optimal although the analysis can be performed relatively reliably on paraffin-embedded tissue. The two species of fragmented DNA are each labeled with a different fluorochrome and hybridized in equal amounts to normal metaphase chromosomes. Images of the metaphase chromosomes are captured with a camera and the relative signal intensities are quantitated along the chromosome. Over- or underrepresentation of tumor signal correlates with amplification or deletion respectively of the hybridized genomic segment.

2.4 Molecular Genetic Techniques

2.4.1 Introduction

It is perhaps not surprising that cancer, which is at heart a genetic disorder, has benefited perhaps the most from the application of a host of new molecular genetic techniques to the analysis of cancer (Fletcher et al. 2001; Thorner et al. 1998). This is especially true of sarcoma diagnosis (Ladanyi et al. 2000). In each case, molecular methods have revealed fundamental features of cancer that are not readily appreciated by standard histopathologic methods. The particular value of these methods, however, is to augment the overall evaluation of a diagnostic tumor biopsy, allowing integration of molecular and morphologic methods in the assessment of the patient's diagnosis, prognosis, and choice of therapy. These methods, then, should be viewed as ancillary diagnostic methods for the diagnosis of cancer. They are *not* standalone diagnostic methods (Fletcher et al. 2001). Each, however, is either in daily use (e.g., PCR) or is rapidly being adopted (e.g., microarrays, proteomics, DNA sequencing). The character of the method and its particular value is addressed below.

2.4.2 PCR and Q-PCR

PCR and its many variants have become mainstays of the molecular workup of any tumor specimen. The applications range from detection of tumor-specific gene translocations (Sorensen et al. 1996) to measurement of expression level of a gene or genes of interest to generation of sufficient amplified DNA to allow sequencing of the product (Eberwine et al. 1992). Routine methods are not qualitative, but are capable of detecting minute amounts of material, such as in the case of minimal residual disease, where 1 cell in a million can typically be detected.

A common use of nonquantitative PCR is for the detection of tumor-specific gene translocations (Barr et al. 1995; Ladanyi and Bridge 2000). In this setting, PCR primers specific for sequences flanking the breakpoint are chosen, such that the amplified product between the primers spans the breakpoint. In this way, only the translocated gene product can be amplified; the untranslocated alleles are not, and normal cells likewise yield no product. The principle behind translocated gene amplification is illustrated in Fig. 2.7, a case of synoviosarcoma with the typical SYT-SSX translocation. By choosing SYT (forward) and SSX (reverse) primers, it can be appreciated that only the SYT-SSX sequence will yield a PCR product. An example of detection of another tumor specific gene translocation from bone marrow is illustrated in Fig. 2.8, where the unique EWS-FLI1 chimeric gene, found only in Ewing's family tumors, is readily detectable by PCR, using primers to EWS (forward) and FLI-1 (reverse). In this way, only the tumor specific chimeric gene is amplified, while ubiquitously expressed EWS is not, for lack of a reverse strand primer. This general method is now routinely used in the analysis of all leukemias and sarcomas, which as a group harbor a particularly high incidence of specific chimeric genes that are readily detected by this method (Barr et al. 1995; Ladanyi and Bridge 2000).

More recently, PCR has been adapted for another specific use: the direct, quantitative measurement of a particular mRNA transcript, which thereby gives a

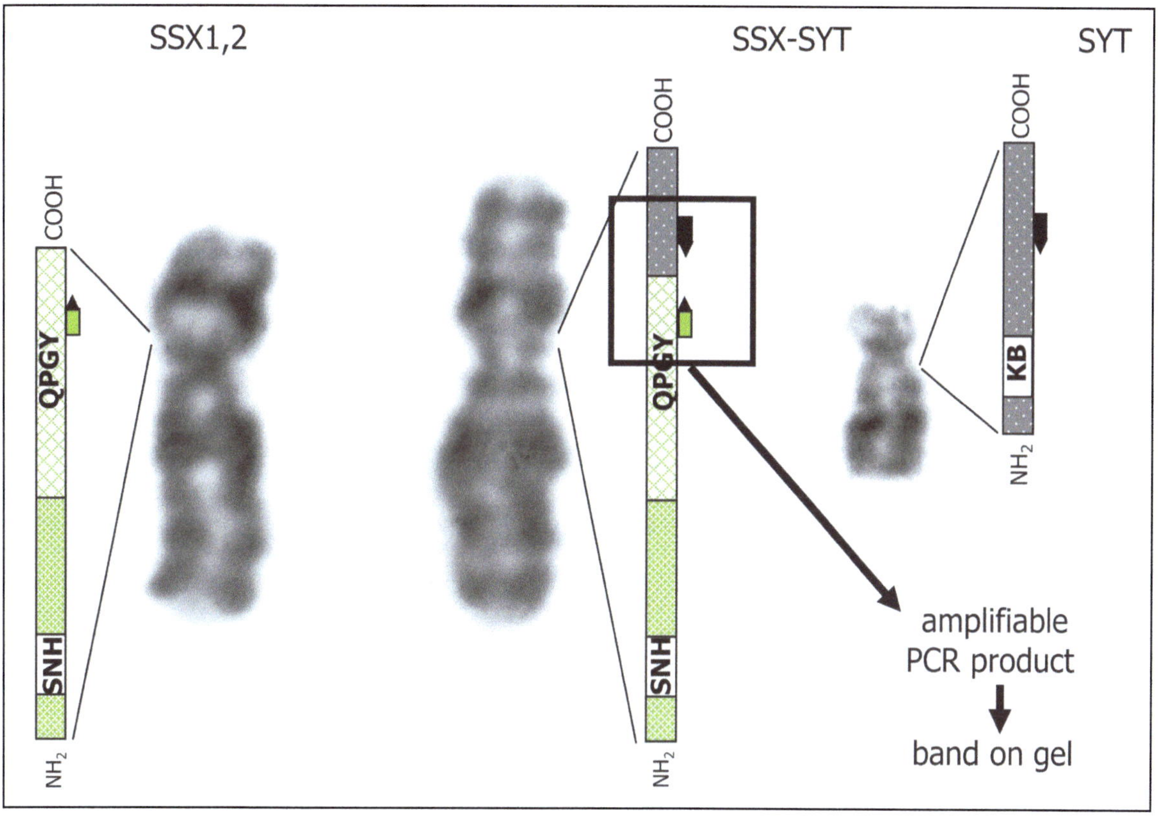

Figure 2.7

PCR reactions for SYT-SSX chimeric gene of synoviosarcoma

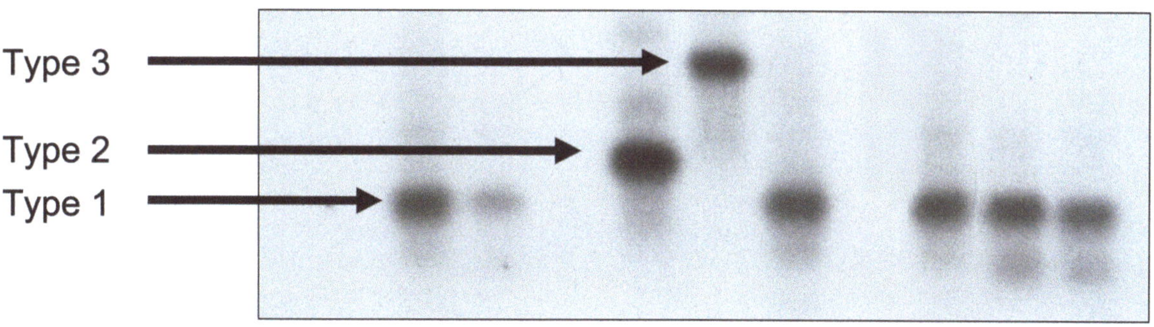

Figure 2.8

Ewing's family tumor PCR for EWS-FLI1 chimeric gene

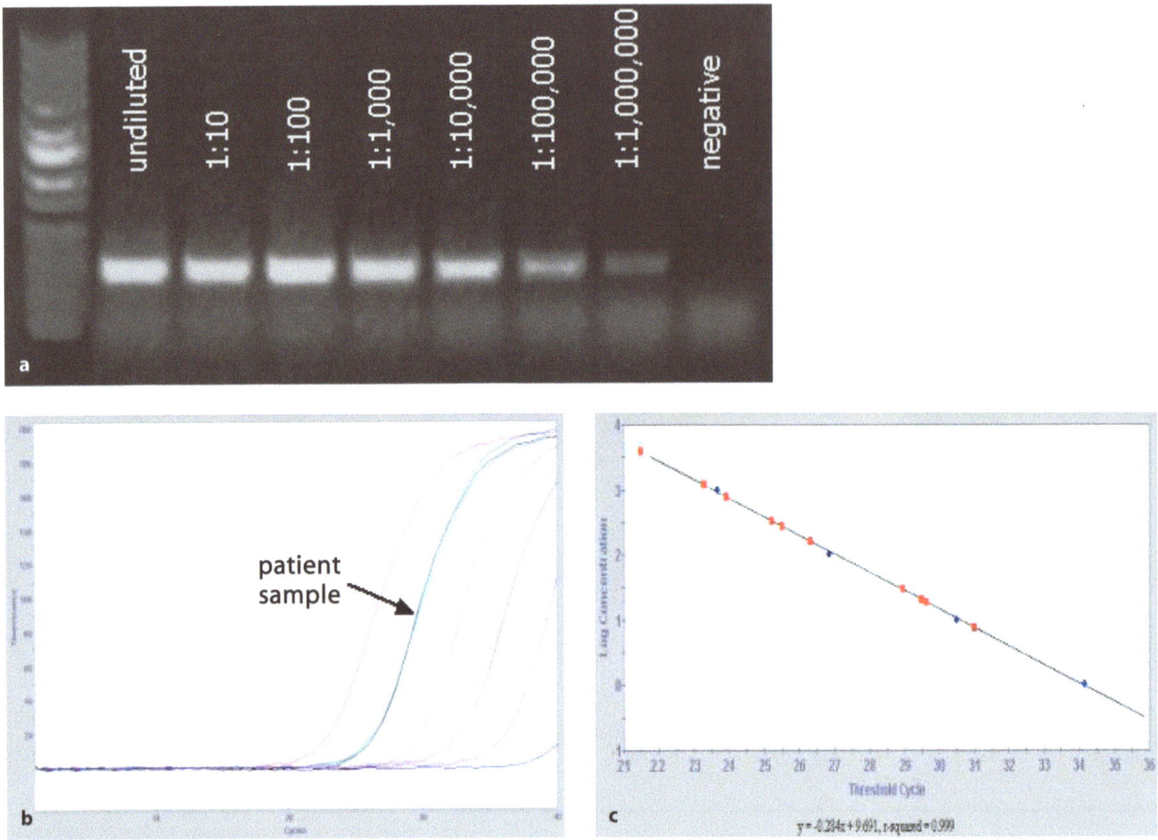

Figure 2.9 a–c

Quantitative PCR

measure of gene expression, analogous to measurement by Northern (RNA) blots, but far faster, cheaper, and practical (Cummings et al. 2002; Freeman et al. 1999; Hill et al. 2003; Hostein et al. 2002; Klein 2002; Peter et al. 2001). Even minute specimens (cytology preps and imprints, fine needle aspirates, frozen sections, and even laser captured cells from tissue sections) can be utilized for quantitative real time PCR (QRT PCR, QPCR). This is useful for any number of purposes, including measurements of both normal and chimeric gene products. Typically, a cycle threshold, or number of PCR cycles before a detectable product appears, is calculated and compared to a positive control standard at various dilutions. By extrapolating to a plot of amount vs. cycle threshold, the same product can be rather precisely measured. An example is shown in Fig. 2.9, where a plot of known control Ct values vs. amount is superimposed on the result of an unknown specimen expressing the same gene. From this, the quantitative expression level of any gene of interest can be deduced.

Although often criticized as being an indirect measure of gene activity, whence it is assumed that only protein levels translated from mRNA transcripts are a valid measure of gene activity, this has not been the case in our studies. In general, we find good agreement between mRNA expression levels and the corresponding protein levels. An example of this is

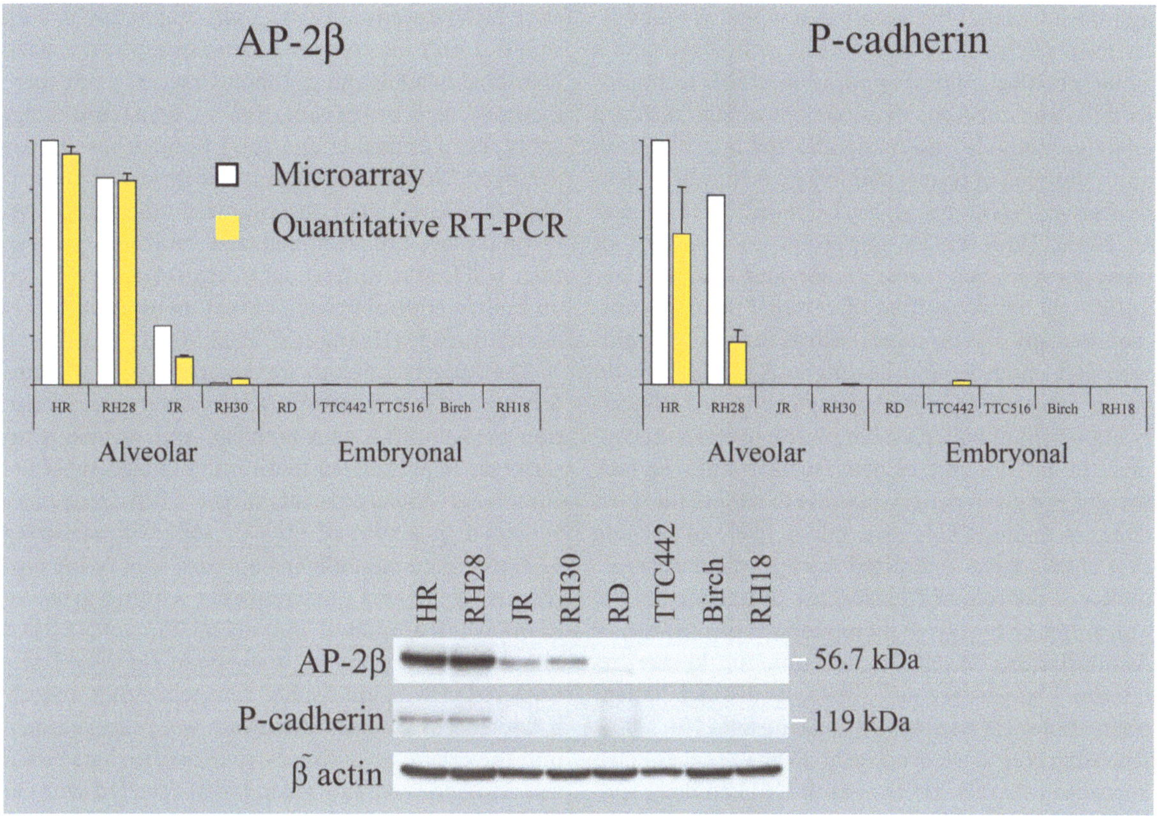

Figure 2.10

Microarray vs. QPCR vs. protein

shown in Fig. 2.10, where a comparison of normalized mRNA expression by microarray and QPCR (upper panel) is compared to protein levels (lower panel) for two genes (AP2β and P cadherin) across several rhabdomyosarcoma tumors. Note the overall close correlation between all three measures.

2.4.3 Microarrays

DNA microarrays are now becoming useful clinical and laboratory research tools, and will almost certainly become important diagnostic tools in the very near future (Diehn et al. 2000; Marx 2000; Ramaswamy et al. 2002). Over the past decade, they have moved from use in "discovery" based research to clinical application (Bhattacharjee et al. 2001; Chen et al. 2002; Garber et al. 2001; Lapointe et al. 2004; Lossos et al. 2002; Nielsen et al. 2002; Nutt et al. 2003; Perou et al. 1999; Pomeroy et al. 2002; Ramaswamy et al. 2003; Shipp et al. 2002; Singh et al. 2002; van de Vijver et al. 2002; Weigelt et al. 2003; Yeang et al. 2001). As sufficient amounts of data are amassed, and suitable experience is gleaned, the massive genomic databases generated by microarrays and related genomic technology will effectively become the equivalent of clinical laboratory "normal values," except that each dataset will contain thousands of datapoints per sample. This, in turn, requires a fundamentally different approach to data interpretation, one that is unfamiliar to most clinicians and clinical pathologists. As a result, practical clinical application of this technology will depend on the development of standardized analytic methods and guidelines for interpretation and validation of results within a given tumor system or disease (Peterson et al. 2003; Simon 2003; Simon et al. 2003). However, an important consequence of cross-comparisons across tumor and disease categories will be recognition of certain "themes" common to many disease states, such as the role of angiogenesis in both wound healing and tumor growth. For diseases where control of angiogenesis is clinically important, it will, for example, be useful to recognize the relative role of neovascularization, or lack thereof, in a given patient, in order to choose the most effective therapy. This principle is likely to become ever more cogent as directed therapy mandates evaluation of the role of a given gene or pathway in the use, or not, of a targeted therapy, much like the recent demonstration of efficacy, or not, for kinase inhibitors like Gleevec and Iressa, in distinct patient populations (DeMatteo 2002; Demetri 2001, 2002; Duensing et al. 2004; Lynch et al. 2004; Paez et al. 2004; Sordella et al. 2004; Tuveson et al. 2001). In these specific examples, both *expression* of the kinase, and *mutation* of the kinase domain, have been found to be important. Both parameters can be evaluated with microarray technology, and it is therefore likely that such assays will become part of the upfront evaluation of patients prior to treatment. This paradigm is likely to be utilized for many if not most of the new generation of directed therapies now being introduced into oncology and medicine in general (Arteaga 2004; Marx 2004; Stratton et al. 2004).

Microarrays are already being used to advantage in clinical and translational research on human tumors, with fairly impressive results (Chen et al. 2002; Ramaswamy and Golub 2002; Yeang et al. 2001). It is already obvious that they provide powerful diagnostic information that has in some cases validated preexisting tumor classes, but, perhaps more significantly, has identified heterogeneity in classical diagnostic groups that has led to the identification of new tumor classification or the identification of subgroups with important clinical import (Alizadeh et al. 2000; Hans et al. 2004; Rosenwald et al. 2002; Staudt 2002). Both superior and inferior prognostic groups have been identified in adult and childhood cancers using these methods, and re-classification of some molecular subtypes of leukemia and solid tumors has already occurred. This is likely to continue for many years, as important, previously unrecognized molecular classes of tumors are identified and validated. This, in turn, will lead to differential treatment groups, based on known clinical behaviors that mandate more selective therapy (Huang et al. 2002; Wright et al. 2003).

The basic technology for microarrays is straightforward: a labeled cDNA made by reverse transcription using mRNA as a template and reverse transcriptase is hybridized to an immobilized substrate containing thousands of target DNA sequences arranged in a grid of dots or squares, measuring 5–25 μm in greatest dimension; each spot or tile represents a gene, or a short sequence within a gene. An example of a spotted microarray (a) and a tiled oligonucleotide array (b) is shown in Fig. 2.11. These captured cDNAs are readily detected, either directly if fluorescent labeled nucleotides were incorporated into the cDNA, or indirectly if a label such as biotin was incorporated and secondarily detected with an avidin-fluorochrome conjugate. Either way, the identity and amount of the cDNA can then be measured on the basis of fluorescence intensity per target sequence. In the case of spotted cDNA (or the newer 50–60mer oligonucleotide) arrays, a competitive hybridization is employed, resulting in a ratio of red to green fluorescence. If both control and tumor sample express the gene, a yellow (e.g., an admixture of the two) is detected. If neither expresses the gene, there is no fluorescence (e.g., black). Depending on intensity and ratio, the relative fold change can be calculated for any given gene or target sequence. Typical densities of current microarrays, both spotted and in situ synthesized (e.g., Affymetrix GeneChips), is essentially the entire transcriptome (~40,000 expressed sequences).

Currently the two major uses of microarrays are for assessment of the expressed genome, or transcriptome, or gene expression profiling, or resequencing of DNA, for mutational analysis (as in p53), and, potentially more importantly, for high density

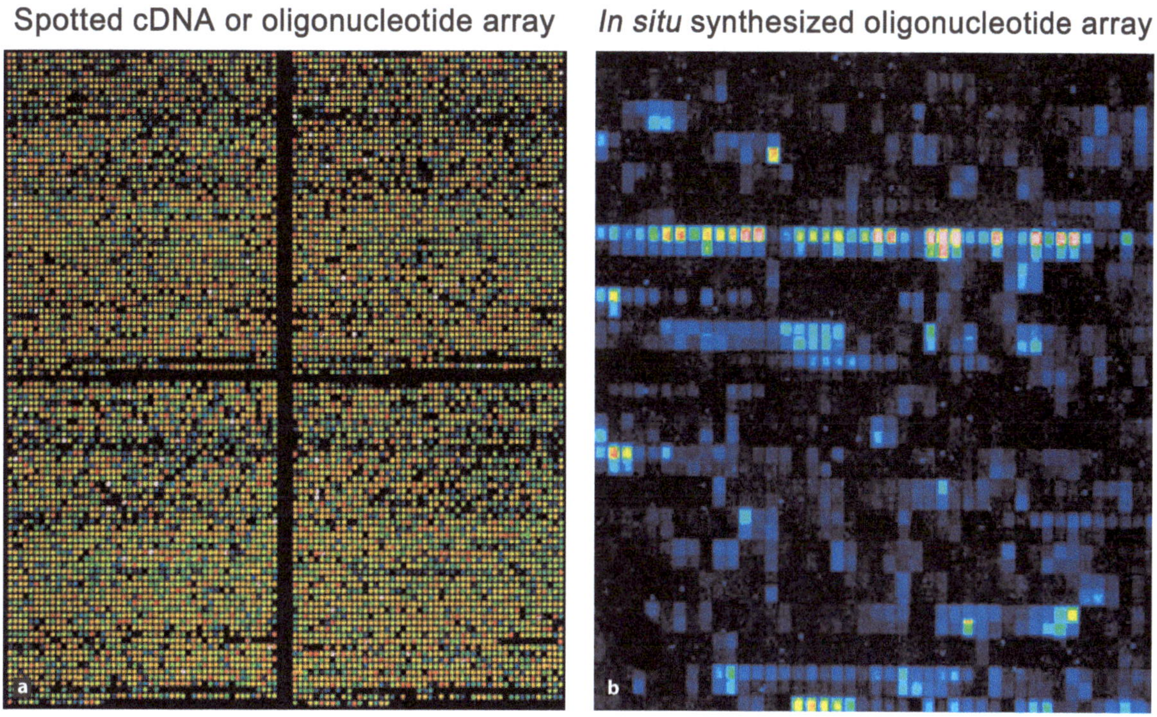

Figure 2.11 a,b

Spotted vs. oligonucleotide microarrays. **a** Spotted cDNA or oligonucleotide array. **b** In situ synthesized oligonucleotide array

polymorphism, or SNP (single nucleotide polymorphism) analysis. An example of an SNP chip is shown in Fig. 2.12, where progressively smaller tiling of distinct nucleotides used for sequence determination is illustrated. The latter use is particularly interesting, as the density of SNP arrays as of this writing has increased to 600,000 SNPs across the entire genome. That means one SNP every 6 kb. More importantly, given the haplotype block structure of the human genome, that translates to more than 125,000 independent tests per genome, which is also larger than the projected number of haplotype blocks in the human genome. This in turn means that each haplotype block will have multiple tagged SNPs identified in each block, which in turn translates to a remarkably precise and inexpensive estimate of the haplotype block structure of the individual in question. Current estimates are that at a cost of a few thousand dollars, a haplotype map of an individual can be created with perhaps 80% or better accuracy. This "HapMap," so called, just a few years ago cost millions of dollars. Now we are confronted with the reality that it will likely not be unreasonable to assess the entire structural genome from such data, at a fraction of the original cost of such haplotype maps.

The interpretation of data from microarrays, as noted above, has created an urgent need for tools that enable the user intelligently to interpret their data. The methods used are largely unprecedented in biomedical research, having previously been the domain of high energy physicists and pattern recognition mathematicians. Even that is insufficient to evaluate the reliability and reproducibility of such data. Thus, a new field of bioinformatics has emerged that incorporates high-dimensional data analysis with standard statistical analytic tools, in an effort to render

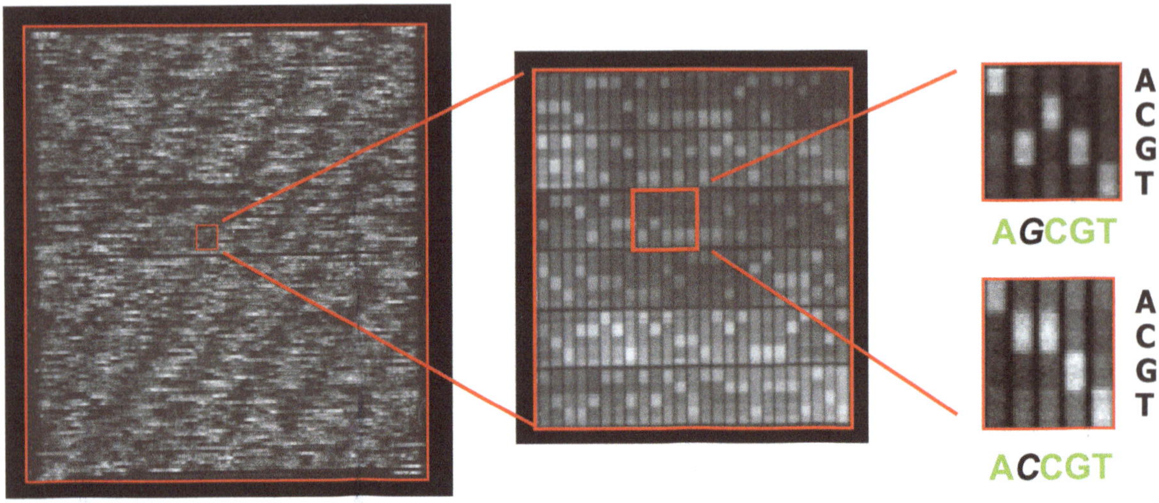

Figure 2.12

Sequencing arrays for DNA sequence determination

these complex datasets comprehensible and reliable (Bassett et al. 1999; Diehn et al. 2000; Eisen et al. 1999; Ermolaeva et al. 1998; Hughes et al. 2000; Lee et al. 2003; Ochs et al. 2004; Peterson and Ringner 2003; Simon 2003; Tamayo et al. 1999; Wittes et al. 1999). Many software packages have been introduced over the past decade, notably Cluster (matrix analysis) and TreeView (hierarchical clustering) (Eisen and Brown 1999). Commercial packages have also been introduced (e.g., GeneSpring) and a host of proprietary packages offered by NCBI, NCI, NIH and many investigators. An example of the latter is illustrated in Fig. 2.13, which illustrates the flow of data analysis, from raw data to final interpretation, in the proprietary software developed at USC Keck School of Medicine. Figure 2.14 shows a typical principal component analysis, one of many methods useful in interpreting these complex datasets. In this case, a diagnostically useful clustering of different solid tumors of childhood is presented, based solely on gene expression profile, derived from an unsupervised learning algorithm. Remarkably, the results of this method both confirm conventional wisdom in most cases. In other cases, expression profiling has identified misclassified cases due to subjective criteria used in the original evaluation of the tumor. In other cases, new molecular subgroups, with distinct genetic features and differing clinical behavior, have been identified. This, in turn, has led to a realization that this method can be a powerful pre-treatment tool for predicting prognosis of an individual patient, and thus better choice of appropriate conventional therapy. There is also the very real possibility of choosing a new, directed therapy based on these data, as discussed above.

An important consideration in the analysis of microarray data is the problem of "noise," or variable levels of fluorescence of a given spot or tile on the microarray (James et al. 2004). Even when control sequences are spiked into the hybridization mixture at known concentrations and hybridized to their complementary sequences that have been incorporated onto the microarray, there is nonetheless significant variation in intensity from array to array, and even within an array for specific genes. In some cases, gene replicates (2X or 3X) are incorporated and the signal averaged to compute an expression value. In other cases, particularly Affymetrix GeneChips, genes may be represented with two or more sequences, based on the UniGene database. Either way, the known vari-

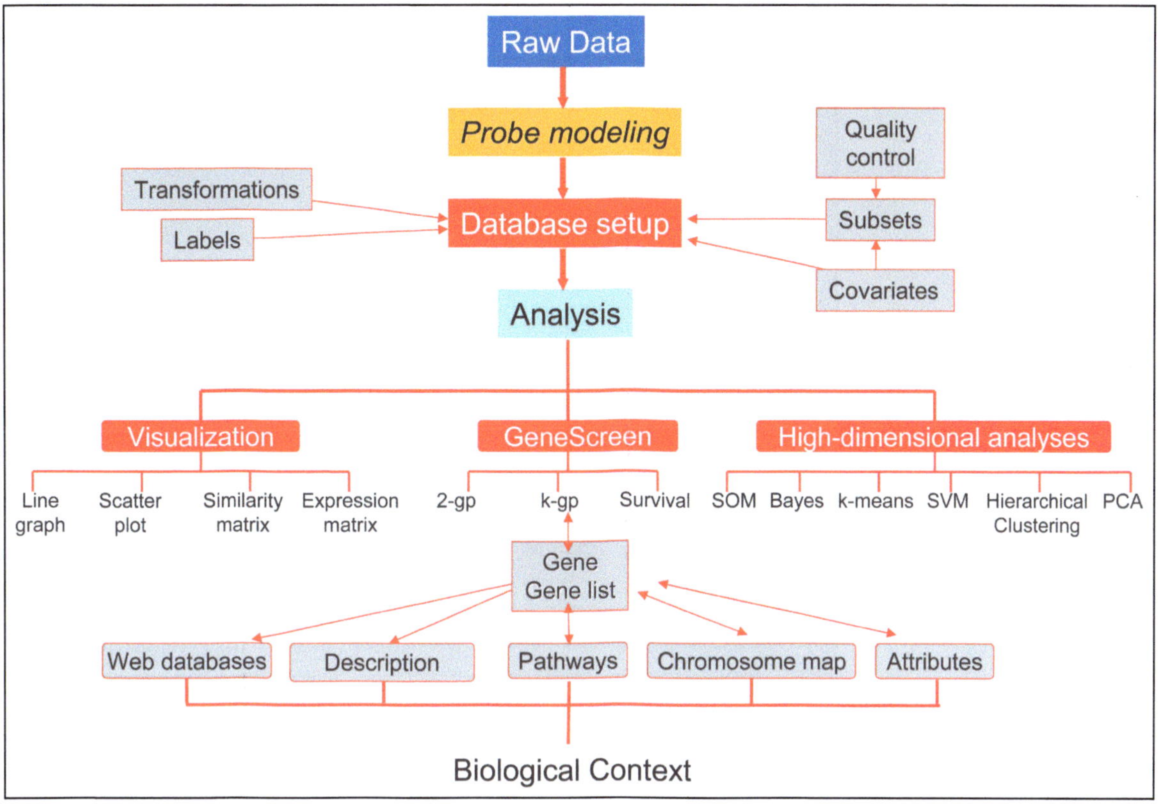

Figure 2.13

Data flow for microarray analysis

ability of quantitative values derived from microarrays has led to an appreciation of the importance of validation. Specifically, an independent measure is necessary to confirm candidate gene expression values. A common method is QPCR, described above and illustrated in Fig. 2.10, where good correlation between microarray expression values, QPCR values, and protein (by Western blot) is seen. Alternatively, one may wish to evaluate protein expression values as the more relevant surrogate expression value. This, however, is not necessarily a 1:1 comparison, for many reasons (mRNA half-life, protein half-life, post-translational modifications, etc.). Nonetheless, there is an emerging consensus that mRNA expression values, whether derived from microarrays or QPCR, should be validated at the protein level (Freeman et al. 1999). This, in turn, is driving rapid adoption of methods to measure proteins in complex mixtures, a field broadly termed "proteomics."

2.4.4 Proteomics

Proteomics is a term to describe a group of technologies that generally utilize mass spectrometry as the final common pathway for analysis of data (Persidis 1998). However, there is no clear consensus on either how to prepare the sample for mass spectrometry, how to measure individual proteins, or not, or even whether sequencing for protein identification is necessary (Baak et al. 2003; Blackstock et al. 1999; Clarke et al. 2003; Conrads et al. 2003; Petricoin et al. 2002a; Rosenblatt et al. 2004; Wulfkuhle et al. 2003). Despite

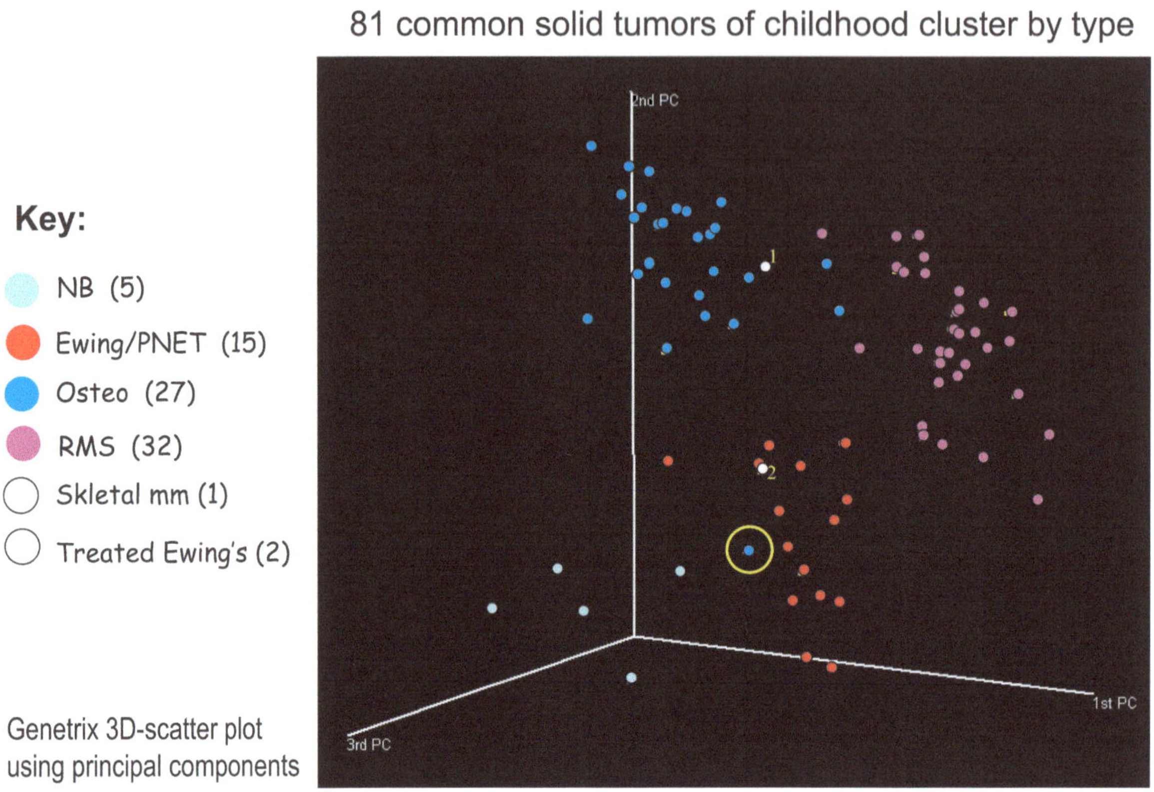

Figure 2.14
Principal component analysis of microarray data

these caveats, the clinical and research utility of this broad technology has excited the interest of both scientists and clinicians, not to mention institutions and granting authorities, who have invested millions of dollars in new proteomic facilities. Unfortunately, much of that investment has not led to clinically useful core resources, as the technology has evolved so rapidly over the past decade as to be almost unrecognizable (Berndt et al. 1999; Nelson et al. 2000; Yanagida et al. 2000). Among other developments, high throughput preparative methods such as SELDI (selective elution and laser desorption and ionization) TOF (time of flight) mass spectrometry have been commercialized by Ciphergen as a method for clinical application of the technology (Merchant et al. 2000; Yip et al. 2002). An example of a typical SELDI TOF proteomic analysis is illustrated in Fig. 2.15, where a series of protein peaks at a molecular weight (or more specifically, mass to charge, M/Z) of 8,300, are seen in one sample, an IL8 control of mw 8,300 that is used here to calibrate the mass spectrometer and provide a reference point for unknowns. This is obviously broadly applicable in the analysis of suspected metastatic, or even early stage, cancer. In fact, this method was utilized by Petricoin and Liotta to analyze serum from a cohort of pre-clinical ovarian cancer patients (Petricoin et al. 2002b). The resulting landmark paper has been widely hailed as a breakthrough in the early diagnosis of cancer. However, there is widespread concern that the results were more likely the result of an artifact (Diamandis 2004; Sorace et al. 2003). It is thus encouraging confirmato-

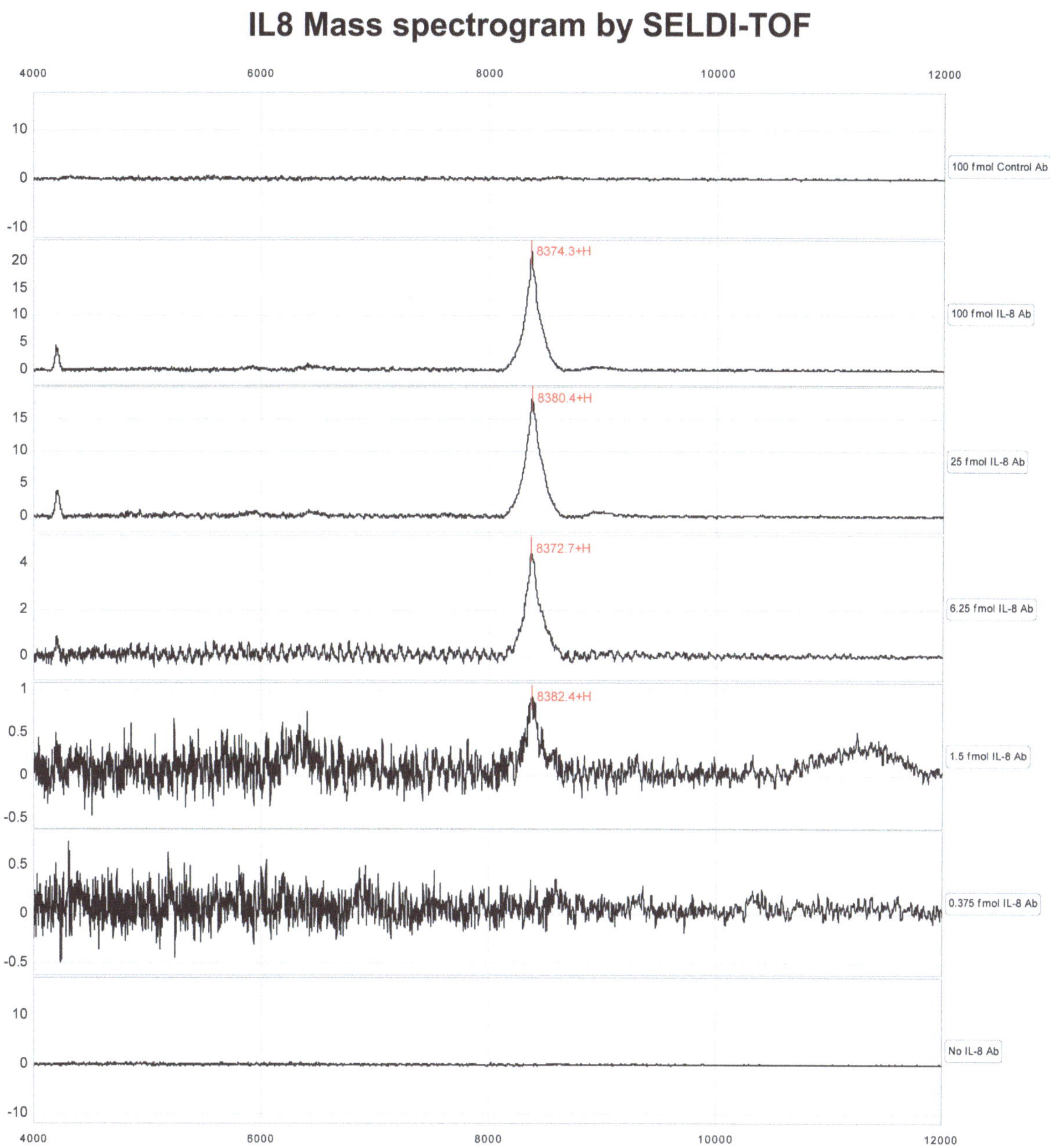

Figure 2.15

SELDI-TOF protein mass spectrogram. Spectrogram courtesy of Ciphergen, Inc.

ry, multi-institutional studies have recently appeared, confirming the utility of this method (Ahmed et al. 2004; Zhang et al. 2004).

SELDI-TOF and similar MS methods rely on pattern recognition, not direct protein or peptide sequencing. Consequently, there is increasing interest in using these methods to screen for differences, but then identifying the suspect proteins by tandem mass spectrometry, or MS-MS, with a quadrapole detector capable of doing real time peptide fragment sequencing. When these short sequences are matched with ever more complete libraries of peptide sequences and the parent proteins in which they are found, it becomes possible to precisely identify the candidate protein peak. This is the method used on more recent publications cited above. Although attractive as a confirmatory method, this technology is not currently a viable clinical tool, given the limited throughput and high cost of the necessary sample pre-processing, typically using liquid chromatography. Thus, most clinical efforts to date have used a higher throughput method such as SELDI TOF MS to identify recurring protein peaks in serum, which have then been subjected to a low throughput method, typically tandem mass spectrometry, to identify by sequencing selected peaks, or, if greater than about 4,000 Da, proteolytic fragments thereof. Clinical utility, in contrast, requires a drastic reduction in complexity and cost from that of tandem mass spectrometry. Surprisingly, that is readily done.

The tension between high throughput and the need for identity lies at the heart of proteomic analysis of cancer. The realization that older technologies such as ELISA assays are a cost-effective, reproducible, readily accepted derivate method of identifying tumor-associated proteins means that proteins identified by mass spec. methods can be reduced to practice as ELISA or similar assays, *if* suitable antibodies are available or can be produced. Fortunately, this is true of most proteins, and suggests that serum protein cancer biomarkers will likely be implemented in cancer management as ELISA or derivative methods. Once such an antibody is available, the inherent ability of ELISA assays to address virtually all these issues makes it an attractive practical method to screen serum for tumor associated proteins – just as it is currently used to detect even scant amounts of viral antigens in HIV, for example. It thus appears that clinical proteomics may well eventuate in a new generation of tumor-associated ELISA assays. The analogy to PSA in prostate cancer and CA125 in ovarian cancer is obvious. The difference is that proteomic analysis prior to development of an ELISA will consider all possible proteins in serum (or tissue, for that matter), and select those that show the strongest correlation with disease. It is likely that no one marker will be sufficient, just as has been found in DNA microarrays. Rather, a small number of proteins (typically $n<20$) will suffice to constitute a cancer "signature."

There is great interest in the ability of these cancer signatures routinely to diagnose, and even predict, disease course and outcome in cancer patients. In fact, both gene and protein cancer signatures, or "biomarkers," are the focus of the NCI in its effort to reduce or eliminate the pain and suffering from cancer. How well the clinical application of these methods will achieve this goal is the subject of intense debate. It is almost certainly too early to say with certainty, but it is intuitively obvious that this is a far better solution than any single biomarker, and certainly likely to be better than current methods. As an obvious comparison, PSA for prostate cancer is far better than nothing, but not in and of itself diagnostic of cancer. It correlates with, but does not confirm, prostate cancer. One can imagine that if a battery of PSA-like markers, each with a 95% probability of detecting cancer, were employed in tandem, the likelihood of diagnosing cancer would approach 100%. This, then, is the promise of cancer signatures derived from the current generation of genomic and proteomic studies now underway.

2.4.5 Conclusion

It should be apparent from the preceding that the diagnostic evaluation of a cancer patient, or suspected cancer patient, is undergoing a remarkable transformation. The impact of the diagnostic methods described herein has not yet been generally felt in oncology, but it will be. It is also influencing the way pathologists approach cancer diagnosis: no longer is a routine H&E section of formalin fixed, paraffin embedded tissue sufficient. Likewise, simple immunohistochemistry of tumor sections is inadequate; by then, the diagnosis of cancer is clear. Only the outlook and likely response to therapy is unclear. The need for early, pre-symptomatic diagnosis of both primary and metastatic disease will certainly engender a new generation of laboratory based diagnostics that will be wedded to current methods of tumor evaluation. The result is likely to be a far more informative and reliable diagnostic evaluation of the cancer patient, *if* oncologists, surgeons, and pathologists can agree on the most informative methods and actually adopt them. That is the real challenge facing the cancer treatment community as the immense amount of new but unconfirmed data from genomic technology floods the cancer literature. How well this is done, and how critically, and at what cost, will largely determine how significant an impact these technologies will have.

References

Ahmed N, Barker G, Oliva KT et al. (2004) Proteomic-based identification of haptoglobin-1 precursor as a novel circulating biomarker of ovarian cancer. Br J Cancer 91(1):129–140

Alizadeh AA, Eisen MB, Davis RE et al. (2000) Distinct types of diffuse large B-cell lymphoma identified by gene expression profiling. Nature 403(6769):503–511

Arteaga CL (2004) Selecting the right patient for tumor therapy. Nat Med 10(6):577–578

Baak JP, Path FR, Hermsen MA et al. (2003) Genomics and proteomics in cancer. Eur J Cancer 39(9):1199–1215

Barr FG, Chatten J, D'Cruz CM et al. (1995) Molecular assays for chromosomal translocations in the diagnosis of pediatric soft tissue sarcomas. JAMA 273:553–557

Bassett DE Jr, Eisen MB, Boguski MS (1999) Gene expression informatics – it's all in your mine. Nat Genet 21 (1 Suppl): 51–55

Bayani J, Squire JA (2001) Advances in the detection of chromosomal aberrations using spectral karyotyping. Clin Genet 59(2):65–73

Bayani J, Squire JA (2002a) Spectral karyotyping. Methods Mol Biol 204:85–104

Bayani JM, Squire JA (2002b) Applications of SKY in cancer cytogenetics. Cancer Invest 20(3):373–386

Bayani J, Thorner P, Zielenska M et al. (1995) Application of a simplified comparative genomic hybridization technique to screen for gene amplification in pediatric solid tumors. Pediatr Pathol Lab Med 15(6):831–844

Berndt P, Hobohm U, Langen H (1999) Reliable automatic protein identification from matrix-assisted laser desorption/ionization mass spectrometric peptide fingerprints. Electrophoresis 20(18):3521–3526

Bhattacharjee A, Richards WG, Staunton J et al. (2001) Classification of human lung carcinomas by mRNA expression profiling reveals distinct adenocarcinoma subclasses. Proc Natl Acad Sci USA 98(24):13790–13795

Blackstock WP, Weir MP (1999) Proteomics: quantitative and physical mapping of cellular proteins. Trends Biotechnol 17(3):121–127

Brandt BH (2002) Molecular diagnostics of solid malignant tumours. Clin Lab 48(11–12):605–615

Bridge J, Liu J, Weibolt V et al. (2000) Novel genomic imbalances in embryonal rhabdomyosarcoma revealed by comparative genomic hybridization and fluorescence in situ hybridization: An Intergroup Rhabdomyosarcoma Study. Genes Chromosomes Cancer 27:337–344

Carr KM, Rosenblatt K, Petricoin EF et al. (2004) Genomic and proteomic approaches for studying human cancer: prospects for true patient-tailored therapy. Hum Genomics 1(2):134–140

Chan JK (2000) Advances in immunohistochemistry: impact on surgical pathology practice. Semin Diagn Pathol 17(3): 170–177

Chen X, Cheung ST, So S et al. (2002) Gene expression patterns in human liver cancers. Mol Biol Cell 13(6):1929–1939

Clarke W, Zhang Z, Chan DW (2003) The application of clinical proteomics to cancer and other diseases. Clin Chem Lab Med 41(12):1562–1570

Coindre JM (2003) Immunohistochemistry in the diagnosis of soft tissue tumours. Histopathology 43(1):1–16

Conrads TP, Zhou M, Petricoin EF 3rd et al. (2003) Cancer diagnosis using proteomic patterns. Expert Rev Mol Diagn 3(4):411–420

Cordon-Cardo C (2001) Applications of molecular diagnostics: solid tumor genetics can determine clinical treatment protocols. Mod Pathol 14(3):254–257

Cui S, Hano H, Harada T et al. (1999) Evaluation of new monoclonal anti-MyoD1 and anti-myogenin antibodies for the diagnosis of rhabdomyosarcoma. Pathol Int 49(1):62–68

Cummings TJ, Brown NM, Stenzel TT (2002) TaqMan junction probes and the reverse transcriptase polymerase chain reaction: detection of alveolar rhabdomyosarcoma, synovial sarcoma, and desmoplastic small round cell tumor. Ann Clin Lab Sci 32(3):219–224

DeMatteo RP (2002) The GIST of targeted cancer therapy: a tumor (gastrointestinal stromal tumor), a mutated gene (c-kit), and a molecular inhibitor (STI571). Ann Surg Oncol 9(9):831–839

Demetri GD (2001) Targeting c-kit mutations in solid tumors: scientific rationale and novel therapeutic options. Semin Oncol 28 (5 Suppl 17):19–26

Demetri GD (2002) Targeting the molecular pathophysiology of gastrointestinal stromal tumors with imatinib. Mechanisms, successes, and challenges to rational drug development. Hematol Oncol Clin North Am 16(5):1115–1124

Devoe K, Weidner N (2000) Immunohistochemistry of small round-cell tumors. Semin Diagn Pathol 17(3):216–224

Diamandis EP (2004) OvaCheck: doubts voiced soon after publication. Nature 430(7000):611

Dias P, Parham DM, Shapiro DN et al. (1990) Myogenic regulatory protein (MyoD1) expression in childhood solid tumors: Diagnostic utility in rhabdomyosarcoma. Am J Pathol 137:1283–1291

Dickman P (1987) Electron microscopy for diagnosis of tumors in children. In: Rosenberg HS, Bernstein J (eds) Perspectives in pediatric pathology, vol 9. S. Karger, Basel, pp 171–213

Diehn M, Alizadeh AA, Brown PO (2000) Examining the living genome in health and disease with DNA microarrays. JAMA 283(17):2298–2299

Duensing A, Medeiros F, McConarty B et al. (2004) Mechanisms of oncogenic KIT signal transduction in primary gastrointestinal stromal tumors (GISTs). Oncogene 23(22): 3999–4006

Eberwine J, Yeh H, Miyashiro K et al. (1992) Analysis of gene expression in single live neurons. Proc Natl Acad Sci USA 89(7):3010–3014

Eisen MB, Brown PO (1999) DNA arrays for analysis of gene expression. Methods Enzymol 303:179–205

Erlandson RA, Cordon CC (1988) Neoplasms of complex or uncertain histogenesis. In: Azar HA (ed) Pathology of human neoplasms. An atlas of diagnostic electron microscopy and immunohistochemistry. Raven Press, New York,

Ermolaeva O, Rastogi M, Pruitt KD et al. (1998) Data management and analysis for gene expression arrays. Nat Genet 20(1):19–23

Fletcher CD, Fletcher JA, Cin PD et al. (2001) Diagnostic gold standard for soft tissue tumours: morphology or molecular genetics? Histopathology 39(1):100–103

Fletcher JA (2004) Molecular biology and cytogenetics of soft tissue sarcomas: relevance for targeted therapies. Cancer Treat Res 120:99–116

Freeman WM, Walker SJ, Vrana KE (1999) Quantitative RT-PCR: pitfalls and potential. Biotechniques 26(1):112–122, 124–125

Garber ME, Troyanskaya OG, Schluens K et al. (2001) Diversity of gene expression in adenocarcinoma of the lung. Proc Natl Acad Sci USA 98(24):13784–13789

Ghadially FN (1985) Diagnostic electron microscopy of tumours. Butterworths, London

Hans CP, Weisenburger DD, Greiner TC et al. (2004) Confirmation of the molecular classification of diffuse large B-cell lymphoma by immunohistochemistry using a tissue microarray. Blood 103(1):275–282

Hattinger CM, Potschger U, Tarkkanen M et al. (2002) Prognostic impact of chromosomal aberrations in Ewing tumours. Br J Cancer 86(11):1763–1769

Hicks J, Mierau G (2004) The spectrum of pediatric tumors in infancy, childhood and adolescence: a comprehensive review with emphasis on special techniques in diagnosis. Ultrastruct Pathol (in press)

Hill DA, Riedley SE, Patel AR et al. (2003) Real-time polymerase chain reaction as an aid for the detection of SYT-SSX1 and SYT-SSX2 transcripts in fresh and archival pediatric synovial sarcoma specimens: report of 25 cases from St. Jude Children's Research Hospital. Pediatr Dev Pathol 6(1):24–34

Hostein I, Menard A, Bui BN et al. (2002) Molecular detection of the synovial sarcoma translocation t(X;18) by real-time polymerase chain reaction in paraffin-embedded material. Diagn Mol Pathol 11(1):16–21

Huang JZ, Sanger WG, Greiner TC et al. (2002) The t(14;18) defines a unique subset of diffuse large B-cell lymphoma with a germinal center B-cell gene expression profile. Blood 99(7):2285–2290

Hughes S, Lim G, Beheshti B et al. (2004) Use of whole genome amplification and comparative genomic hybridisation to detect chromosomal copy number alterations in cell line material and tumour tissue. Cytogenet Genome Res 105(1): 18–24

Hughes TR, Marton MJ, Jones AR et al. (2000) Functional discovery via a compendium of expression profiles. Cell 102:109–126

Jaffer S, Bleiweiss IJ (2004) Beyond hematoxylin and eosin – the role of immunohistochemistry in surgical pathology. Cancer Invest 22(3):445–465

James AC, Veitch JG, Zareh AR et al. (2004) Sensitivity and specificity of five abundance estimators for high-density oligonucleotide microarrays. Bioinformatics 20(7):1060–1065

Klein D (2002) Quantification using real-time PCR technology: applications and limitations. Trends Mol Med 8(6):257–260

Knuutila S (2004) Cytogenetics and molecular pathology in cancer diagnostics. Ann Med 36(3):162–171

Ladanyi M (1995) The emerging molecular genetics of sarcoma translocations. Diagn Mol Pathol 4(3):162–173

Ladanyi M, Bridge JA (2000) Contribution of molecular genetic data to the classification of sarcomas. Hum Pathol 31(5):532–538

Lapointe J, Li C, Higgins JP et al. (2004) Gene expression profiling identifies clinically relevant subtypes of prostate cancer. Proc Natl Acad Sci USA 101(3):811–816

Lee Y, Lee CK (2003) Classification of multiple cancer types by multicategory support vector machines using gene expression data. Bioinformatics 19(9):1132–1139

Liehr T, Claussen U (2002) Current developments in human molecular cytogenetic techniques. Curr Mol Med 2(3): 283–297

Liehr T, Starke H, Weise A et al. (2004) Multicolor FISH probe sets and their applications. Histol Histopathol 19(1):229–237

Llombart-Bosch A, Contesso G, Peydro-Olaya A (1996) Histology, immunohistochemistry, and electron microscopy of small round cell tumors of bone. Semin Diagn Pathol 13(3):153–170

Lombardi L, Orazi A (1988) Electron microscopy in an oncologic institution. Diagnostic usefulness in surgical pathology. Tumori 74(5):531–535

Lossos IS, Alizadeh AA, Diehn M et al. (2002) Transformation of follicular lymphoma to diffuse large-cell lymphoma: alternative patterns with increased or decreased expression of c-myc and its regulated genes. Proc Natl Acad Sci USA 99(13):8886–8891

Lynch TJ, Bell DW, Sordella R et al. (2004) Activating mutations in the epidermal growth factor receptor underlying responsiveness of non-small-cell lung cancer to gefitinib. N Engl J Med 350(21):2129–2139

Marx J (2000) DNA arrays reveal cancer in its many forms. Science 289:1670–1672

Marx J (2004) Medicine. Why a new cancer drug works well, in some patients. Science 304(5671):658–659

Mathew P, Valentine MB, Bowman LC et al. (2001) Detection of MYCN gene amplification in neuroblastoma by fluorescence in situ hybridization: a pediatric oncology group study. Neoplasia 3(2):105–109

Mawad JK, Mackagy B, Raymond AK et al. (1994) Electron microscopy in the diagnosis of small round cell tumors of bone. Ultrastruct Pathol 18:263–268

Merchant M, Weinberger SR (2000) Recent advancements in surface-enhanced laser desorption/ionization-time of flight-mass spectrometry. Electrophoresis 21(6):1164–1177

Millar BC, Moore JE (2004) Molecular diagnostics: current options. Methods Mol Biol 266:139–166

Monforte-Munoz H, Lopez-Terrada D, Affendie H et al. (1999) Documentation of EWS gene rearrangements by fluorescence in-situ hybridization (FISH) in frozen sections of Ewing's sarcoma-peripheral primitive neuroectodermal tumor. Am J Surg Pathol 23(3):309–315

Nelson RW, Nedelkov D, Tubbs KA (2000) Biosensor chip mass spectrometry: a chip-based proteomics approach. Electrophoresis 21(6):1155–1163

Nielsen TO, West RB, Linn SC et al. (2002) Molecular characterisation of soft tissue tumours: a gene expression study. Lancet 359(9314):1301–1307

Nutt CL, Mani DR, Betensky RA et al. (2003) Gene expression-based classification of malignant gliomas correlates better with survival than histological classification. Cancer Res 63(7):1602–1607

Ochs MF, Moloshok TD, Bidaut G et al. (2004) Bayesian decomposition: analyzing microarray data within a biological context. Ann N Y Acad Sci 1020:212–226

Paez JG, Janne PA, Lee JC et al. (2004) EGFR mutations in lung cancer: correlation with clinical response to gefitinib therapy. Science 304(5676):1497–1500

Pandita A, Zielenska M, Thorner P et al. (1999) Application of comparative genomic hybridization, spectral karyotyping, and microarray analysis in the identification of subtype-specific patterns of genomic changes in rhabdomyosarcoma. Neoplasia 1(3):262–275

Papadimitriou JC, Nikitakis N, Armand R (2004) Immunohistochemical studies in the differential diagnosis of small round cell soft tissue tumors. Arkh Patol 66(2):31–36

Perou CM, Jeffrey SS, van de Rijn M et al. (1999) Distinctive gene expression patterns in human mammary epithelial cells and breast cancers. Proc Natl Acad Sci USA 96(16): 9212–9217

Persidis A (1998) Proteomics. Nat Biotechnol 16(4):393–394

Peter M, Gilbert E, Delattre O (2001) A multiplex real-time pcr assay for the detection of gene fusions observed in solid tumors. Lab Invest 81(6):905–912

Peterson C, Ringner M (2003) Analyzing tumor gene expression profiles. Artif Intell Med 28(1):59–74

Petricoin EF, Ardekani AM, Hitt BA et al. (2002a) Use of proteomic patterns in serum to identify ovarian cancer. Lancet 359(9306):572–577

Petricoin EF, Zoon KC, Kohn EC et al. (2002b) Clinical proteomics: translating benchside promise into bedside reality. Nat Rev Drug Discov 1(9):683–695

Peydro-Olaya A, Llombart-Bosch A, Carda-Batalla C et al. (2003) Electron microscopy and other ancillary techniques in the diagnosis of small round cell tumors. Semin Diagn Pathol 20(1):25–45

Pomeroy SL, Tamayo P, Gaasenbeek M et al. (2002) Prediction of central nervous system embryonal tumour outcome based on gene expression. Nature 415(6870):436–442

Ramaswamy S, Golub TR (2002) DNA microarrays in clinical oncology. J Clin Oncol 20(7):1932–1941

Ramaswamy S, Ross KN, Lander ES et al. (2003) A molecular signature of metastasis in primary solid tumors. Nat Genet 33(1):49–54

Rosenblatt KP, Bryant-Greenwood P, Killian JK et al. (2004) Serum proteomics in cancer diagnosis and management. Annu Rev Med 55:97–112

Rosenwald A, Staudt LM (2002) Clinical translation of gene expression profiling in lymphomas and leukemias. Semin Oncol 29(3):258–263

Sandberg AA, Bridge JA (1994) The cytogenetics of bone and soft tissue tumors. R.G. Landes Co., Austin

Shipp MA, Ross KN, Tamayo P et al. (2002) Diffuse large B-cell lymphoma outcome prediction by gene-expression profiling and supervised machine learning. Nat Med 8(1):68–74

Simon R (2003) Diagnostic and prognostic prediction using gene expression profiles in high-dimensional microarray data. Br J Cancer 89(9):1599–1604

Simon R, Radmacher MD, Dobbin K et al. (2003) Pitfalls in the use of DNA microarray data for diagnostic and prognostic classification. J Natl Cancer Inst 95(1):14–18

Singh D, Febbo PG, Ross K et al. (2002) Gene expression correlates of clinical prostate cancer behavior. Cancer Cell 1(2):203–209

Sorace JM, Zhan M (2003) A data review and re-assessment of ovarian cancer serum proteomic profiling. BMC Bioinformatics 4(1):24

Sordella R, Bell DW, Haber DA et al. (2004) Gefitinib-sensitizing EGFR mutations in lung cancer activate anti-apoptotic pathways. Science 305(5687):1163–1167

Sorensen PHB, Triche TJ (1996) Gene fusions encoding chimaeric transcription factors in solid tumours. Semin Cancer Biol 7:3–14

Staudt LM (2002) Gene expression profiling of lymphoid malignancies. Annu Rev Med 53:303–318

Stratton MR, Futreal PA (2004) Cancer: understanding the target. Nature 430(6995):30

Suster S (2000) Recent advances in the application of immunohistochemical markers for the diagnosis of soft tissue tumors. Semin Diagn Pathol 17(3):225–235

Tamayo P, Slonim D, Mesirov J et al. (1999) Interpreting patterns of gene expression with self-organizing maps: methods and application to hematopoietic differentiation. Proc Natl Acad Sci USA 96(6):2907–2912

Thorner PS, Squire JA (1998) Molecular genetics in the diagnosis and prognosis of solid pediatric tumors. Pediatr Dev Pathol 1(5):337–365

Tonon G, Roschke A, Stover K et al. (2000) Spectral karyotyping combined with locus-specific FISH simultaneously defines genes and chromosomes involved in chromosomal translocations. Genes Chromosomes Cancer 27(4):418–423

Triche TJ, Hicks J, Sorensen P (2005) Molecular pathology of pediatric malignancies. In: Pizzo P, Poplack D (eds) Principles and practice of pediatric oncology, 5 edn. JP Lippincott, Philadelphia

Tuveson DA, Willis NA, Jacks T et al. (2001) STI571 inactivation of the gastrointestinal stromal tumor c-KIT oncoprotein: biological and clinical implications. Oncogene 20(36):5054–5058

van de Vijver MJ, He YD, van't Veer LJ et al. (2002) A gene-expression signature as a predictor of survival in breast cancer. N Engl J Med 347(25):1999–2009

van Haelst UJ (1986) Em in the study of soft tissue tumors: diagnosis/differential diagnosis and histogenesis. Monogr Ser Eur Org Res Treat Cancer 16(71):71–91

Weber-Hall S, Anderson J, McManus A et al. (1996) Gains, losses, and amplification of genomic material in rhabdomyosarcoma analyzed by comparative genomic hybridization. Cancer Res 56(14):3220–3224

Weigelt B, Glas AM, Wessels LF et al. (2003) Gene expression profiles of primary breast tumors maintained in distant metastases. Proc Natl Acad Sci USA 100(26):15901–15905

Went PT, Dirnhofer S, Bundi M et al. (2004) Prevalence of KIT expression in human tumors. J Clin Oncol 22(22):4514–4522

Wittes J, Friedman HP (1999) Searching for evidence of altered gene expression: a comment on statistical analysis of microarray data [editorial; comment]. J Natl Cancer Inst 91(5):400–401

Wright G, Tan B, Rosenwald A et al. (2003) A gene expression-based method to diagnose clinically distinct subgroups of diffuse large B cell lymphoma. Proc Natl Acad Sci USA 100(17):9991–9996

Wulfkuhle JD, Paweletz CP, Steeg PS et al. (2003) Proteomic approaches to the diagnosis, treatment, and monitoring of cancer. Adv Exp Med Biol 532:59–68

Yanagida M, Miura Y, Yagasaki K et al. (2000) Matrix assisted laser desorption/ionization-time of flight-mass spectrometry analysis of proteins detected by anti-phosphotyrosine antibody on two-dimensional gels of fibroblast cell lysates after tumor necrosis factor-alpha stimulation [in process citation]. Electrophoresis 21(9):1890–1898

Yeang CH, Ramaswamy S, Tamayo P et al. (2001) Molecular classification of multiple tumor types. Bioinformatics 17 Suppl 1:S316–322

Yip TT, Lomas L (2002) SELDI ProteinChip array in oncoproteomic research. Technol Cancer Res Treat 1(4):273–280

Zhang FF, Murata-Collins JL, Gaytan P et al. (2000) Twenty-four-color spectral karyotyping reveals chromosome aberrations in cytogenetically normal acute myeloid leukemia. Genes Chromosomes Cancer 28(3):318–328

Zhang Z, Bast RC Jr, Yu Y et al. (2004) Three biomarkers identified from serum proteomic analysis for the detection of early stage ovarian cancer. Cancer Res 64(16):5882–5890

Diagnostic Imaging of Pediatric Bone and Soft Tissue Sarcomas

Thomas D. Henry, Mary E. McCarville,
Fredric A. Hoffer

Contents

3.1 Introduction

The role of the radiologist in the diagnosis and treatment of the pediatric patient with a bone or soft tissue sarcoma continues to evolve. Initial imaging studies help guide the radiologic work-up and select those patients for whom image-guided biopsy of the primary tumor and metastatic lesions is indicated. After initiation of therapy, attention shifts to the notoriously difficult task of assessing tumor response. Theoretically, the radiologist may remain involved for years following diagnosis, monitoring for recurrent disease and the development of second tumors, and potentially treating disease using techniques such as radiofrequency ablation and tumor localization for surgical resection of recurrences. The goals of this chapter are to describe the imaging concepts involved in the evaluation of these patients and to provide an overview of the more commonly encountered tumors, with additional attention to the pertinent rarer entities.

3.2 Initial Evaluation of Bone and Soft Tissue Sarcomas

The initial challenge for the radiologist is to distinguish lesions with benign imaging characteristics from those with aggressive features. Many benign tumors of bone have such classically described radiographic appearances that plain film alone may be diagnostic. In these cases, further radiologic work-up is not warranted, as it can lead to confusion and unnecessary biopsy. Most masses will have non-specific plain film findings requiring further evaluation with

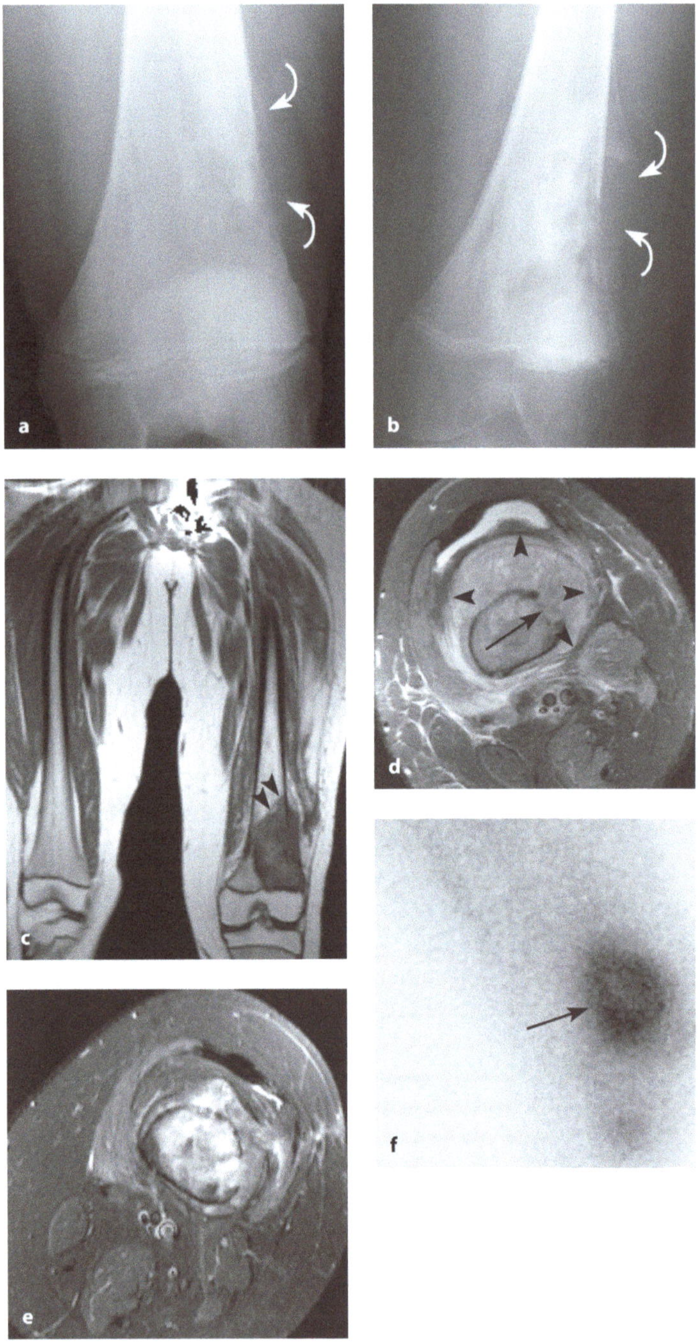

Figure 3.1 a–f

Osteosarcoma. **a** Initial AP knee radiograph of 15-year-old boy complaining of left knee pain for several months. Note poorly defined involvement of the metaphysis. Laterally there are proximal and distal periosteal reactions broken through by a soft tissue mass. The two triangles of periosteal reaction are called Codman's triangles (*arrows*). **b** Three months later, after completing 12 weeks of chemotherapy, the soft tissue tumor margins and Codman's triangle (*arrow*) are now more defined and sclerotic as is expected with maturation. Also note the increased sclerosis within the intramedullary metaphyseal mass. **c** Coronal T1 MR is most helpful in determining the extent of intramedullary osteosarcoma (*arrowheads*), which is confined to the distal left metaphysis in this case. **d** Axial STIR image is most helpful in determining the soft tissue extent of the osteosarcoma. A section through distal left femur demonstrates a large soft tissue component (*arrowheads*) of the mass doubling the normal diameter of the bone. The tumor probably originated near the lateral cortex, which is broken through (*arrow*). The peripheral areas of highest signal represent surrounding subcutaneous and muscle edema and a femoral patellar joint effusion. **e** Axial STIR image taken at the same level as the prior image after 12 weeks of chemotherapy; the soft tissue mass is markedly smaller and there is now increased signal within the metaphyseal and soft tissue components of the tumor, representing areas of necrosis. **f** Thallium-201 scan demonstrates intense "donut" sign of decreased central activity in the region of the left distal femoral tumor (*arrow*). This sign is a predictor of poor outcome

cross sectional imaging techniques. It is important to realize that although the magnetic resonance (MR) features of a particular tumor at presentation offer much valuable information, it is only in rare cases that these characteristics are diagnostic (Bloem et al. 1997). Tissue diagnosis is essential for determining appropriate therapy.

3.3 Imaging Techniques for Evaluating the Primary Tumor

Various examples of primary bone sarcomas, soft tissue sarcomas, and their mimics are shown in Figs. 3.1–3.27. Plain radiographs are the essential starting point, and generally the first study obtained by the referring physician upon patient presentation (Fig. 3.1 a). At least two perpendicular views should be obtained of any suspected mass. MR imaging has largely supplanted computed tomography (CT) in the evaluation of primary bone and soft tissue sarcomas due to its superior definition of soft tissues and its multiplanar capabilities. However, CT remains useful and is admittedly far more sensitive in detecting calcification (Fig. 3.8 a) (Kransdorf et al. 1993). Although of limited use in the evaluation of bone tumors, ultrasound plays an important adjunct role in characterizing soft tissue masses, especially with sarcomas located superficially or in the pelvis or scrotum (Varma 1999). Additionally, ultrasound is a valuable tool of the interventionalist for tumor localization, biopsy (Fig. 3.15 b), and image-guided ablation (Fig. 3.23 b).

MR imaging should be performed in at least two orthogonal planes (Fletcher 1997). Small volume coils or flexible coils provide optimal signal but may be impractical with large tumors or in imaging the lower extremities of patients who cannot extend the knee joint (Fletcher 1997). When imaging bone sarcomas, longitudinal images of the whole bone are essential in order to exclude skip lesions (Figs. 3.2, 3.3). Either the coronal or sagittal plane can be used, with sagittal preferred for the humerus in order to avoid phase artifacts related to the chest (Hoffer 2002). T1, T2-fat saturation (FS), and short tau inversion recovery (STIR) sequences all effectively detect marrow disease (Figs. 3.1 c, 3.2, 3.3, 3.10, 3.15 c). Transverse T2 and gadolinium-enhanced T1 sequences are useful for assessing the soft tissue component and defining tumor vascularity and relationship to adjacent structures (Figs. 3.1 d, 3.10 a) (Lang et al. 1998). Postcontrast T1 images also allow better definition of necrot-

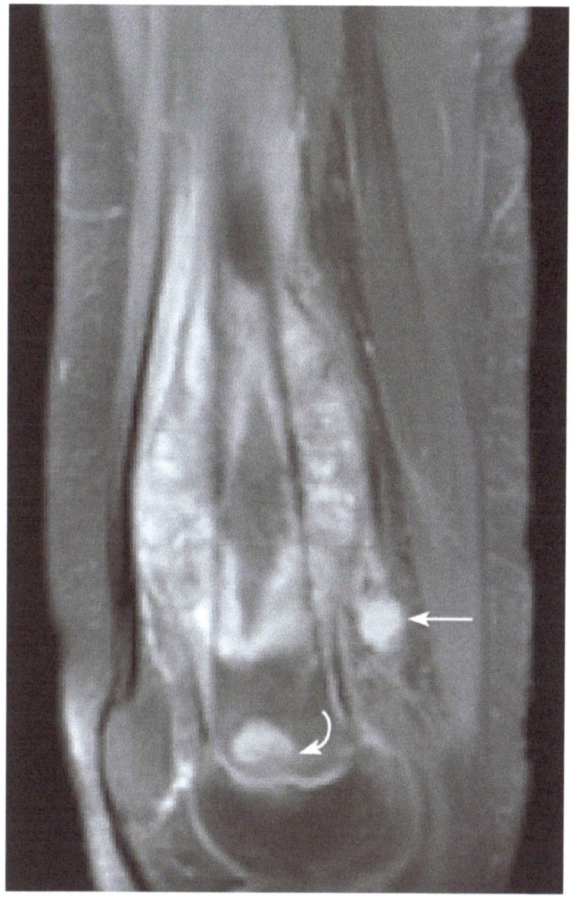

Figure 3.2

Osteosarcoma. This 12-year-old boy developed metastases while on treatment. Note the primary tumor margins in the soft tissue mass match the intramedullary primary tumor involvement on this postcontrast T1 sagittal MR. However, there is a separate distal metaphyseal skip metastasis (*curved arrow*) and a popliteal lymph node metastasis (*straight arrow*) confirmed by pathology after limb salvage

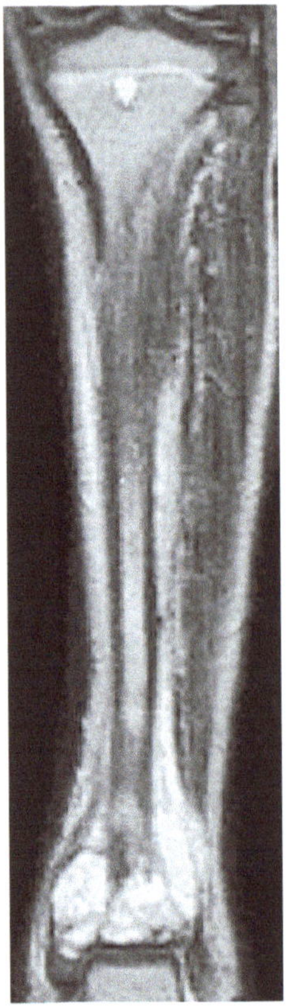

Figure 3.3

Osteosarcoma. This 6-year-old boy has a left tibial osteosarcoma primary tumor and proximal left metaphyseal skip metastasis noted on coronal STIR MR. This emphasizes the importance of imaging the whole bone. The patient later died of his disease

ic regions (Figs. 3.9c, 3.11b, 3.26) and help identify intra-articular involvement (Schima et al. 1994). Both T1- and T2-weighted images can be obtained using fast spin echo (FSE), gradient echo (GE), or spin echo (SE) technique with or without fat suppression.

Although not routinely performed during the initial radiologic work-up of bone and soft tissue sarcomas, fluorine-18-fluorodeoxyglucose positron emission tomography (18-FDG PET) can reliably predict whether a musculoskeletal lesion is benign or malignant based upon the tumor's standardized uptake value (SUV), a quantified measure of the avidity of the lesion for the radiolabeled glucose analog (Feldman et al. 2003). Questions concerning the appropriate SUV cut-off value persist, but generally speaking those lesions with an SUV greater than 2.0 are malignant (aggressive), and those below 2.0 are benign (Feldman et al. 2003).

3.4 Staging

3.4.1 Local Extent of the Tumor

Imaging in longitudinal planes allows for the most accurate measurement of tumor extent (Figs. 3.1c, 3.2, 3.3), which is especially important when considering the option of limb-sparing surgery in a patient with a bone sarcoma (Fletcher 1997; Hoffer 2002). For soft tissue sarcomas, the anatomic site will determine the extent of surgical resection and the need for additional therapies. Preoperative imaging also will guide the decision to obtain biopsy versus proceeding with primary resection of tumor (Herzog et al. 2003).

For bone sarcomas, epiphyseal extension needs to be accurately determined. If all abnormal epiphyseal signal is considered tumor, then sensitivity for detecting epiphyseal involvement reaches 100%, but specificity falls to 40–60% (Hoffer et al. 2000). The accuracy is improved when one can reliably distinguish edema from tumor. Tumor should be dark on T1, bright on STIR, enhance inhomogeneously, and disrupt the normal architecture (Hoffer et al. 2000). Peritumoral edema (Figs. 3.1d, 3.7e), which may result from venous or lymphatic compression as well as from vasodilation with increased hydrostatic pressure, tends to give an intermediate signal on T1, may be bright on STIR, may enhance with contrast, and should not alter the normal architecture (Hoffer et al. 2000). Dynamic enhanced MR imaging (DEMRI) (Fig. 3.6) can offer objective insight into the nature of peritumoral abnormal signal (differentiating tumor from edema and hematopoietic marrow), but is less accurate than static MR in determining epiphyseal extension (Hoffer et al. 2000). In all cases when intercalary resection is considered, it is imperative to repeat the MR near the time of surgery to ensure that no epiphyseal invasion has occurred.

Some MR findings of bone sarcomas are non-specific, with signal overlap seen between viable tumor, necrotic tissue, hemorrhage, and edema (Figs. 3.4b, 3.8b, 3.9c,d). For this reason, various pulse sequences and imaging techniques must be employed. The highly T2-weighted STIR sequence inherently suppresses fat and maximizes tumor contrast, but gener-

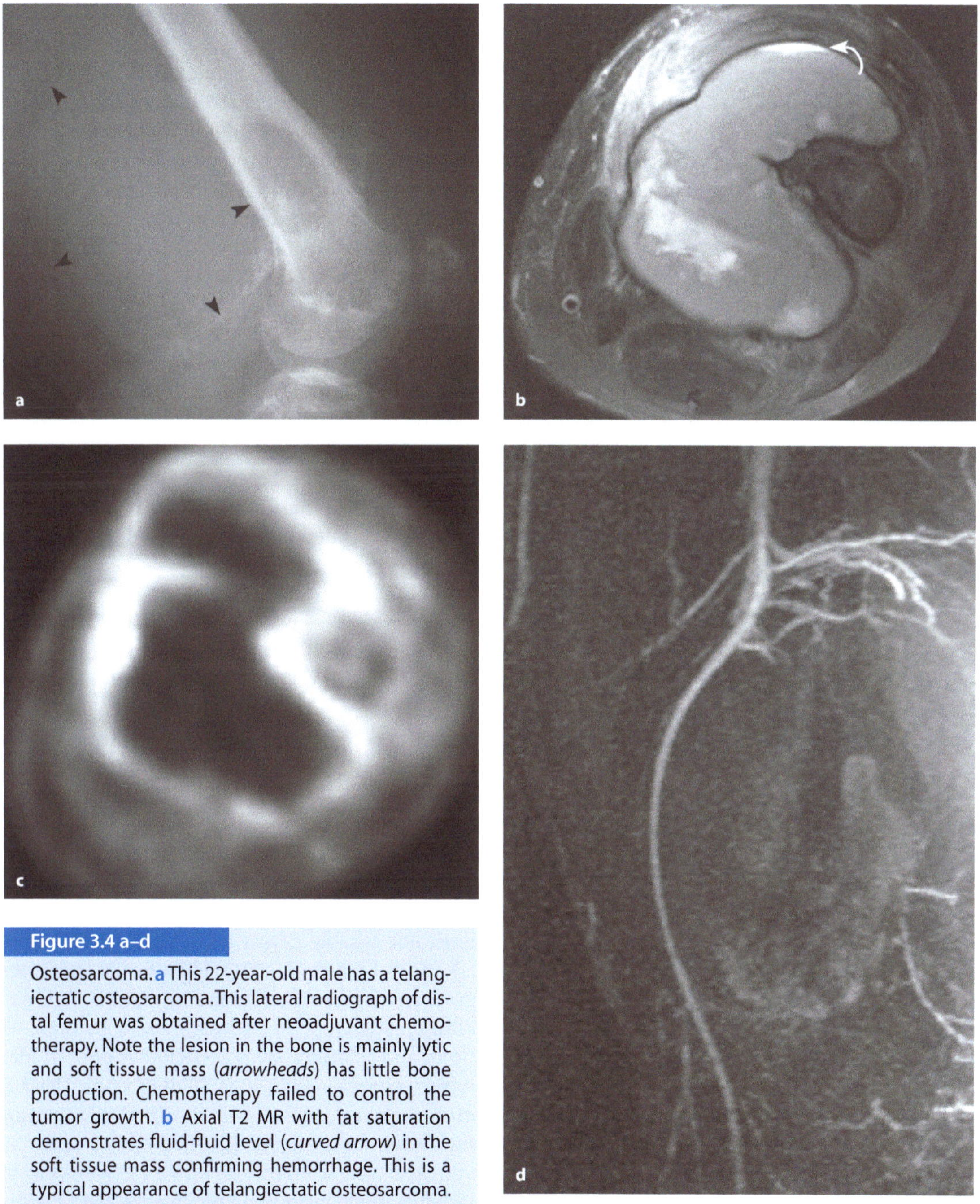

Figure 3.4 a–d

Osteosarcoma. a This 22-year-old male has a telangiectatic osteosarcoma. This lateral radiograph of distal femur was obtained after neoadjuvant chemotherapy. Note the lesion in the bone is mainly lytic and soft tissue mass (*arrowheads*) has little bone production. Chemotherapy failed to control the tumor growth. b Axial T2 MR with fat saturation demonstrates fluid-fluid level (*curved arrow*) in the soft tissue mass confirming hemorrhage. This is a typical appearance of telangiectatic osteosarcoma. c Axial F-18 FDG positron emission tomogram (PET) demonstrates that only the edges of the tumor (*bright signal uptake*) are viable. d MR arteriography shows displacement of the popliteal artery. A later phase MR venogram showed occlusion of the popliteal vein. The leg was amputated and the vessels were found to be encased by tumor

ally overestimates tumor extent in the presence of edema (Hoffer 2002). Additional sequences such as static and dynamic contrast-enhanced T1-weighted images often provide useful distinguishing information. A technique which can be used to differentiate marrow invasion from other processes is "in and out of phase" MR imaging. This technique takes advantage of the different signals of fat and water on specific sequences to aid in the distinction between malignant and benign marrow processes. Most neoplasms replace fat, bone, and hematopoietic elements in marrow, whereas most non-neoplastic abnormalities, whether trauma, infection, ischemia, or marrow hyperplasia, do not (Disler et al. 1997).

Most soft tissue sarcomas appear as heterogeneously enhancing, deep-seated masses with T1 signal similar to skeletal muscle and heterogeneous, hyperintense T2 signal (van der Woude et al. 1994). Characteristics vary depending upon the amount of necrosis and hemorrhage contained (Hanna and Fletcher 1995). Fat can be easily identified. Tumors greater than 5 cm regardless of location are considered to have a poorer prognosis, and are treated more aggressively (Levine 1999). Identification of involvement of neighboring neurovascular structures is vital in determining resectability of the lesion. Conventional angiography has largely been replaced by CT or MR angiography for this purpose (Fig. 3.4 d). Only rarely do soft tissue sarcomas invade adjacent bone and bone marrow (Fenstermacher 2003). When the MR findings are equivocal, 18-FDG PET scanning may increase the specificity of disease extent (Bredella et al. 2002).

3.4.2 Detection of Metastatic Disease

Bone sarcomas most often metastasize to the lungs, bone, and bone marrow, in descending order of frequency (Fletcher 1997). Lymph nodes are rarely involved (Enneking et al. 1980). When bone metastasis does occur with osteosarcoma, it is more common to find a skip lesion in the same bone (Figs. 3.2, 3.3) than involvement of a second bone (Hoffer 2002). Ewing sarcoma and small cell osteosarcoma are the tumors most likely to present with distant osseous metastases (Hoffer 2002).

Rhabdomyosarcoma (RMS) metastasizes to lung, liver, bone marrow, bone, lymph nodes, and brain (Gurney et al. 1995; Koscielniak et al. 1992; Parasuraman et al. 1999; Raney et al. 1988). Imaging of regional lymph nodes is much more important in the staging of RMS (Figs. 3.14 a,b, 3.17 b–d) than of non-rhabdomyosarcomas (NRSTS). Primary tumors of the extremities, paratesticular region, and perineum have the highest incidence of nodal metastasis at diagnosis (Feldman et al. 2003).

Chest CT is the standard for evaluating patients with sarcomas for the presence of pulmonary metastases. It is essential to perform CT before the patient receives anesthesia because any resultant atelectasis may be mistaken for or may obscure metastatic disease (Hoffer 2002). Atelectasis generally appears as linear density in the dependent portion of the lung, in contrast to the typically rounded shape of metastatic foci, but considerable overlap in appearance exists. Occasionally patients will be scanned in both the supine and prone position in order to help differentiate between these processes, as atelectatic lung may reexpand when the affected lung is no longer in the dependent position, while metastatic lesions will persist. Conventional scintigraphy with Tc 99m MDP has been the accepted modality for identifying skeletal metastases at presentation, but is limited by relatively low sensitivity (62–89 %) (Daldrup-Link et al. 2001). Additionally, skeletal scintigraphy identifies metastases at a fairly late stage (after osteoblastic reaction has occurred), has inherently poor anatomic detail even with SPECT multiplanar capabilities, and does not reliably detect lesions smaller than 5 mm (Daldrup-Link et al. 2001). The normal epiphyses of growing children and adolescents have high osteoblastic activity, often masking tumor in these locations, and scintigraphy is notoriously poor at identifying vertebral metastases (Bloem et al. 1997; Daldrup-Link et al. 2001). These limitations have spurred the search for more reliable methods of tumor staging, with whole body MR and PET scanning both showing much promise (Antoch et al. 2003; Daldrup-Link et al. 2001; Mazumdar et al. 2002).

MR imaging allows direct visualization of bone marrow, which is the earliest site of neoplastic cell infiltration in the setting of skeletal metastasis (Daldrup-Link et al. 2001). In the past, long scanning times (up to 1 h) and poor image quality have been major obstacles to the use of whole body MR imaging for staging; however, recent technical advances have resulted in head to toe scan times as short as 15 min, with improved image resolution and fewer artifacts (Lauenstein et al. 2002). Turbo STIR and fast gradient echo T1 out of phase sequences used in conjunction appear to offer a good compromise of fast scanning time and high accuracy in differentiating metastases from fatty or hematopoietic marrow. These MRI techniques have also been shown to reliably identify hepatic, lymphatic, and even the larger pulmonary metastases (Lauenstein et al. 2002).

Fluorine-18-fluorodeoxyglucose PET scanning uses a glucose analog to identify regions of increased metabolism, providing a functional rather than a morphologic indicator of nodal metastasis and early marrow infiltration (Fig. 3.16) (Daldrup-Link et al. 2001). Past limitations of PET have included lack of availability and reimbursement, as well as poor anatomic resolution (Daldrup-Link et al. 2001). The introduction of hybrid PET/CT technology has addressed much of the latter problem, and availability is expected to increase as reimbursement is granted for new uses. PET has been shown in one study to be more accurate at staging tumors in adults than whole body MRI, although MR proved more reliable in identifying hepatic and osseous metastases (Antoch et al. 2003). Anatomic site of bone metastases also seems to be an important factor in detection, with PET more often missing lesions in the skull (due to masking by brain activity), MR in the small and flat bones, and skeletal scintigraphy the spine (Daldrup-Link et al. 2001). Lymphoscintigraphy and intraoperative mapping with sentinel node biopsy (Fig. 3.17 c–d) are valuable adjuncts in identifying lymphatic spread in some cases, and appear to detect smaller nodal metastases than PET (Feldman et al. 2003; Havenga et al. 2003).

3.5 Criteria for Evaluating Treatment Response

In osteosarcoma and Ewing sarcoma, initial tumor response to therapy is the strongest predictor of relapse, recurrence, feasibility of limb-salvage surgery, and overall survival (Gherlinzoni et al. 1992; Meyers et al. 1992; Winkler et al. 1988). Identifying the poor responders early helps facilitate a more fluid approach to treatment based upon constant modification and integration of therapeutic modalities using the most current indicators of treatment efficacy. Ewing sarcoma typically presents with a soft tissue component which can be fairly easily measured during the treatment course (Fig. 3.10 a, b). Osteosarcomas, on the other hand, predominantly involve the bone and tend to ossify rather than shrink when treated (Fig. 3.1 a, b), presenting a specific challenge in objectively determining tumor response to therapy. Several modalities have been proposed to assess response, with many often conflicting variables competing for influence, including accuracy, cost, time, availability, invasiveness, and need for sedation. The ability of each modality to accurately distinguish treatment-associated soft tissue changes from viable tumor is of paramount importance, and quite controversial.

Static MR imaging of sarcomas is notoriously nonspecific in patients during and after neoadjuvant chemotherapy. MR signal of viable tumor, neighboring edema and necrosis can overlap considerably, and differentiating between good and poor responders often involves reliance upon subjective parameters (van der Woude et al. 1994). Chemotherapy itself has variable effects on marrow signal, while patients receiving GCSF demonstrate the signal characteristics of increased hematopoiesis (Fletcher et al. 1993). These include decreased T1 and increased T2 signal, findings which can simulate metastatic disease (Fletcher 1997). These persistent problems have spurred many investigations to explore newer MR techniques as well as other modalities.

Dynamic enhanced MR imaging (DEMRI) has been investigated as a tool for both evaluating the response of bone sarcomas to neoadjuvant chemotherapy and identifying tumors that are likely to fail treatment (Reddick et al. 1999; Reddick et al. 2001). This technique is especially valuable in imaging osteosarcomas, since one cannot rely on tumor shrinkage to determine response. DEMRI involves selecting a desired slice in one plane and acquiring multiple consecutive images during contrast injection, demonstrating the enhancement characteristics of the tumor. The value of DEMRI lies in its ability to assess tumor microvascularity indirectly and non-invasively by using contrast agents to measure changes in tumor microcirculation at multiple intervals during treatment (Reddick et al. 1999, 2001). Rapid disappearance of intratumoral vessels is associated with good response to chemotherapy, persistence of vascularity with poor response (Reddick et al. 2001). Several methods of analyzing the data generated have been used; one of these, DVM, equally weighs both the ICAR (a measure of the rate of contrast agent accumulation in the vasculature and in the tumor interstitial spaces) and ME (the measure of the total accumulation of contrast agent in these spaces) to generate a quantitative value of contrast accumulation in the region of interest (ROI) selected by the radiologist, yielding a calculated percent tumor necrosis. Ninety percent necrosis has traditionally been considered indicative of good response, but prior to DEMRI this information was only reliably available in cases of patients with surgically resected tumors completing neoadjuvant chemotherapy (Reddick et al. 2001; Rosen et al. 1982). Additionally, there is hope that this technology can be used to assess chemotherapy access in individual tumors, and even applied toward customizing drug delivery systems to patients based upon specific tumor microcirculation characteristics (Taylor and Reddick 2000).

Nuclear medicine techniques have also been utilized to assess tumor response to therapy. Avidity of osteosarcoma for Tc 99m MDP changes little during therapy regardless of therapeutic response, but thallium-201 avidity usually decreases in tumors that respond to chemotherapy (Kaste et al. 2001). Thallium has great affinity for cellular activity and does not normally concentrate in normal bone or marrow, so increased avidity indicates increased cellular activity in the tumor (Kaste et al. 2001). Sestamibi is an equal alternative to thallium for determining viability of the tumor. F-18 FDG-PET (Figs. 3.4c, 3.8c, 3.12c) offers the same metabolic information as thallium and sestamibi scintigraphy with better spatial resolution and less radiation. The role of PET scanning in assessment of the response of pediatric bone sarcomas to chemotherapy remains to be elucidated, but it does appear that decreased activity (quantified as the standardized uptake value) following neoadjuvant chemotherapy is indicative of good histologic response (Franzius and Schober 2003; Hawkins et al. 2002). To date, only small studies have been conducted on the pediatric population.

Color Doppler flow imaging (CDFI) can be used to assess the soft tissue component of a tumor as well as evaluate tumor blood supply and intratumoral vascularity (Fig. 3.19b). In capable hands, this modality offers a safe and readily available method for assessing response to chemotherapy (van der Woude et al. 1994). However, only tumors with a significant soft tissue component and vascularity can be accurately assessed, and a significant overlap exists between the Doppler characteristics of tumors judged good and poor responders (van der Woude et al. 1994). Angiography will likewise demonstrate tumor vascularity but is invasive and qualitative, and therefore generally not an accepted modality in this respect (van der Woude et al. 1994).

Primary soft tissue sarcomas can be serially measured on imaging studies, allowing relatively precise and reproducible assessment of response. However, these measurements become more complicated as the number of metastatic foci increases. The latest attempt to standardize criteria produced RECIST, which unfortunately did not specifically consider pediatric tumors when it was formulated (McHugh and Kao 2003). Despite this obvious limitation, RECIST has been applied to the pediatric population, and its strict reliance on size as the primary factor determining response has caused several problems (McHugh and Kao 2003). Among these, issues of consistency and interchangeability of equipment and modalities on serial studies have raised particular questions. Ultrasound and MRI are routinely used in pediatrics and have the advantage over CT of not exposing the patient to ionizing radiation, but under the RECIST system the same modality must be used for all measurements and ultrasound is not allowed (McHugh and Kao 2003). Disagreements regarding the optimal measurement techniques also persist, with some investigators advocating two- or three-dimensional measurements, while the criteria call for the single greatest diameter (McHugh and Kao 2003). The peculiar behaviors of certain pediatric tumors also confound criteria created for adults. For example, it is known that some pediatric sarcomas are partially cystic or necrotic at presentation, which would exclude them from the response assessment by the RECIST criteria. However, such tumors have been observed to both shrink and expand with treatment, which argues for their inclusion as measurable lesions (McHugh and Kao 2003). Additionally, functional imaging is excluded from RECIST despite the ability of 18-FDG PET scanning to identify tumor response in the absence (or preceding) tumor shrinkage (Smith 1998).

3.6 Outcome Criteria

Percentage tumor necrosis induced by chemotherapy generally has been predictive of disease free survival (DFS) (Reddick et al. 1999). This relevant association relies on the concept that if there is contrast access, then there is chemotherapy access: if one can reach the tumor, so can the other. Highly vascular and highly permeable tumors will have higher regional access at initiation of therapy, and therefore be more susceptible to the cytotoxic effects of chemotherapeutic agents. Studies of DEMRI and osteosarcoma (Fig. 3.6) have demonstrated improved DFS when tumors have greater initial regional access (as demonstrated by tumor enhancement characteristics, described above in the section on response) (Reddick et al. 2001). Likewise, greater reduction in regional access after treatment has been shown to be predictive of improved outcome (Reddick et al. 2001). DEMRI therefore appears to offer a much more objective assessment of response than static MR, with direct implications regarding outcome in patients with osteosarcoma (Reddick et al. 2001). DEMRI performed at presentation of tumors in the Ewing sarcoma family has not been found to be predictive of outcome (Hoffer 2002).

Thallium-201 can be useful in predicting event-free survival (EFS) for patients with non-metastatic osteosarcoma (Kaste et al. 2001). A characteristic pattern of intense peripheral uptake of radioisotope with central photopenia has been called the donut pattern of avidity (Fig. 3.1 f), and is associated with poor prognosis when seen at presentation (3 year EFS of 63% when present at week zero, compared with 94% when the donut is absent) (Kaste et al. 2001). This pattern is postulated to be related to overpacking of tumor cells or central tumor ischemia (Kaste et al. 2001). FDG-PET has been investigated as a prognostic indicator of both bone and soft tissue sarcomas, with tumors with larger standardized uptake values (SUVs) at initial imaging shown to have a significantly poorer prognosis (both overall survival and EFS) (Eary et al. 2002; Franzius et al. 2002). These findings are not surprising, since higher SUVs are seen with more metabolically active tumors.

3.7 Biopsy of the Primary Lesion

Image-guided percutaneous biopsy is the preferred method for obtaining tissue for pathological diagnosis of a soft tissue mass that is over 5 cm in diameter. Ultrasound is the preferred method of guidance for soft tissue sarcomas due to its real time image generation, lack of ionizing radiation, and good display of anatomic detail, including any neighboring vessels (Figs. 3.15 b, 3.19 b). Fluoroscopy is the imaging guidance of choice for biopsying bone lesions of the extremities. CT is generally best suited for biopsy of pelvic and spinal bone tumors as well as lung metastases. Smaller lesions may benefit from initial surgical resection, avoiding the possibility of needle tract tumor spread. When percutaneous biopsy is performed, the needle tract should be resected at the time of definitive surgery. It is imperative to obtain an adequate core of tissue for the various molecular, immunohistochemical, and cytogenetic studies which are required for diagnosis; therefore multiple passes of the needle are performed. Needle localization technique is useful in finding small primary or recur-

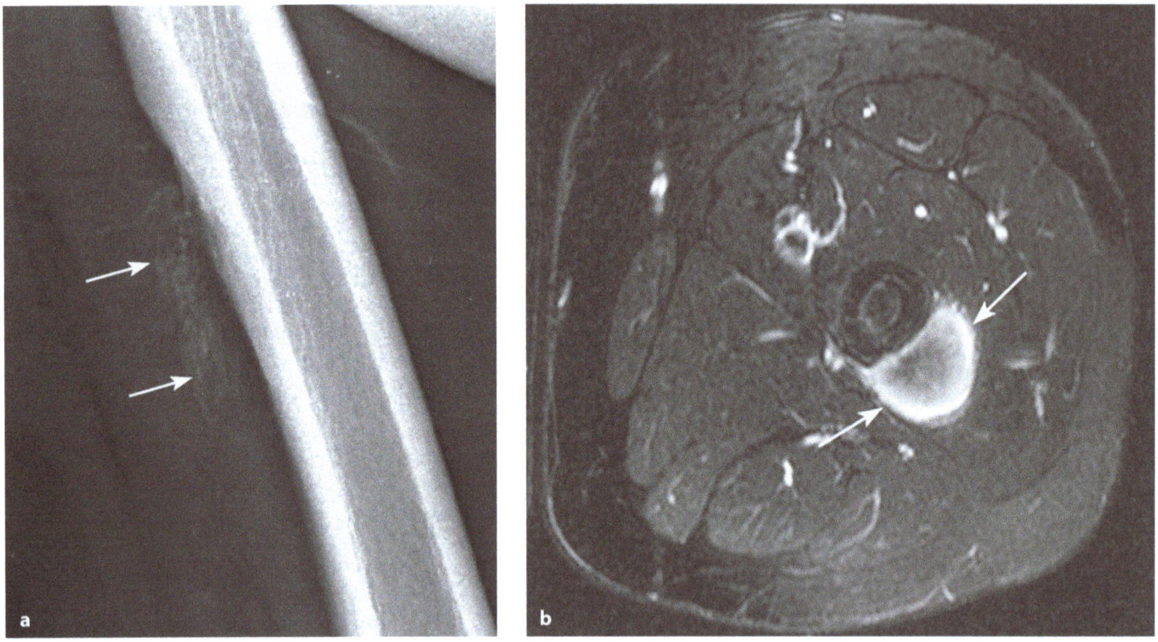

Figure 3.5 a, b

Osteosarcoma. a This 17-year-old boy had adenocarcinoma of the colon resected and later developed leg pain. Lateral radiograph of the mid left femur demonstrates a posterior periosteal reaction and soft tissue calcification or ossification (*arrows*). b The center of this periosteal lesion (*arrows*) is dark on this axial T2-weighted fat suppressed MR due to the ossification. The lesion is attached to the periosteum but does not involve the medullary cavity of the femur. Percutaneous biopsy of the left calf revealed a high grade periosteal osteosarcoma

rent soft tissue sarcomas. Additionally, this technique can be combined with thoracoscopy for the resection of small lung nodules, which would be difficult or impossible for the surgeon to locate during thoracotomy, thus sparing the patient the more invasive procedure (Hardaway et al. 2000).

3.8 Imaging Characteristics of Specific Tumors

3.8.1 Bone Sarcomas

3.8.1.1 Osteosarcoma

Eighty percent of osteosarcomas occur in tubular bones, with 50–75% occurring about the knee (Resnick and Greenway 1996). The radiographic pattern is variable, but typically is characterized by a poorly defined metaphyseal lesion originating in the medullary space, with new bone production, cortical breakthrough, periosteal reaction, and associated soft tissue mass (Fig. 3.1). One may see a characteristic Codman's triangle or the classic sunburst appearance of new bone formation within the surrounding soft tissues. A pathologic fracture occasionally occurs (Resnick and Greenway 1996). Skeletal scintigraphy demonstrates diffuse increased uptake within the primary tumor and metastases, as well as reliably identifying skip lesions greater than 5 mm (Bloem 1997). CT offers additional detail, especially of the cortex, but MR is the preferred modality for identifying the intra- and extraosseous extent of tumor, including skip lesions in the same bone and involvement of neighboring neurovascular structures (Fig. 3.4 d) (Resnick and Greenway 1996). For this

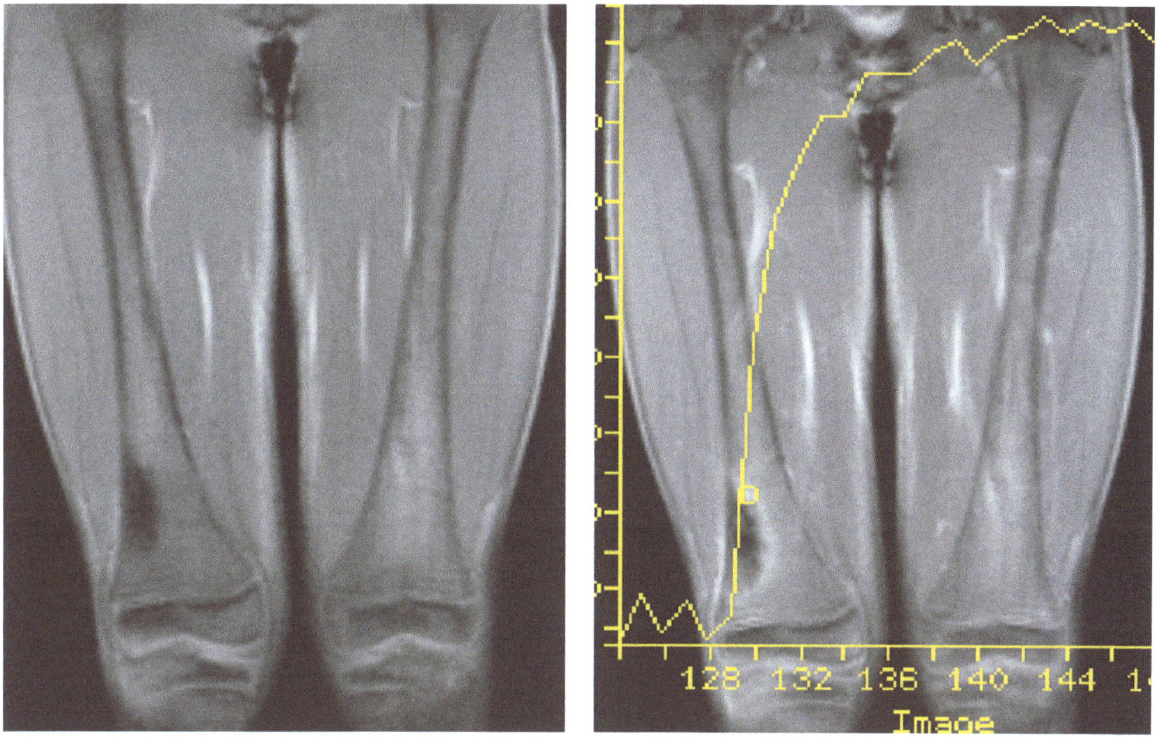

Figure 3.6

Osteosarcoma. This is the first and last coronal image of a DEMRI (dynamic contrast enhanced MR image) with an overlying time intensity curve of the region of interest representing the circle within the rim of the osteosarcoma. The briskly enhancing tumor is represented by a high ICAR (initial contrast accumulation rate) or slope, and the amount of enhancement is represented by the maximum intensity or the top of the curve

reason, it is important to include T1-weighted images of the entire involved bone (Figs. 3.2, 3.3) (Bloem 1997). The extent of intramedullary tumor is most sensitively determined by STIR, but most specifically by T1-weighted sequences. Although distinguishing peritumoral intramedullary edema from tumor can be challenging, more rapid enhancement with dynamic enhanced MR imaging (Fig. 3.6) and alteration of architecture favor tumor over edema (Bloem 1997; Hoffer 2002). Soft tissue edema in itself is a non-specific feature shared by malignant disease (Figs. 3.1 d, 3.7 e), osteomyelitis (Fig. 3.11), and more aggressive benign entities such as Langerhans cell histiocytosis. The existence of an associated soft tissue mass is a more helpful finding in distinguishing between malignant and benign processes (Fletcher 1997). The presence of an effusion suggests, but does not diagnose, joint involvement (Bloem 1997). Several variants of osteosarcoma occur in the pediatric population. The telangiectatic variety of osteosarcoma usually involves the metaphysis of long tubular bones, most often the femur. The notable characteristic is osteolysis, producing cystic cavities filled with blood, which is responsible for the fluid-fluid levels seen on T2-weighted MR sequences (Fig. 3.4) (Hoffer 2002). High signal on T1-weighted imaging is also characteristic, representing this tumor's methemoglobin component (Bloem 1997). These lesions are often expansile and can be confused with aneurysmal bone cysts (ABC) and giant cell tumors of bone

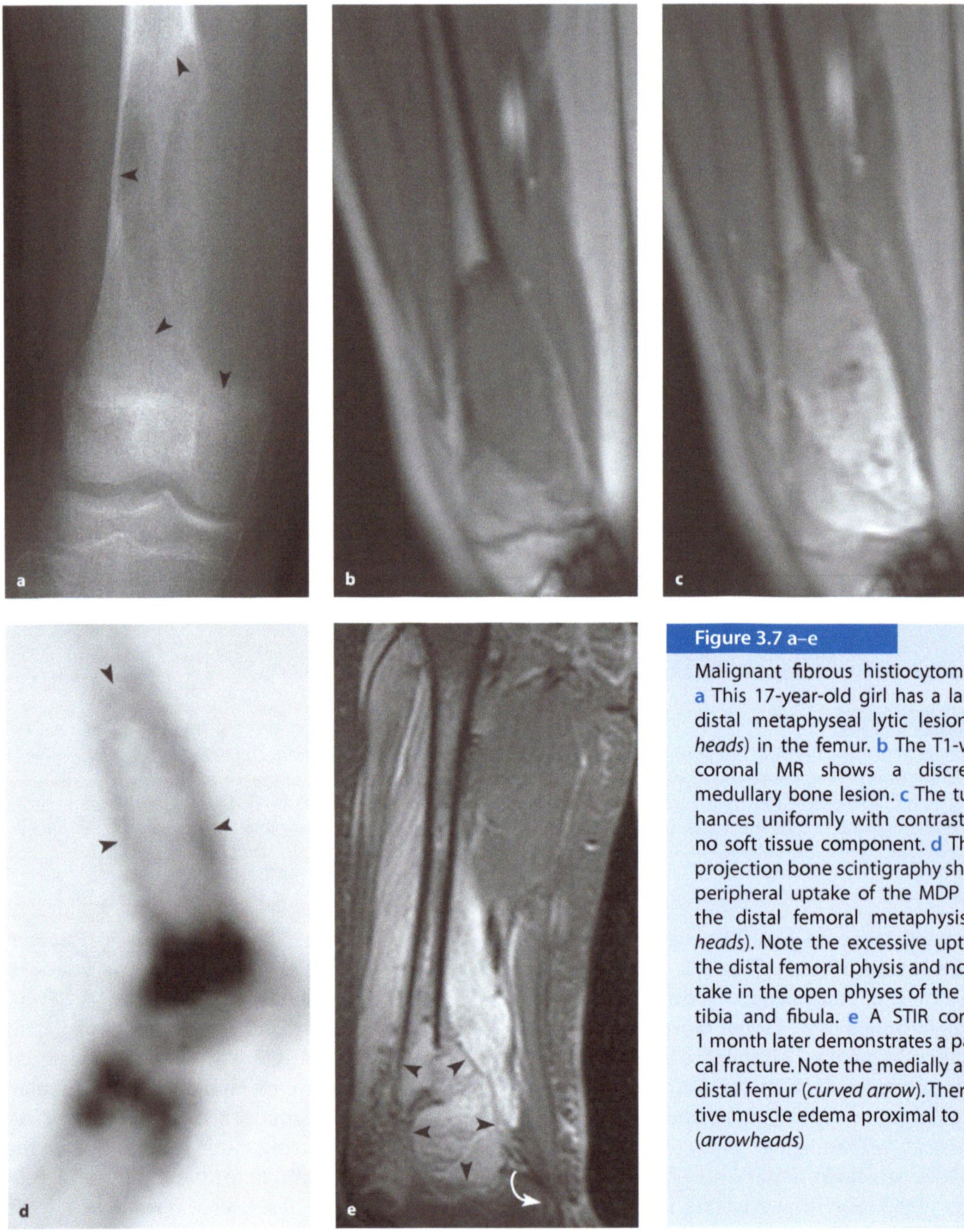

Figure 3.7 a–e

Malignant fibrous histiocytoma (MFH). a This 17-year-old girl has a large right distal metaphyseal lytic lesion (*arrowheads*) in the femur. b The T1-weighted coronal MR shows a discrete dark medullary bone lesion. c The tumor enhances uniformly with contrast and has no soft tissue component. d The lateral projection bone scintigraphy shows only peripheral uptake of the MDP agent in the distal femoral metaphysis (*arrowheads*). Note the excessive uptake near the distal femoral physis and normal uptake in the open physes of the proximal tibia and fibula. e A STIR coronal MR 1 month later demonstrates a pathological fracture. Note the medially angulated distal femur (*curved arrow*). There is reactive muscle edema proximal to the mass (*arrowheads*)

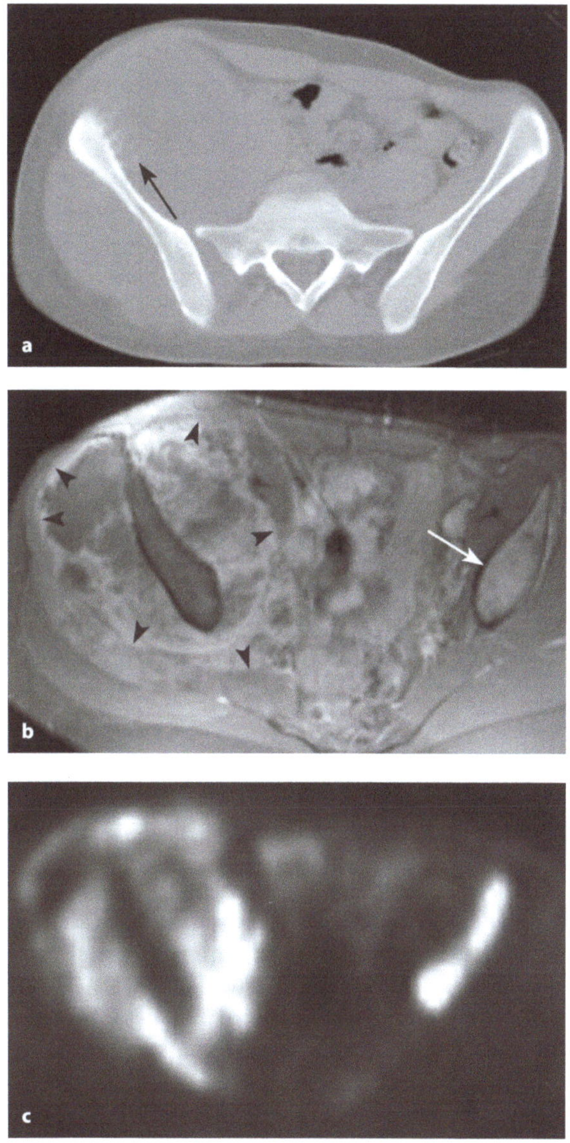

Figure 3.8 a–c

Chondrosarcoma. a This 18-year-old female presented with an advanced stage pelvic mass as demonstrated by this non-contrast CT. Note the partial calcification (*arrow*) of the soft tissue mass medial to right iliac bone. Calcification is seen with chondrosarcoma but is difficult to distinguish by imaging from the ossification in osteosarcoma. b This axial contrast-enhanced T1-weighted MR image demonstrates markedly abnormal low signal throughout the right iliac bone, suggesting necrosis. The associated large, heterogeneously enhancing soft tissue mass (*arrowheads*) lifts the iliacus and gluteal musculature off of the involved bone. Note the additional enhancing tumor involving the marrow space of the left iliac bone (*arrow*) with very little soft tissue component. Percutaneous biopsy of the viable portions of the right iliac soft mass and left iliac bone marrow revealed chondrosarcoma. c Axial FDG-PET obtained at same level as image b; note bright metabolic activity corresponding to the rim of the right iliac soft tissue component, the lack of activity within the dead right iliac bone, and the increased activity in the left iliac bone representing tumor infiltration

(Resnick and Greenway 1996). The rare periosteal osteosarcoma (Fig. 3.5) generally affects tubular long bones of adolescents and young adults (Resnick and Greenway 1996). In contrast to parosteal osteosarcoma, when occurring in the distal femur, it typically arises from the anterior, medial, or lateral surface of the metaphysis (Resnick and Greenway 1996). The lesion is generally small and may contain radiating osseous spicules extending into the overlying soft tissues (Resnick and Greenway 1996). Rapid enhancement with intravenous contrast administration is a common feature of this and all other osteosarcomas (Fig. 3.6). Malignant fibrous histiocytoma (MFH), when it occurs in bone, can mimic osteosarcoma (Fig. 3.7).

3.8.1.2 Chondrosarcoma

Conventional chondrosarcoma most commonly affects the metaphyseal portions of long tubular bones, particularly the femur, and the iliac bones (Fig. 3.8) (Resnick and Greenway 1996). Plain films reveal an expansile osteolytic lesion with periosteal new bone formation and varying degrees of calcification, depending upon the amount of chondroid matrix that is present (Manaster 2002; Resnick and Greenway 1996). Endosteal thickening is occasionally present, a finding also seen with Ewing sarcoma (Manaster 2002). Cortical breakthrough and wide zones of transition are seen with high grade lesions, but most chondrosarcomas are slow growing and less aggressive, remaining asymptomatic until they are quite large (Manaster 2002; Resnick and Greenway 1996). Radionuclide scanning helps identify metabolically active peripheral osteochondromas threatening malignant transformation. CT accurately assesses the intraosseous and soft tissue extent. MR imaging typically reveals an enhancing homogeneous or inhomogeneous tumor with high T2 signal. Local invasion and distant metastases are known to occur with higher grade tumors (Resnick and Greenway 1996).

3.8.1.3 Ewing Sarcoma of Bone

Ewing sarcoma most commonly affects the long tubular bones of the lower extremities, typically the distal femoral metadiaphysis or metaphysis (Hoffer 2002). Pure diaphyseal involvement is less common, and isolated epiphyseal disease is rare (Miller and Hoffer 2001; Resnick and Greenway 1996). Other primary sites include the humerus, vertebral bodies, and flat bones of the pelvis and thorax. In contrast to osteosarcoma and giant cell tumor, Ewing sarcoma generally does not cross cartilage boundaries (Bloem 1997). Radiographically, this is an aggressive appearing lesion (Figs. 3.9, 3.10) with an ill-defined permeative pattern of bone destruction and large soft tissue mass (Miller and Hoffer 2001). If imaged early before the soft tissue component is well formed, an expansile lytic medullary process with associated soft tissue edema will be seen, and the lesion may be mistaken for eosinophilic granuloma or acute osteomyelitis (Fig. 3.11) (Hoffer 2002). Left untreated, Ewing sarcoma often develops the classic lamellated onion skin appearance of multiple reactive periosteal layers (Fig. 3.9a) surrounding the intramedullary tumor. The periosteal reaction can also take the form of "hair on end" bony spicules formed at right angles to the parent bone, similar to the sunburst pattern of osteosarcoma (Hoffer 2002; Resnick and Greenway 1996). If the intramedullary portion of the tumor outgrows its blood supply, it may become necrotic, mimicking a subacute osteomyelitis with intramedullary abscess (Figs. 3.9, 3.11) (Hoffer 2002). Whole body skeletal scintigraphy is useful for identifying bone metastases, although subject to the limitations previously discussed. MR imaging of the primary lesion is preferred to CT due to its superior ability to characterize the tumor's soft tissue component and relationship to neighboring structures (Fig. 3.9) (Miller and Hoffer 2001). Like osteosarcoma, the medullary extent is optimally evaluated with T1-weighted coronal images of the entire bone, with fat saturation technique and gadolinium enhancement routinely implemented (Miller and Hoffer 2001). The heavily T2-weighted STIR sequence is useful in the evaluation of the soft tissue component, but may overestimate both the tumor's intramedullary and soft tissue extent due to the presence of bright edema (Fletcher 1997; Hoffer 2002). Whole body MR and PET scanning are under active investigation for their potential in one step staging of primary tumor and metastases, but results from larger studies are not yet available.

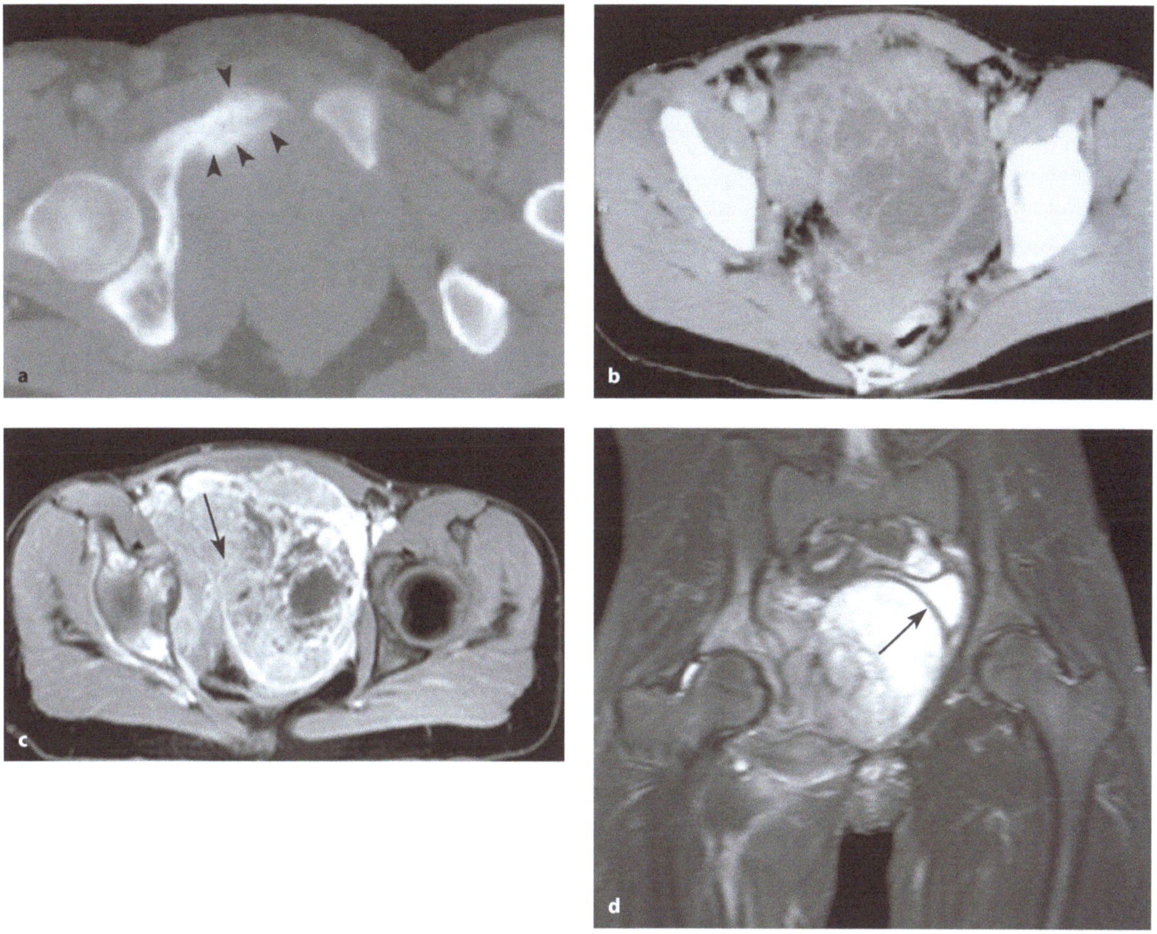

Figure 3.9 a–d

Ewing sarcoma. **a** This 15 year old had right-sided pelvic mass and pain. CT shows R pubic bone periosteal new bone formation (*arrowheads*) typical of Ewing sarcoma. **b** CT appearance suggests sarcoma botryoides (rhabdomyosarcoma). However, this is simply a Ewing sarcoma which is seminecrotic, pushing on the bladder rather than invading it. **c** This axial T1-weighted gadolinium enhanced MR shows the right pelvic lesion and large soft tissue mass. The viable portion to the right was percutaneously biopsied (*arrow* depicts needle path) revealing the diagnosis and t(11;22). **d** Coronal STIR MR shows the right pelvic bone Ewing sarcoma extending into the soft tissue and displacing the right bladder wall (*arrow*) to the left. The necrotic portion of the mass and the urine in the bladder are very bright

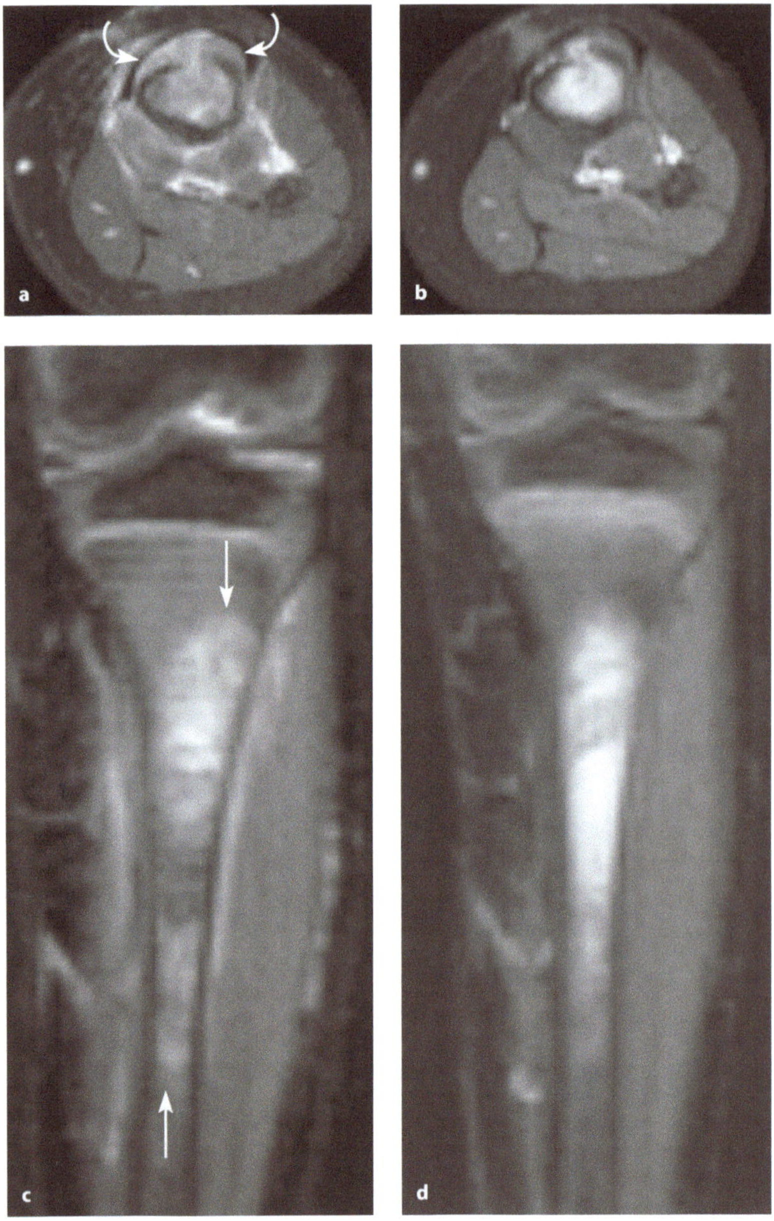

Figure 3.10 a–d

Ewing sarcoma. **a** Axial contrast-enhanced T1-weighted MR of proximal tibial metaphysis of a 7-year-old boy with Ewing sarcoma. Enhancing tumor fills marrow space and breaks through the cortex anteriorly. Note the anterior soft tissue mass. **b** Axial contrast-enhanced T1-weighted MR obtained 7 weeks later shows the soft tissue component of the tumor has substantially decreased. **c** The initial coronal STIR MR demonstrates the medullary tumor (*arrows*) as increased signal within the proximal tibia. The proximal physis and epiphysis are not involved. **d** Coronal STIR 7 weeks after diagnosis demonstrates a brighter signal within the intramedullary tumor suggesting tumor necrosis

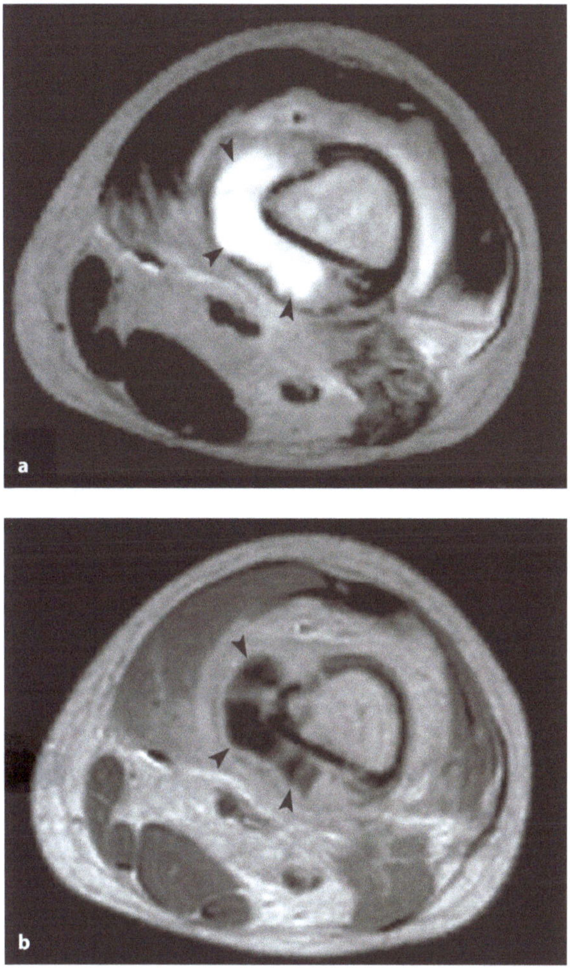

Figure 3.11 a,b

Osteomyelitis. a This 7-year-old girl with suspected malignant tumor had this axial T2-weighted MR of the distal left femur that demonstrated a bright subperiosteal fluid collection (*arrowheads*) but no soft tissue mass. Fat rather than tumor surrounds the anterior lateral portion of the femur. b This axial T1-weighted MR with gadolinium enhancement demonstrates the dark unenhanced subperiosteal abscess (*arrowheads*), which was aspirated at the time of the biopsy. The subperiosteal aspiration and medullary bone biopsy revealed osteomyelitis from *Staphylococcus aureus*. Osteomyelitis can mimic a Ewing sarcoma

3.8.2 Soft Tissue Sarcomas

3.8.2.1 Differentiating Benign from Malignant Soft Tissue Lesions

Soft tissue sarcomas are a diverse group of tumors, and the first challenge is to distinguish them from benign lesions. In neonates, malignant soft tissue sarcomas are often initially misdiagnosed as vascular anomalies, which are the most common congenital soft tissue masses (McCarville et al. 1999; Teo et al. 2000). The key in distinguishing vascular anomalies from sarcomas is in identifying the flow characteristics, predominance of tissue versus vascular components, and enhancement characteristics with contrast administration. Fast flow vascular anomalies include hemangiomas (Fig. 3.20) and arteriovenous malformations. If the lesion is tissue predominant then hemangioma is favored, but sarcomas may have fast flow and tissue predominance as well (Fig. 3.19). One study has demonstrated that the MR findings of lobulation, septation, and high T2 signal with central low signal-intensity dot strongly favor hemangioma over sarcoma (Teo et al. 2000). Of the slow flow lesions, enhancement with intravenous contrast administration favors a venous malformation (cavernous hemangioma), while a non-enhancing lesion is most likely a lymphatic malformation such as lymphangioma or cystic hygroma (Meyer et al. 1991). Complex cystic and solid structures offer additional challenges, but the use of multiple MR pulse sequences and contrast administration significantly improves specificity (Ma et al. 1998). For example, infantile fibrosarcoma with its necrotic, cystic spaces has been confused with a lymphatic malformation.

Other benign entities which may mimic soft tissue sarcomas include desmoid tumors (aggressive fibromatosis), lipomas, hematomas, cysts and abscesses. In general, benign lesions tend to be more homogeneous and smoothly marginated than malignant tumors, and they rarely invade adjacent structures. Desmoid tumors, however, are the benign tumors most often misdiagnosed as malignant, due to their generally aggressive, infiltrative nature and tendency to recur locally (Berquist et al. 1990; Fenstermacher 2003). Desmoids have a characteristic dual MR appearance (Fig. 3.21) with the fibrous portion appearing as a low signal on T1- and T2-weighted sequences, and the fibroblastic portion appearing isointense to muscle on T1, hyperintense on T2, and demonstrating enhancement with gadolinium. Desmoid tumors that are mostly or entirely fibroblastic can mimic a sarcoma (Fenstermacher 2003). Hematomas can be difficult to differentiate from hemorrhagic tumor, but the finding of a tumor nodule or rim of tumor can suggest the diagnosis (Kransdorf et al. 1993). Abscesses can be distinguished on MR imaging by a characteristic well-defined border and rim with centrally decreased signal intensity on T1- and bright fluid signal intensity on T2-weighted sequences (Schlesinger and Hernandez 1992).

3.8.2.2 Soft Tissue Ewing Sarcoma Family of Tumors

Ewing's sarcoma family of tumors (ESFT) are primarily tumors of children and adolescents which may arise in bone or soft tissue. When it occurs in the skeleton, PNET has aggressive characteristics mimicking Ewing sarcoma including bone destruction and soft tissue mass (Fig. 3.12) (Knisely 2003). ESFT can arise as a soft tissue mass in the pelvis, with metastases common at presentation (Knisely 2003). Desmoplastic small round cell tumor (DSRCT) (Fig. 3.13) most often presents as an abdominal mass in adolescent or young adult males (Herzog et al. 2003). Prognosis is generally poor due to the presence of widespread metastases which make surgical resection impossible (Herzog et al. 2003).

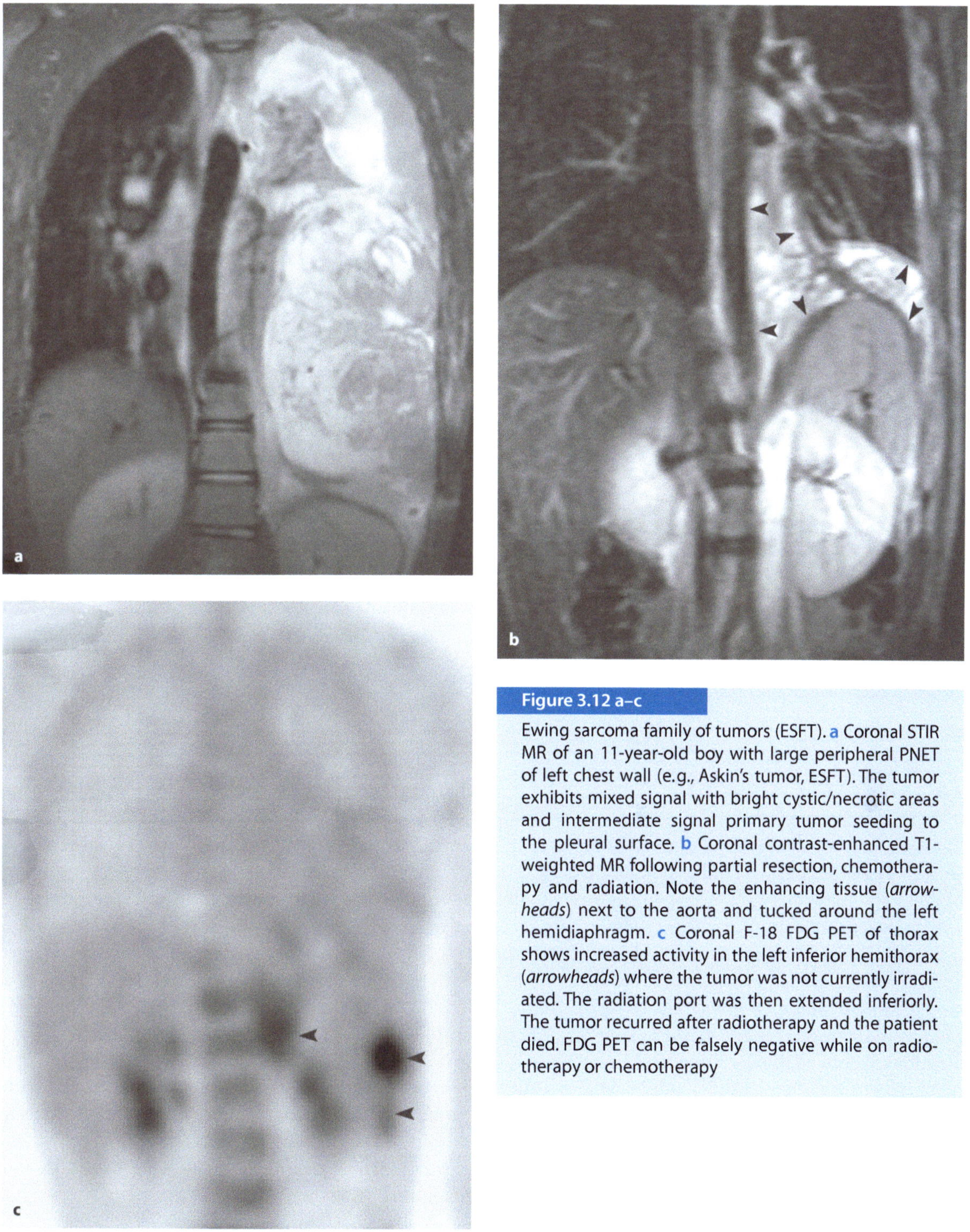

Figure 3.12 a–c

Ewing sarcoma family of tumors (ESFT). **a** Coronal STIR MR of an 11-year-old boy with large peripheral PNET of left chest wall (e.g., Askin's tumor, ESFT). The tumor exhibits mixed signal with bright cystic/necrotic areas and intermediate signal primary tumor seeding to the pleural surface. **b** Coronal contrast-enhanced T1-weighted MR following partial resection, chemotherapy and radiation. Note the enhancing tissue (*arrowheads*) next to the aorta and tucked around the left hemidiaphragm. **c** Coronal F-18 FDG PET of thorax shows increased activity in the left inferior hemithorax (*arrowheads*) where the tumor was not currently irradiated. The radiation port was then extended inferiorly. The tumor recurred after radiotherapy and the patient died. FDG PET can be falsely negative while on radiotherapy or chemotherapy

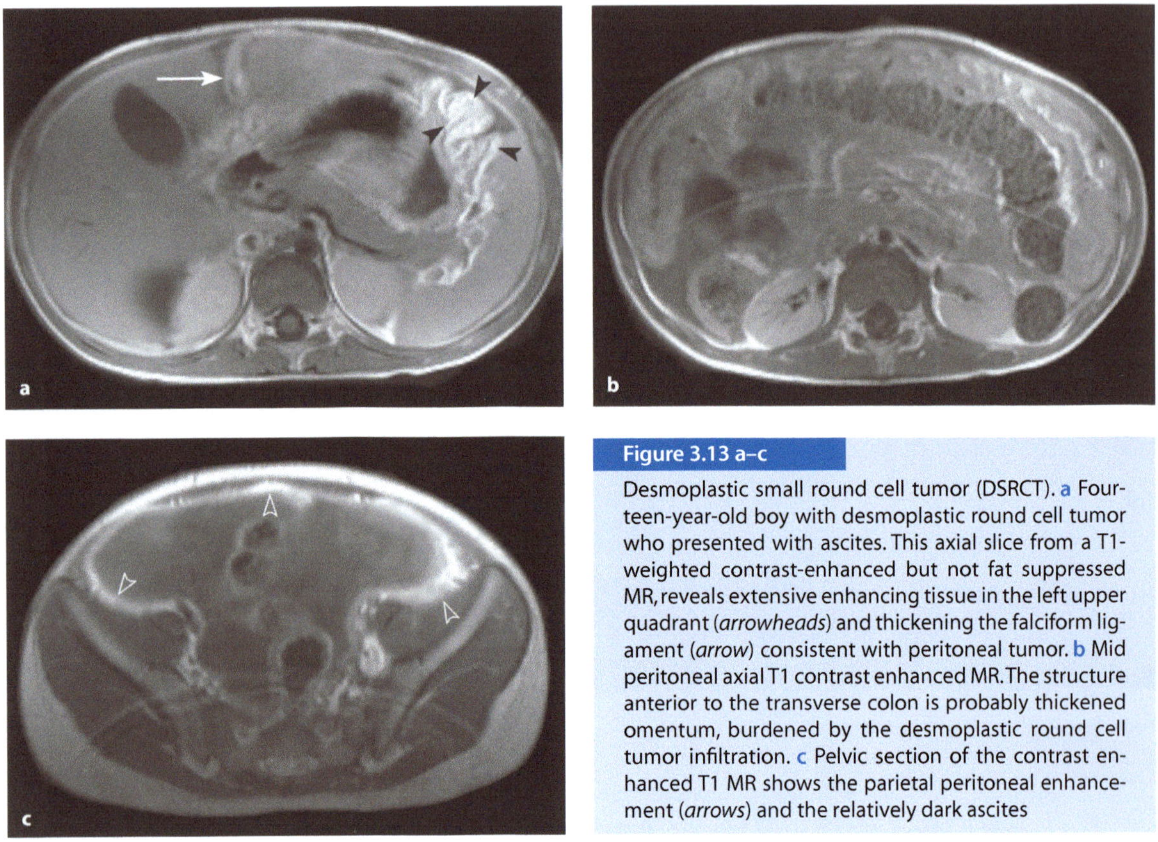

Figure 3.13 a–c

Desmoplastic small round cell tumor (DSRCT). a Fourteen-year-old boy with desmoplastic round cell tumor who presented with ascites. This axial slice from a T1-weighted contrast-enhanced but not fat suppressed MR, reveals extensive enhancing tissue in the left upper quadrant (*arrowheads*) and thickening the falciform ligament (*arrow*) consistent with peritoneal tumor. b Mid peritoneal axial T1 contrast enhanced MR. The structure anterior to the transverse colon is probably thickened omentum, burdened by the desmoplastic round cell tumor infiltration. c Pelvic section of the contrast enhanced T1 MR shows the parietal peritoneal enhancement (*arrows*) and the relatively dark ascites

3.8.2.3 Rhabdomyosarcoma

Representing approximately 5% of all pediatric cancers, rhabdomyosarcoma (RMS) (Figs. 3.14–3.19) is a highly heterogeneous tumor that arises in virtually any tissue or organ other than bone (McCarville et al. 2001). Tumors arising in the extremities, perineum, and paratesticular region are more likely to have regional lymph node involvement at presentation (Figs. 3.14–3.16) (Herzog et al. 2003). Tumors in these locations as well as those arising in the cranial, parameningeal sites, the trunk, bladder and prostate (Fig. 3.18) are considered to have a less favorable outcome (McCarville et al. 2001). A more favorable prognosis is seen in patients with tumors arising from non-parameningeal head and neck sites, the orbit, and eyelid (Fig. 3.17), the genitourinary system other than prostate or bladder, and the biliary tract (McCarville et al. 2001; Raney 2002). CT and MR will demonstrate a heterogeneous, solid or partially cystic and necrotic soft tissue mass. Depending upon aggressiveness, the tumor may be well circumscribed or locally infiltrating, but bone is rarely invaded (McCarville et al. 1999). MR signal is non-specific, as with most soft tissue sarcomas, and will generally be isointense or slightly hyperintense to muscle on T1, with high signal on T2-weighted images (Fig. 3.18) (McCarville et al. 1999; Yang et al. 1997). Heterogeneous enhancement of viable tumor is seen with gadolinium administration. Ultrasound distinguishes solid and cystic components of tumor and assesses vascularity of both the rhabdomyosarcoma and neighboring tissues (Fig. 3.19b).

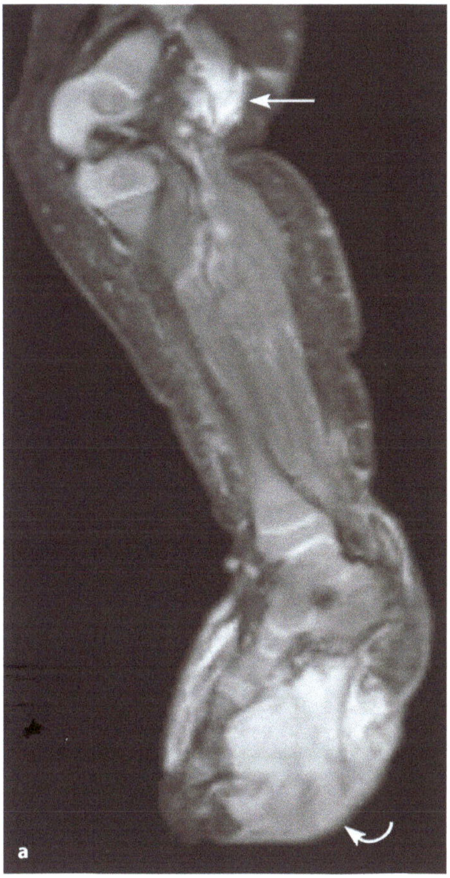

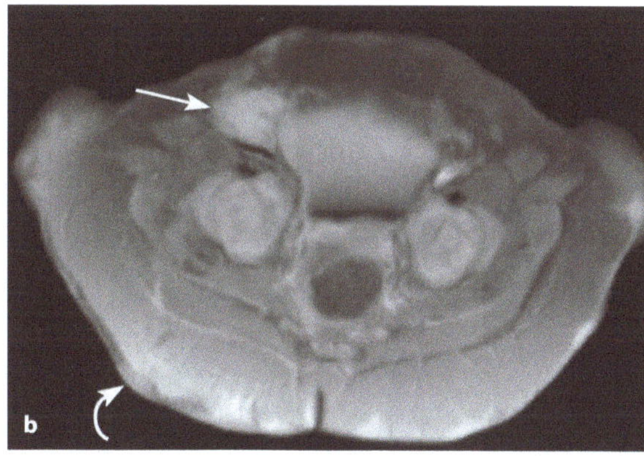

Figure 3.14 a, b

Rhabdomyosarcoma. **a** One-month-old girl with rapidly enlarging foot mass noted at birth. Biopsy revealed alveolar rhabdomyosarcoma. Sagittal fat suppressed contrast-enhanced T1-weighted MR image demonstrates the large solid rhabdomyosarcoma (*curved arrow*) on the plantar aspect of the right foot. Also note the popliteal pathology (*straight arrow*). **b** Axial fat suppressed contrast-enhanced T1-weighted MR image of the pelvis shows bulky right external iliac adenopathy (*straight arrow*), metastatic from the primary site. Also note one of the many subcutaneous nodules (*curved arrow*) proven to be metastases. Neonatal rhabdomyosarcoma is typically aggressive and approximately half of patients present with widespread metastatic disease

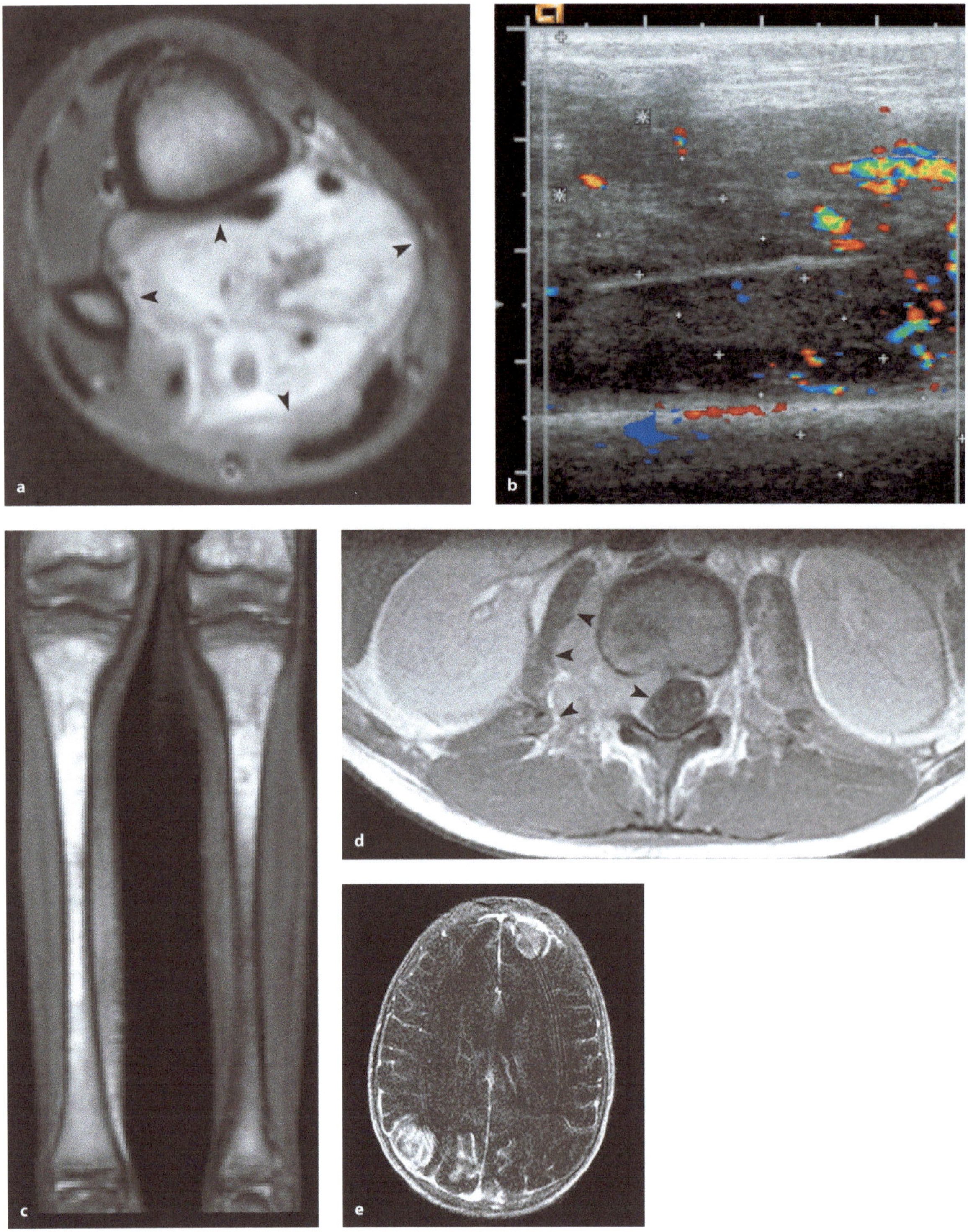

◀ **Figure 3.15 a–e**

Rhabdomyosarcoma. **a** This 7-year-old girl presented with a systemic illness and leg mass. Axial STIR MR demonstrates the primary right calf mass (*arrowheads*). Note the bright signal in the tibia. **b** Percutaneous biopsy of calf mass guided with ultrasound revealed t(2;13) on PCR from fresh 15G core biopsy material. **c** Coronal STIR MR reveals bright signal suggesting diffuse marrow disease confirmed by routine bone marrow biopsy and aspirate which documented a 94% tumor burden in the marrow. **d** Axial T1 with gadolinium enhancement lumbar spine shows vertebral metastasis with extradural tumor (*arrowheads*) encroaching on spinal canal. **e** T1-weighted axial MR of the brain with non-contrast image subtracted from gadolinium contrast image demonstrating brain metastases 18 months after diagnosis. The rhabdomyosarcoma metastases were confirmed by biopsy

Figure 3.16

Rhabdomyosarcoma. This 11 year old has bone marrow packed with alveolar rhabdomyosarcoma with an unknown primary. This fluorine-18 FDG PET maximum intensity projected (MIP) image shows the left calf primary site (*arrow*), diffuse increase in bone marrow uptake, and soft tissue, breast and lymph node metastases

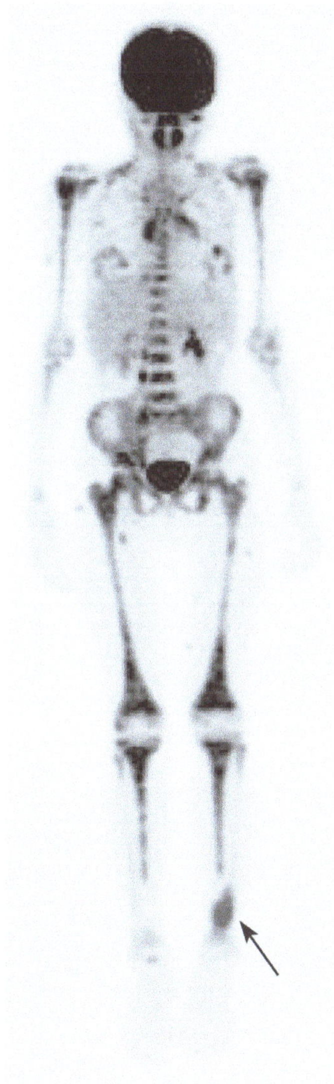

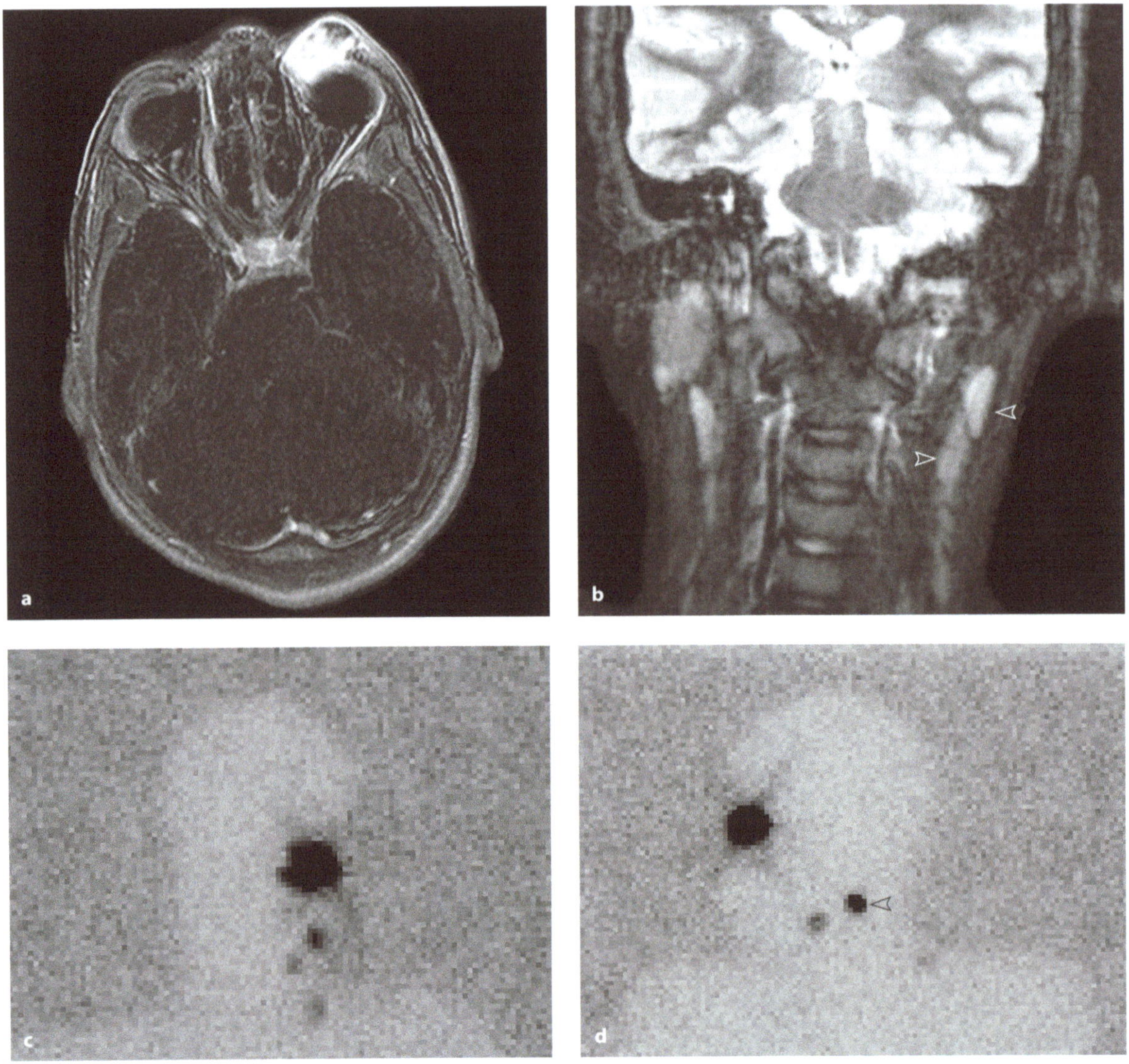

Figure 3.17 a–d

Rhabdomyosarcoma. a This 11-year-old girl has a left preorbital rhabdomyosarcoma as seen on this postcontrast subtracted axial T1 MR image. b There are prominent cervical lymph nodes (*arrows*) on the STIR MR. Which lymph node is apt to be metastatic? c Lymphoscintigraphy was performed by injecting filtered technetium-99m sulfur colloid at the primary left preorbital rhabdomyosarcoma site. Frontal view of head and neck was performed with a cobalt source placed behind the patient to silhouette the patient's head. The largest most intense signal is where the agent was injected. Three lymph nodes in the left neck first took up the sulfur colloid. d Lateral view of lymphoscintigraphy shows the injection site around the left orbital rhabdomyosarcoma as the largest signal intensity. Two left cervical nodes and one left supraclavicular node are demonstrated. Biopsy of the posterior cervical node (*arrow*) demonstrated no tumor

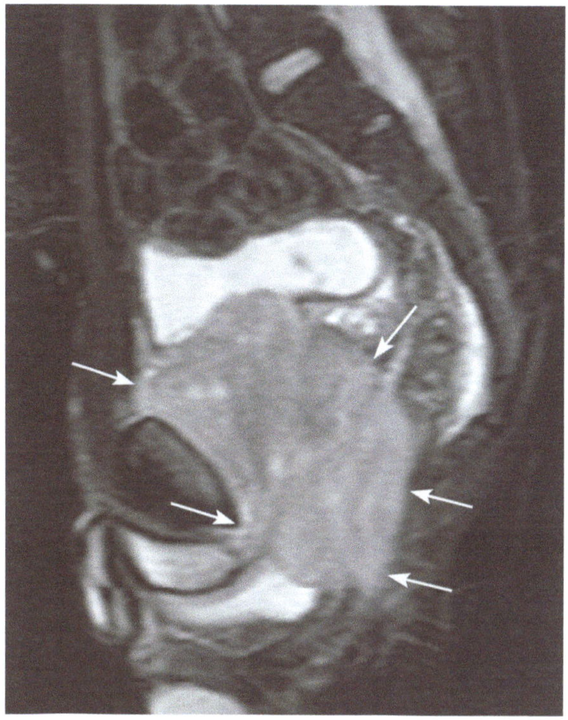

Figure 3.18

Rhabdomyosarcoma. Nineteen year old with urinary obstruction had a sagittal STIR MR revealing a prostatic rhabdomyosarcoma (*arrows*) between the bladder and the penis

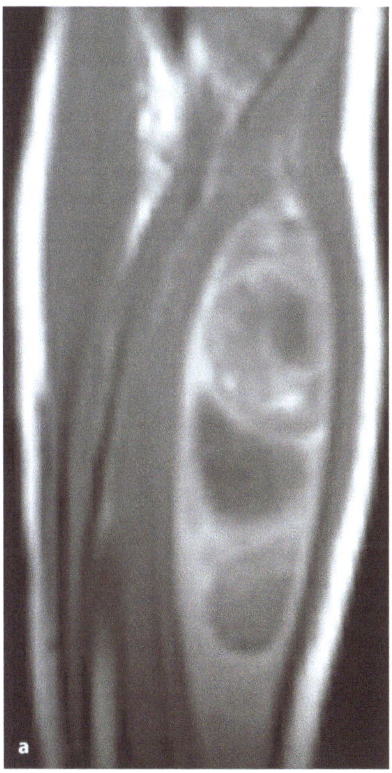

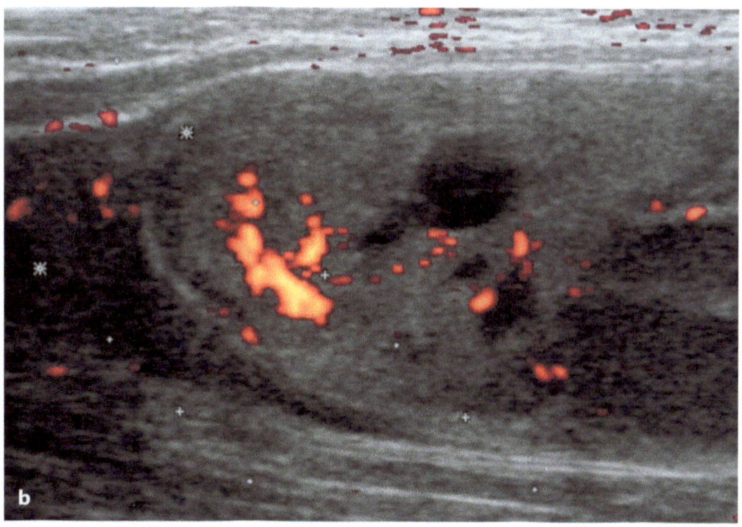

Figure 3.19 a, b

Rhabdomyosarcoma. **a** Initial contrast-enhanced T1 coronal image of palpable soft tissue mass in the proximal forearm of a 6-year-old boy, first noticed 2 months earlier after trauma. **b** Power Doppler ultrasound of soft tissue mass right forearm taken during needle biopsy. The superior pole of the tumor is highly vascular and more echogenic; the more inferior portion is less echogenic, suggesting necrosis or hemorrhage

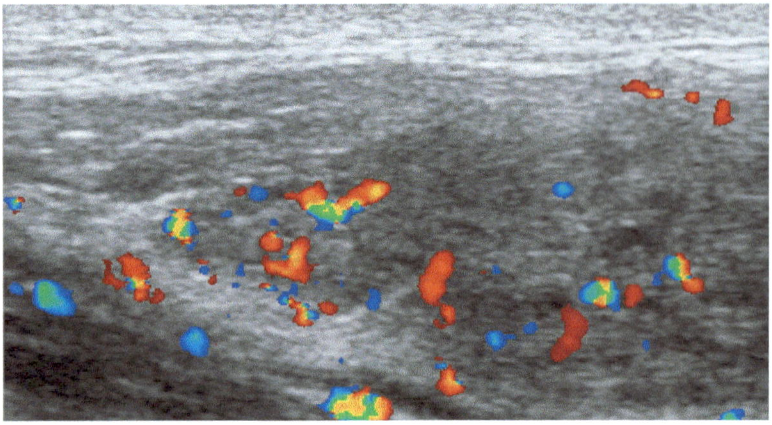

Figure 3.20

Hemangioma. This 16 year old has a vascular soft tissue mass of the arm as demonstrated on this color flow Doppler US. This lesion has fast flow and tissue predominance consistent with hemangioma. Although this patient is older than expected for this lesion, pathology from a percutaneous biopsy confirmed hemangioma. No treatment was indicated

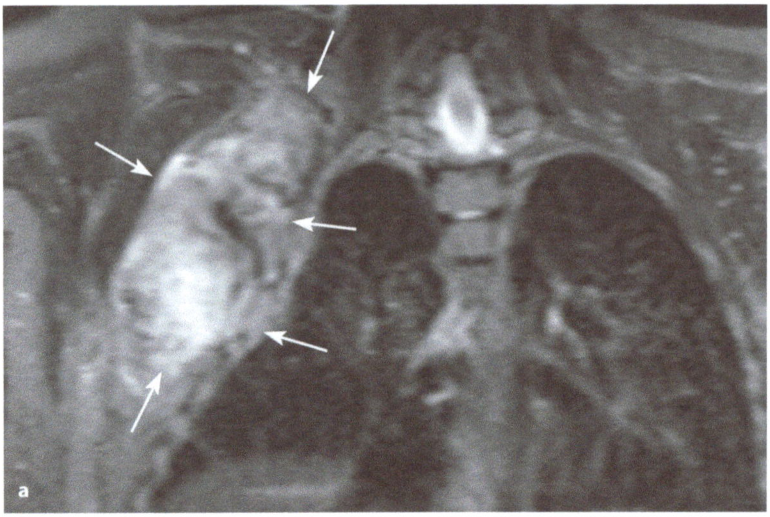

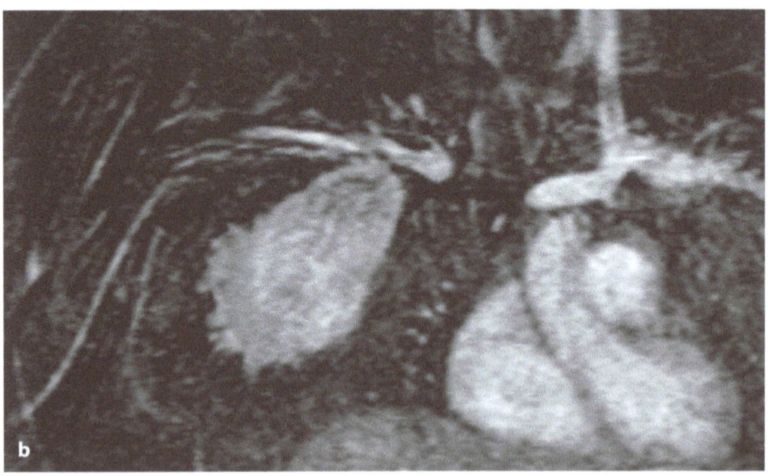

Figure 3.21 a, b

Desmoid tumor. **a** Twelve-year-old body with right axillary mass (*arrow*). On MR the central portion is dark on STIR, representing fibrosis, and most of the lesion is bright consistent with fibroblastic disease. This pattern is typical for desmoid tumor (aggressive fibromatosis), which was later proven by percutaneous biopsy and resection. **b** Contrast enhanced coronal T1 MR with subtraction of non-contrast series shows more uniform enhancement of this active desmoid tumor

3.8.2.4 Non-rhabdomyosarcoma Soft Tissue Sarcomas

The non-rhabdomyosarcoma soft tissue sarcomas (NRSTS) (Figs. 3.22–3.27) include a heterogeneous group of tumors of mesenchymal origin. Although each type occurs rarely in comparison with RMS, together they comprise approximately 60% of all pediatric soft tissue sarcomas (Herzog et al. 2003). The extremities, especially lower, account for approximately 50% of cases, followed in frequency by head and neck sites, trunk, and abdomen (Herzog et al. 2003). Treatment and prognosis vary according to histology and other factors. Many of these sarcomas share similar imaging characteristics; therefore we will limit our discussion to those entities with more specific features.

3.8.2.4.1 Synovial Sarcoma

Synovial sarcoma (Figs. 3.22, 3.23) is the most common NRSTS occurring in children and adolescents (McCarville et al. 2002). Although primarily a tumor of the extremities arising from the bursae, joint capsules, and tendon sheaths near large joints, synovial sarcoma can occur virtually anywhere, including locations distant from joint spaces (Coffin 1997). Fewer than 10% are intra-articular (Campanacci 1990; Coffin 1997; Jones et al. 1993). The majority of tumors present as large (greater than 5 cm), deep-seated, often painful, soft tissue masses of the lower extremities (Jones et al. 1993). Approximately one-third contain calcifications visible on plain film (Cadman et al. 1965; Jones et al. 1993). A study of 34 patients found that 71% of synovial sarcomas were contiguous with bone or associated with cortical thinning or marrow invasion at the time of discovery (Jones et al. 1993). This finding may help to distinguish synovial sarcoma from most other soft tissue sarcomas, which rarely invade bone (Sundaram and McLeod 1990). Distant metastases often involve the lungs (Fig. 3.23). MR imaging is essential and can be fairly specific; however, a high percentage of the smaller tumors are initially misdiagnosed as benign lesions such as hematoma, ganglion cyst, or Baker's cyst due to their frequently lobulated, well-defined margins and tendency to displace, rather than invade, surrounding soft tissue structures (Berquist et al. 1990; Jones et al. 1993). Signal is predominantly hypointense to muscle on T1-weighted images, with frequent areas of hyperintensity due to hemorrhage, and internal septations (Fujimoto et al. 1997; Jones et al. 1993). A T2 "triple signal" with areas hypo-, iso-, and hyperintense relative to fat has been described, corresponding pathologically to regions of solid and fibrous tissue, hemorrhage, and necrosis within the tumor (McCarville et al. 2002; Jones et al. 1993). A characteristic fluid-fluid level representing various stages of hemorrhage is seen in approximately 18% of cases (Jones et al. 1993). This finding in a soft tissue mass should im-

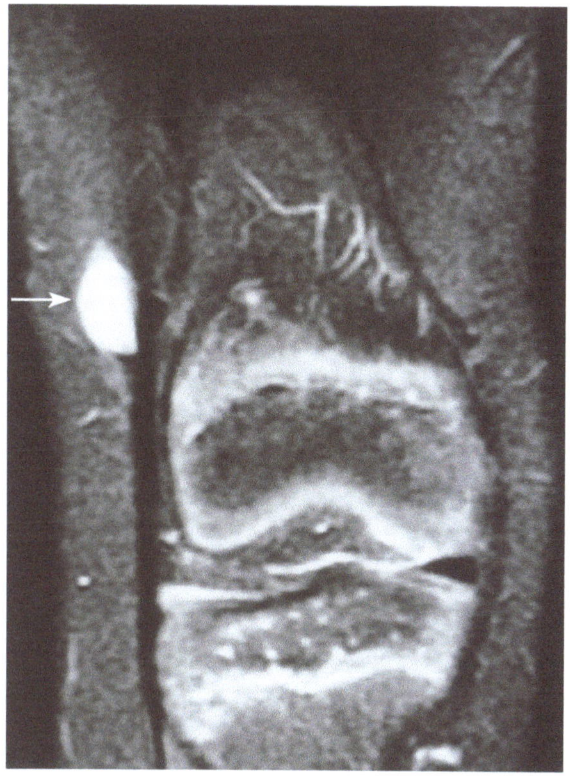

Figure 3.22

Synovial sarcoma. Six-year-old girl with synovial sarcoma. This STIR coronal MR image shows a cystic mass (*arrow*) adjacent to the medial collateral ligament. Synovial sarcomas often occur near joints and are commonly cystic as shown here

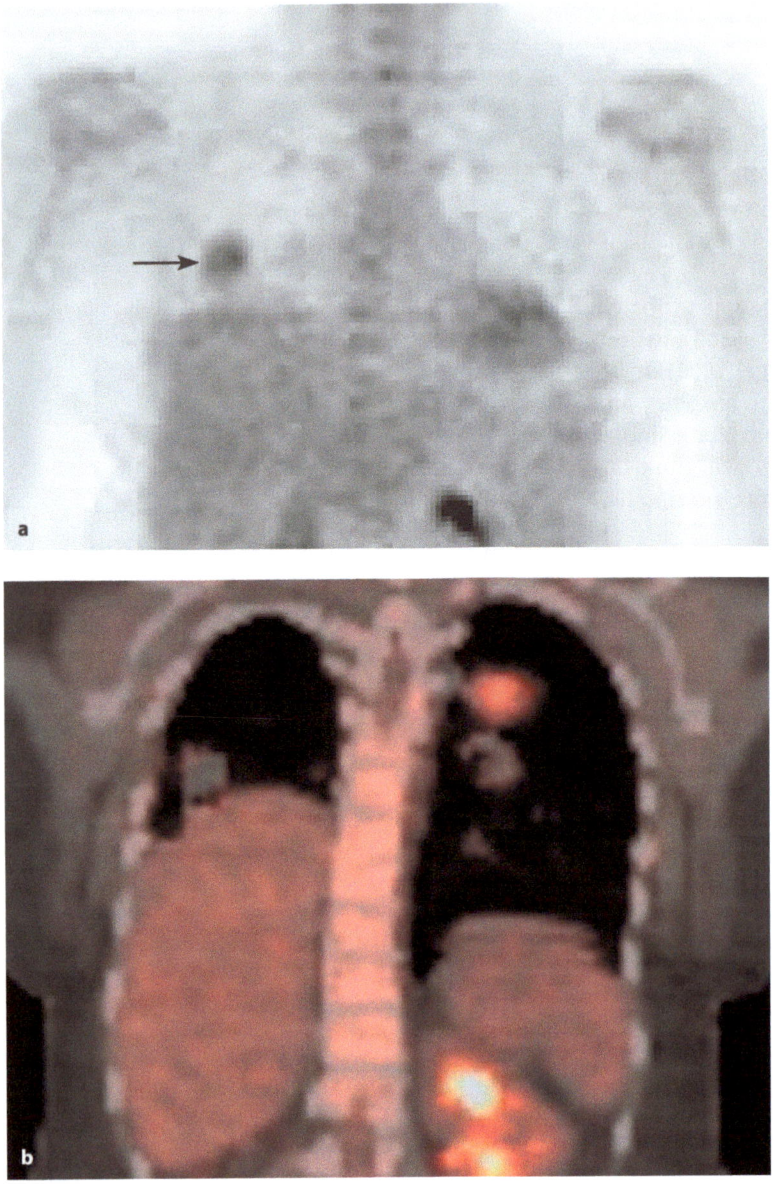

Figure 3.23 a, b

Synovial sarcoma. **a** Fluorine-18 FDG PET frontal view of chest shows an active pulmonary metastasis (*arrow*) from synovial sarcoma to right lower lobe. **b** PET/CT fusion image after radiofrequency ablation of right lower lobe metastasis demonstrates "gray-cold" right lower lobe lesion and new, "red-hot" left upper lobe lesion

mediately suggest the diagnosis of synovial sarcoma, malignant fibrous histiocytoma (MFH), or venous or lymphatic malformation. Synovial sarcoma should be considered in any child or adolescent with a soft tissue mass with the characteristic MR findings, regardless of the location, and the diagnosis should also be considered in any well-defined, hemorrhagic, and inhomogeneous soft tissue mass arising near a joint space (Fujimoto et al. 1997; Jones et al. 1993). The distinct monophasic and biphasic histologic types of synovial sarcoma cannot be differentiated with MR imaging (Jones et al. 1993).

3.8.2.4.2 Congenital Fibrosarcoma

Congenital, or infantile, fibrosarcoma occurs in the first 5 years of life and is the most common soft tissue sarcoma of infants (Herzog et al. 2003; McCarville et al. 1999). Radiographs show a rapidly enlarging soft tissue mass, sometimes with adjacent bone deformity due to mass effect, but rarely bone invasion (Pousti et al. 1998). Calcifications may be present (Lee et al. 1996). MR (Fig. 3.24) demonstrates mixed solid and cystic components, as well as a fluid-fluid level if hemorrhage is present (McCarville et al. 1999). Angiography will demonstrate the markedly disorganized vessels and large draining veins that are characteristic of this tumor (Lee et al. 1996; Vinnicombe and Hall 1994).

3.8.2.4.3 Hemangiopericytoma

Five to 10% of hemangiopericytomas occur in the pediatric population (Enzinger 1988; Rodriguez-Galindo et al. 2000). The typical clinical presentation is of a firm or rubbery, frequently mobile and painless subcutaneous mass occurring in the extremities, head and neck region, or trunk (McCarville et al. 1999). Plain film may demonstrate calcific stippling within the soft tissue mass (Hoey et al. 1998). Bone invasion occasionally occurs and peripheral enhancement is common, both features readily identified with contrast-enhanced CT (McCarville et al. 1999). MR findings (Figs. 3.25, 3.26) are non-specific, with solid and cystic components, enhancement, and occasionally a hemorrhagic fluid-fluid level seen (McCarville et al. 1999). Arteriography demonstrates hypervascularity with large feeding arteries, but in contrast to fibrosarcoma, no large draining veins (McCarville et al. 1999). Ultrasound demonstrates a well-circumscribed, hypoechoic lesion with a heterogeneous echotexture (Bosch et al. 1998). In an infant the differential should include infantile fibrosarcoma and RMS (Herzog et al. 2003). Malignancy is determined by the presence of metastases or local recurrence rather than histology, and maturation to hemangioma has been documented following chemotherapy (Bosch et al. 1998; Rodriguez-Galindo et al. 2000).

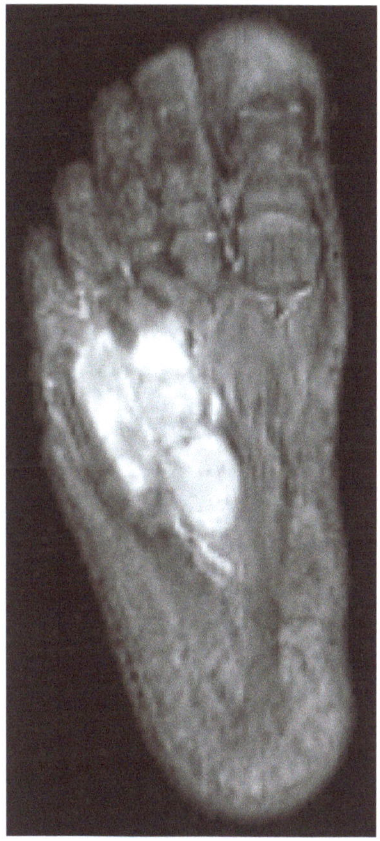

Figure 3.24

Fibrosarcoma. Two-year-old boy with persistent fibrosarcoma after attempted resection. Long axis STIR examination demonstrates the bright tumor in the plantar surface of the right foot. Repeat percutaneous biopsy revealed viable tumor

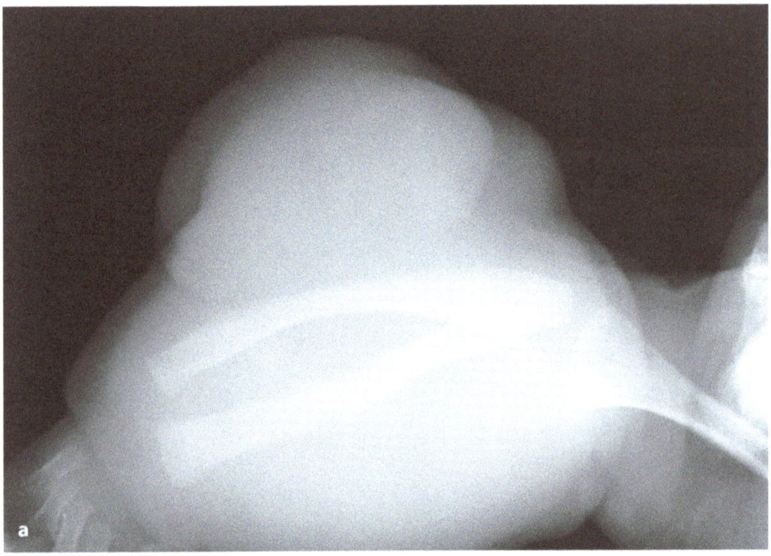

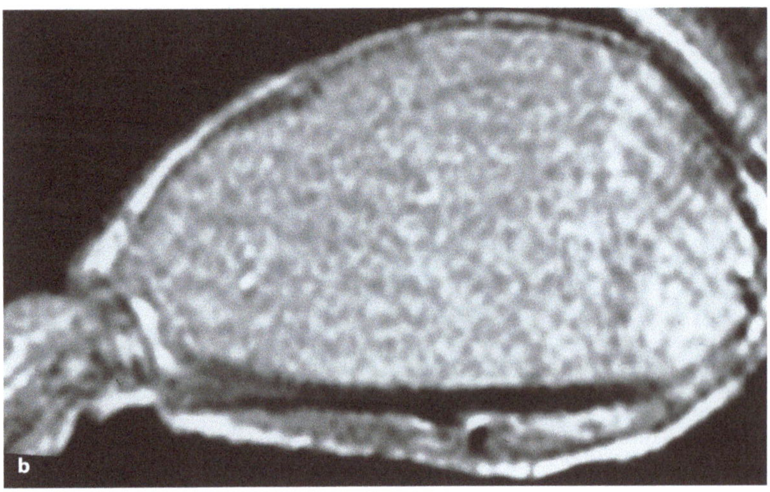

Figure 3.25 a, b

Hemangiopericytoma. **a** One-week-old girl born with right forearm mass that was biopsy proven infantile hemangiopericytoma. Plain film of the forearm shows a large, lobulated soft-tissue mass without calcification or obvious bone destruction. **b** Sagittal contrast-enhanced T1-weighted MR image shows the solid nature of this soft tissue mass. Infantile hemangiopericytomas have a more benign outcome than their adult counterpart and are treated with surgical resection alone unless residual tumor is present

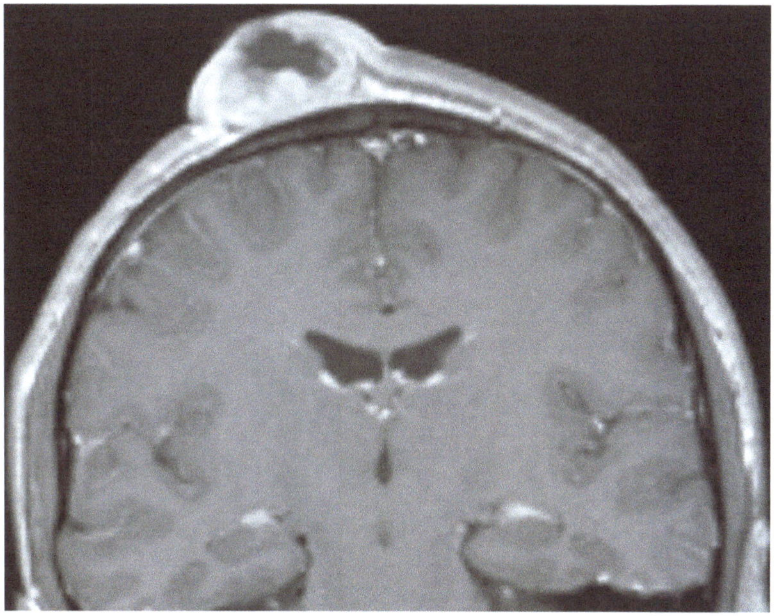

Figure 3.26

Hemangiopericytoma. Twenty-year-old male complaining of 3-month history of scalp swelling. Coronal enhanced T1-weighted MR demonstrates inhomogeneous enhancing soft tissue mass with central hypointense necrotic or cystic area. The underlying calvarium was not involved. Biopsy revealed hemangiopericytoma and the patient was treated with radiation and wide surgical excision

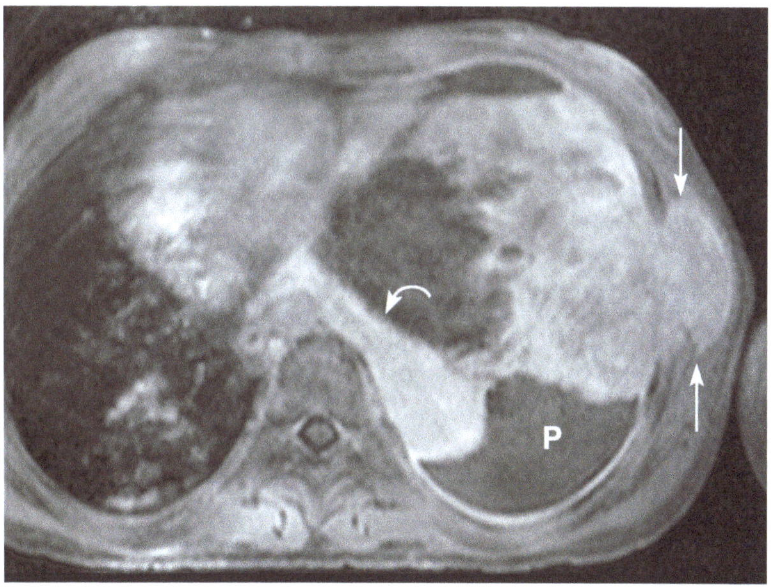

Figure 3.27

Malignant peripheral nerve sheath tumor (MPNST). This 13-year-old girl has neurofibromatosis (NF1) and presented with anemia and shortness of breath. This axial contrast enhanced MR demonstrates a chest wall mass (*straight arrows*) extending into the left hemithorax. There is collapsed lung (*curved arrow*) and pleural effusion (*P*). The medial portion of the mass was necrotic and bleeding. A percutaneous biopsy revealed MPNST. The mass responded only to resection

3.8.2.4.4 Malignant Peripheral Nerve Sheath Tumors (MPNST)

Malignant peripheral nerve sheath tumors comprise 5–10% of all pediatric NRSTS, typically arising as deep soft tissue masses of the lower extremities or trunk (McCarville et al. 1999). Patients with neurofibromatosis type 1 (NF-1) are at particularly high risk; therefore it is imperative that they be closely monitored for malignant transformation of neurofibromas, clinically manifested by rapid growth, development of irregular shape, or visible changes of the overlying skin (Khoo and Foo 1994; Riccardi and Powell 1989). Patients who develop de novo neurofibrosarcomas tend to be older than those with NF-1 (Bhargava et al. 1997). CT demonstrates an enhancing homogeneous soft tissue mass which may invade adjacent bone. Both calcifications and intratumoral cavities have been described (McCarville et al. 1999). MR imaging is non-specific (Fig. 3.27), but in general the tumor is isointense to muscle on T1-weighted images and heterogeneous with areas of high signal and infiltrative margins on T2 (McCarville et al. 1999). MR may also demonstrate the close relationship of the tumor to the nerve. The target sign, a central dark, dense collagen core surrounded by a hyperintense rim of myxomatous tissue on T2-weighted sequences, is seen with benign neurofibromas and with satellite lesions of MPNSTs, but not as the primary neurofibrosarcoma (Laor 2004). Loss of this finding in a known neurofibroma should raise concern for malignant transformation. PET scanning shows promise as an additional screening modality for identifying malignant transformation (Solomon et al. 2001).

3.9 Post-treatment Imaging Concerns

Bones included in the radiation port demonstrate not only characteristics of rickets, but also fibrosis and fatty conversion of marrow (Vogler and Murphy 1988). Radiation osteitis is a dose-related complication of radiotherapy that presents as osteopenia with coarsened trabeculae and occasionally pathologic fracture, usually within 3 years of treatment (Howland et al. 1975; Dalinka and Mazzeo 1985; Bragg et al. 1975). The differential diagnosis generally includes osteomyelitis, recurrent primary tumor, and radiation-induced sarcoma (Bragg et al. 1975). Radiation necrosis is another potential osseous complication of external beam radiation therapy. Characteristic alterations of skeletal muscle due to inflammatory changes, edema, and atrophy are also encountered, and increased signal on T2, STIR, and enhanced T1W images can be seen for over a year after treatment (Fletcher et al. 1990).

Postsurgical imaging presents a particular challenge in the setting of metallic prostheses. With MR imaging, artifact can be reduced by using broad-bandwidth sequences with thin sections (Viano et al. 2000). Routine fat suppression techniques are adversely affected by metal, but STIR and T1-weighted imaging with and without gadolinium, followed by subtraction of the pre-contrast image from the contrast-enhanced image, can be substituted (Viano et al. 2000). Ultrasound and PET are not adversely affected by metal.

Further difficulties are encountered in post-therapeutic image interpretation. In the case of incomplete resection of soft tissue sarcoma, MR imaging has not been demonstrated to be sensitive or specific enough to be used alone to decide whether further resection is warranted (Kaste et al. 2002). Additional modalities and clinical information are required. Second primary tumors (often sarcomas) may occur within or adjacent to the primary sarcoma site in patients who receive larger doses of radiation (Hawkins et al. 1996; Newton et al. 1991). Recommendations for long-term follow-up imaging of these patients are not uniform.

3.10 Radiofrequency Ablation

Radiofrequency ablation (RFA) is a relatively new technique with vast potential in the definitive treatment of distant metastases (Fig. 3.23) as well as in the control of symptoms and local tumor effects. In the adult population, ablation of hepatic and pulmonary metastases has been well described (Livraghi et al. 2003; Dupuy et al. 2000). Additionally, RFA has a promising role in the symptomatic control of painful bone metastases (Dupuy et al. 1998; Schaefer et al. 2002). The applications of these techniques in the pediatric population are currently evolving. Although surgical excision is the preferred treatment of pulmonary metastases from osteosarcoma, the high rate of recurrence (91 %) at both the surgical scar and distant pulmonary sites results in diminishing returns with subsequent thoracotomy (Dupuy et al. 2000). RFA can offer much less invasive follow-up treatment in these patients. A fourth application for RF ablation may be for recurrent local sarcoma in the soft tissue, marginal bone, or regional lymph nodes. RF ablation should substitute for needle localization and tumor resection. The volume of tissue ablated at one session is limited by the proportionate increase in risk of renal insufficiency from tumor lysis, myoglobinuria, and hemoglobinuria. Aggressive hydration during and after RFA helps decrease this risk. Some patients will develop the transient tumor lysis syndrome of fever, pain, nausea, and fatigue after ablation, treated by control of symptoms alone. Other complications include damage to adjacent structures such as thin-walled bile ducts, vessels, bowel and nerves. Nerve injury can be avoided by placing a needle temperature probe and avoiding temperatures at the nerve over 45°C. The probe tract is always carefully burned after each ablation to prevent spread of viable tumor cells (Livraghi et al. 2003; Dupuy et al. 2000).

Acknowledgements. This work was supported in part by Cancer Center Support (CORE) Grant CA 21765 from the National Cancer Institute and by the American Lebanese Syrian Associated Charities (ALSAC).

References

Antoch G, Vogt FM, Freudenberg LS, Nazaradeh F et al. (2003) Whole-body dual-modality PET/CT and whole-body MRI for tumor staging in oncology. JAMA 290(24):3199–3206

Berquist TH, Ehman RL, King BF, Hodgman CG, Ilstrup DM (1990) Value of MR imaging in differentiating benign from malignant soft-tissue masses: study of 95 lesions. AJR Am J Roentgenol 155:1251–1255

Bhargava R, Parham DM, Lasater OE, Chari RS, Chen G, Fletcher BD (1997) MR imaging differentiation of benign and malignant peripheral nerve sheath tumors: use of the target sign. Pediatr Radiol 27:124–129

Bloem JL, van der Woude HJ, Geirnaerdt M, Hogendoorn PC, Taminiau AH, Hermans J (1997) Does magnetic resonance imaging make a difference for patients with musculoskeletal sarcoma? Br J Radiol 70:327–337

Bosch AM, Hack WW, Ekkelkamp S (1998) Congenital hemangiopericytoma: two case reports. Pediatr Surg Int 13:211–212

Bragg DG, Shidnia H, Chu FCH, Higinbotham NL (1975) The clinical and radiographic aspects of radiation osteitis. Radiology 97:103–111

Bredella MA, Caputo GR, Steinbach LS (2002) Value of FDG positron emission tomography in conjunction with MR imaging for evaluating therapy response in patients with musculoskeletal sarcomas. AJR Am J Roentgenol 179:1145–1150

Cadman NL, Soule EH, Kelly PJ (1965) Synovial sarcoma: an analysis of 134 tumors. Cancer 18:613–627

Campanacci M (1990) Bone and soft tissue tumors. Springer-Verlag, New York, pp 998–1012

Coffin CM (1997) Synovial-based tumors and synovial sarcoma. In: Coffin CM, O'Shea PA, Dehner LP (eds) Pediatric soft tissue tumors: a clinical, pathological, and therapeutic approach, 1st edn. Williams & Wilkins, Baltimore, pp 295–310

Daldrup-Link HE, Franzius C, Link TM, Laukamp D, Sciuk J, Jurgens H et al. (2001) Whole-body MR imaging for detection of bone metastases in children and young adults: comparison with skeletal scintigraphy and FDG PET. AJR Am J Roentgenol 177:229–236

Dalinka MK, Mazzeo VP (1985) Complications of radiation therapy. Crit Rev Diagn Imaging 23:235–267

Disler DG, McCauley TR, Ratner LM, Kesack CD, Cooper JA (1997) In-phase and out-of-phase MR imaging of bone marrow: prediction of neoplasia based on the detection of coexistent fat and water. AJR Am J Roentgenol 169:1439–1447

Dupuy DE, Safran H, Mayo-Smith WW, Goldberg SN (1998) Percutaneous radiofrequency ablation of osseous metastatic disease. Radiology 202 (Suppl):146

Dupuy DE, Zagoria RJ, Akerley W, Mayo-Smith WW, Kavanagh PV, Safran H (2000) Radiofrequency ablation of malignancies in the lung. AJR 174:57

Eary JF, O'Sullivan F, Powitan Y, Chandhury KR, Vernon C, Bruckner JD, Conrad EU (2002) Sarcoma tumor FDG uptake measured by PET and patient outcome: a retrospective analysis. Eur J Nucl Med Mol Imaging 29(9):1149–1154

Enneking WF, Spannier SS, Goodman MA (1980) Current concepts review: The surgical staging of musculoskeletal sarcomas. J Bone Joint Surg Am 62:1027

Enzinger FM (1988) Hemangiopericytoma. In: Weiss SW (ed) Soft tissue tumors, 2nd edn. Mosby, St. Louis, pp 596–613

Feldman F, van Heertum R, Manos C (2003) 18FDG PET scanning of benign and malignant musculoskeletal lesions. Skeletal Radiol 32(4):201–208

Fenstermacher MJ (2003) Imaging evaluation of patients with soft tissue sarcoma. Surg Oncol Clin N Am 12:305–332

Fletcher BD (1997) Effects of pediatric cancer therapy on the musculoskeletal system. Pediatr Radiol 27:623–636

Fletcher BD (1997) Imaging pediatric bone sarcomas. Diagnosis and treatment-related issues. Radiol Clin North Am 35:1477–1494

Fletcher BD, Hanna SL, Kun LE (1990) Changes in MR signal intensity and contrast enhancement of therapeutically irradiated soft tissue. Magn Reson Imaging 8:771–777

Fletcher BD, Wall JE, Hanna SL (1993) Effect of hematopoietic growth factors on MR images of bone marrow in children undergoing chemotherapy. Radiology 189:745–751

Franzius C, Bielack S, Flege S, Sciuk J, Jurgens H, Schober O (2002) Prognostic significance of (18)F-FDG and (99m)Tc-methylene diphosphonate uptake in primary osteosarcoma. J Nucl Med 43(8):1012–1017

Franzius C, Schober O (2003) Assessment of therapy response by FDG PET in pediatric patients [review]. Q J Nucl Med 47(1):41–55

Fujimoto K, Hasgimoto S, Abe T, Meno S, Terasaki H, Nishimura H et al. (1997) Synovial sarcoma arising from the chest wall: MR imaging findings. Radiat Med 15:411–414

Gherlinzoni F, Picci P, Bacci G, Campanacci D (1992) Limb-sparing versus amputation in osteosarcoma: correlation between local control, surgical margins, and tumor necrosis – Istituto Rizzoli experience. Ann Oncol 3(Suppl 2):23–27

Gurney JG, Severson RK, Davis S et al. (1995) Incidence of cancer in children in the United States. Cancer 75:2186

Hanna SL, Fletcher BD (1995) MR imaging of malignant soft-tissue tumors [review]. Magn Reson Imaging Clin N Am 3:629–650

Hardaway BW, Hoffer FA, Rao BN (2000) Needle localization of small pediatric tumors for surgical biopsy. Pediatr Radiol 30:318–322

Havenga K, Cobben DC, Oyen WJ, Nienhuijs S, Hoekstra HJ, Ruers TJ, Wobbes T (2003) Fluorodeoxyglucose-positron emission tomography and sentinel lymph node biopsy in staging primary cutaneous melanoma. Eur J Surg Oncol 29(8):662–664

Hawkins DS, Rajendran JG, Conrad EU 3rd, Bruckner JD, Eary JF (2003) Evaluation of chemotherapy response in pediatric bone sarcomas by [F-18]-fluorodeoxy-D-glucose positron emission tomography. Cancer 2002; 94(12):3277–3284. Erratum in: Cancer 97(12):3130

Hawkins MM, Wilson LMK, Burton HS, Potok MHN et al. (1996) Radiotherapy, alkylating agents, and risk of bone cancer after childhood cancer. J Natl Cancer Inst 88:270–278

Herzog CE, Stewart JM, Blakely ML (2003) Pediatric soft tissue sarcomas. Surg Oncol Clin N Am 12:419–447, vii

Hoey SA, Letts RM, Jimeniz C (1998) Infantile hemangiopericytoma of the musculoskeletal system: case report and literature review. J Pediatr Orthop 18:359–362

Hoffer FA (2002) Primary skeletal neoplasms: osteosarcoma and Ewing sarcoma. Top Magn Reson Imaging 13:231–239

Hoffer FA, Nikanorov AY, Reddick WE, Bodner SM, Xiong X, Jones-Wallace D et al. (2000) Accuracy of MR imaging for detecting epiphyseal extension of osteosarcoma. Pediatr Radiol 30:289–298

Howland WJ, Loeffler RK, Starchman DE, Johnson RG (1975) Postirradiation atrophic changes of bone and related complications. Radiology 117:677–685

Jones BC, Sundaram M, Kransdorf MJ (1993) Synovial sarcoma: MR imaging findings in 34 patients. AJR Am J Roentgenol 161:827–830

Kaste SC, Billips C, Tan M, Meyer WH, Parham DM, Rao BN et al. (2001) Thallium bone imaging as an indicator of response and outcome in nonmetastatic primary extremity osteosarcoma. Pediatr Radiol 31:251–256

Kaste SC, Hill A, Conley L, Shidler TJ, Rao BN, Neel MM (2002) Magnetic resonance imaging after incomplete resection of soft tissue sarcoma. Clin Orthop 397:204–211

Khoo AK, Foo CL (1994) Malignant change in cutaneous neurofibromas – case reports. Ann Acad Med Singapore 23: 785–789

Knisely BL (2003) Imaging of the chest: pleura and chest wall. In: Haaga JR (ed) CT and MR imaging of the whole body, 4th edn. Mosby, St Louis, pp 1007–1008

Koscielniak E, Rodury C, Flament F et al. (1992) Metastatic rhabdomyosarcoma and histologically similar tumors in childhood: a retrospective European multicenter analyses. Med Pediatr Oncol 20:209–214

Kransdorf MJ, Jelinek JS, Moser RP Jr (1993) Imaging of soft tissue tumors. Radiol Clin North Am 31:359–372

Lang P, Johnston JO, Arenal-Romero F, Gooding CA (1998) Advances in MR imaging of pediatric musculoskeletal neoplasms. Magn Reson Imaging Clin N Am 6:579–604

Laor T (2004) MR imaging of soft tissue tumors and tumor-like lesions. Pediatr Radiol 34:24–37

Lauenstein TC, Goehde SC, Herborn CU, Treder W, Ruehm SG, Debatin JF et al. (2002) Three-dimensional volumetric interpolated breath-hold MR imaging for whole-body tumor staging in less than 15 minutes: a feasibility study. AJR Am J Roentgenol 179:445–449

Lee MJ, Cairns RA, Munk PL, Poon PY (1996) Congenital-infantile fibrosarcoma: magnetic resonance imaging findings. Can Assoc Radiol J 47:121–125

Levine EA (1999) Prognostic factors in soft tissue sarcoma. Semin Surg Oncol 17:23–32

Livraghi T, Solbiati L, Meloni MF, Gazelle GS, Halpern EF, Goldberg SN (2003) Treatment of focal liver tumors with percutaneous radio-frequency ablation: complications encountered in a multicenter study. Radiology 226:441–451

Ma LD, McCarthy EF, Bluemke DA, Frassica FJ (1998) Differentiation of benign from malignant musculoskeletal lesions using MR imaging: pitfalls in MR evaluation of lesions with a cystic appearance. AJR Am J Roentgenol 170:1251–1258

Manaster BJ (2002) Tumors. In: Thrall JH (ed) Musculoskeletal imaging: the requisites, 2nd edn. Mosby, St Louis, pp 46–74

Mazumdar A, Siegel MJ, Narra V, Luchtman-Jones L (2002) Whole-body fast inversion recovery MR imaging of small cell neoplasms in pediatric patients: a pilot study. AJR Am J Roentgenol 179:1261–1266

McCarville MB, Kaste SC, Pappo AS (1999) Soft-tissue malignancies in infancy. AJR Am J Roentgenol 173:973–977

McCarville MB, Spunt SL, Pappo AS (2001) Rhabdomyosarcoma in pediatric patients: the good, the bad, and the unusual. AJR Am J Roentgenol 176:1563–1569

McCarville MB, Spunt SL, Skapek SX, Pappo AS (2002) Synovial sarcoma in pediatric patients. AJR Am J Roentgenol 179: 797–801

McHugh K, Kao S (2003) Can pediatric radiologists resist RECIST (Response evaluation criteria in solid tumors)? Pediatr Radiol 33:739–743

Meyer JS, Hoffer FA, Mulliken J, Barnes P (1991) MR correlation of the biological classification of soft tissue vascular anomalies. AJR 157:559–564

Meyers PA, Heller G, Healy J et al. (1992) Chemotherapy for non-metastatic osteogenic osteosarcoma: the Memorial Sloan-Kettering experience. J Clin Oncol 10:5–15

Miller SL, Hoffer FA (2001) Malignant and benign bone tumors. Radiol Clin North Am 39:673–699

Moore SG, Bisset GS III, Siegel MJ, Donaldson JS (1991) Pediatric musculoskeletal MR imaging. Radiology 179:345–360

Newton WA, Meadows AT, Shimada H, Bunin GR, Vawter GF (1991) Bone sarcomas as second malignant neoplasms following childhood cancer. Cancer 67:193–201

Parasuraman S, Langston J, Rao BN, Poquette CA, Jenkins JJ, Merchant T et al. (1999) Brain metastases in pediatric Ewing sarcoma and rhabdomyosarcoma: the St. Jude Children's Research Hospital experience. J Pediatr Hematol Oncol 21:370–377

Pousti TJ, Upton J, Loh M, Grier H (1998) Congenital fibrosarcoma of the upper extremity. Plast Reconstr Surg 102:1158–1162

Raney RB (2002) Soft-tissue sarcoma in childhood and adolescence. Curr Oncol Rep 4:291–298

Raney RB, Tefft M, Maurer HM et al. (1988) Disease patterns and survival in children with metastatic soft tissue sarcoma. Cancer 62:1257–1266

Reddick WE, Taylor JS, Fletcher BD (1999) Dynamic MR imaging (DEMRI) of microcirculation in bone sarcoma. J Magn Reson Imaging 10:277–285

Reddick WE, Wang S, Xiong X, Glass JO, Wu S, Kaste SC et al. (2001) Dynamic magnetic resonance imaging of regional contrast access as an additional prognostic factor in pediatric osteosarcoma. Cancer 91:2230–2237

Resnick D, Greenway GD (1996) Tumors and tumor-like lesions of bone: imaging and pathology of specific lesions. In: Resnick D (ed) Bone and joint imaging, 2nd edn. WB Saunders, Philadelphia, pp 1001–1059

Riccardi VM, Powell PP (1989) Neurofibrosarcoma as a complication of von Recklinghausen neurofibromatosis. Neurofibromatosis 2:152–165

Rodriguez-Galindo C, Ramsey K, Jenkins JJ, Poquette CA, Kaste SC et al. (2000) Hemangiopericytoma in children and adults. Cancer 88:198–204

Rosen G, Caparros B, Huvos AG et al. (1982) Preoperative chemotherapy for osteogenic sarcoma: selection of postoperative adjuvant chemotherapy based on the response of the primary tumor to preoperative chemotherapy. Cancer 49:1221–1230

Schaefer O, Lohrmann C, Herling M, Uhrmeister P, Langer M (2002) Combined radiofrequency thermal ablation and percutaneous cementoplasty treatment of a pathologic fracture. J Vasc Inter Radiol 13:1047–1050

Schima W, Amann G, Stiglbauer R et al. (1994) Preoperative staging of osteosarcoma: Efficacy of MR imaging in detecting joint involvement. AJR Am J Roentgenol 163:1171

Schlesinger AE, Hernandez RJ (1992) Diseases of the musculoskeletal system in children: imaging with CT, sonography, and MR. AJR Am J Roentgenol 158:729–741

Smith TA (1998) FDG uptake, tumor characteristics and response to therapy: a review. Nucl Med Commun 19:97–105

Solomon SB, Semih Dogan A, Nicol TL et al. (2001) Positron emission tomography in the detection and management of sarcomatous transformation in neurofibromatosis. Clin Nucl Med 26:525–528

Sundaram M, McLeod RA (1990) MR imaging of tumor and tumor-like lesions of bone and soft tissue. AJR Am J Roentgenol 155:817–824

Taylor JS, Reddick WE (2000) Evolution from empirical dynamic contrast-enhanced magnetic resonance imaging to pharmacokinetic MRI. Adv Drug Deliv Rev 41:91–110

Teo EL, Strouse PJ, Hernandez RJ (2000) MR imaging differentiation of soft-tissue hemangiomas from malignant soft-tissue masses. AJR Am J Roentgenol 174:1623–1628

van der Woude HJ, Bloem JL, Schipper J, Hermans J, Eck-Smit BL, van Oostayen J et al. (1994) Changes in tumor perfusion induced by chemotherapy in bone sarcomas: color Doppler flow imaging compared with contrast-enhanced MR imaging and three-phase bone scintigraphy. Radiology 191:421–431

Varma DG (1999) Optimal radiologic imaging of soft tissue sarcomas. Semin Surg Oncol 17:2–10

Viano AM, Gronemeyer SA, Hoffer FA, Haliloglu M (2000) Improved MR imaging for patients with metallic implants. Magn Reson Imaging 18:287–295

Vinnicombe SJ, Hall CM (1994) Infantile fibrosarcoma: radiological and clinical features. Skeletal Radiol 23:337–341

Vogler JB, Murphy WA (1988) Bone marrow imaging. Radiology 168:679–693

Winkler K, Beron G, Delling G et al. (1988) Neoadjuvant chemotherapy of osteosarcoma: results of a randomized cooperative trial (COSS-82) with salvage chemotherapy based on histologic tumor response. J Clin Oncol 6:329–337

Yang WT, Kwan WH, Li CK, Metreweli C (1997) Imaging of pediatric head and neck rhabdomyosarcomas with emphasis on magnetic resonance imaging and a review of the literature. Pediatr Hematol Oncol 14:243–257

Local Control Issues in Pediatric Bone and Soft Tissue Sarcomas

John C. Breneman, David Rodeberg,
Ruth F. Lavigne, Ken Brown, Eugene S. Wiener

Contents

4.1 Significance of Local Control in Pediatric Sarcomas

The outcome of children with bone and soft tissue sarcomas has improved dramatically over the past few decades with the use of multimodality therapy. The routine use of multiagent chemotherapy has significantly decreased the risk of developing metastatic disease with a corresponding increase in long-term survival. With this improved control of systemic tumor, local control has become a concern in pediatric patients with selected sarcomas such as rhabdomyosarcoma.

The impact of local control on patients and the course of their disease is very significant. Successful control of the primary tumor eliminates a source of clonogenic cells and protects the function of the primary tumor site. Conversely, failure to control local disease can result in lost function of the affected body part, renewed risk of microscopic tumor dissemination, decreased survival rates, and emotional trauma to young patients and their families (Collin et al. 1987).

The favorable cure rates for many of these diseases makes choice of local control measures particularly important. All local control modalities have the potential to cause morbidity, and this risk of harm is often increased in young patients who have not achieved full growth. The general philosophy for treatment of pediatric sarcomas is eradication of local tumor with a minimum of morbidity to function, appearance, potential growth and development.

Multiple factors have contributed to increasingly effective local control with decreasing morbidity. Advances in three-dimensional imaging techniques have improved the ability to visualize and determine the local extent of tumor as well as detect microscopic metastases. New radiation therapy modalities enable radiation oncologists to increase dose to tumor while avoiding surrounding normal structures. Surgical reconstructive techniques have also improved and evolved. New chemotherapy agents and regimens have been developed which improve not only systemic disease control, but help with management of local tumor.

4.2 Background to Local Control Modalities

4.2.1 Patterns of Tumor Growth

Sarcomas are malignant tumors of mesenchymal connective tissue which spread hematogenously along musculo-aponeurotic planes, rather than by lymphatics. As sarcomas grow, surrounding normal tissue is compressed creating a pseudocapsule. A reactive zone surrounds the pseudocapsule consisting of an outer rim of edema, inflammatory cells and small blood vessels. As the malignant mass grows, extensions penetrate into the reactive zones along the perivascular space surrounding the mass. Satellite cells can become separated from the main tumor mass and form tumor satellites in the edematous reactive zone beyond the tumor pseudocapsule. The progressive infiltration and invasion of surrounding tissue combined with the associated edema and inflammation leads to a poorly demarcated boundary between the tumor and its reactive zone.

4.2.2 Surgery

The indications for surgery in the treatment of sarcomas include initial biopsy, resection of the primary tumor, reconstruction after resection and, in some cases, resection of metastatic lesions. Many of these topics will be discussed in more detail for each disease but some general principles applicable to all are outlined below.

4.2.2.1 Biopsy Guidelines

The general principles of biopsy should be followed, including longitudinal incisions, the ability to remove the biopsy tract with the lesion at the time of surgical excision, avoidance of neurovascular structures and a direct route to the tumor through muscles rather than retracting them. Although the tissue diagnosis can often be made by fine needle aspiration or core needle biopsy, an open incisional biopsy of the primary site is recommended in children to obtain enough tissue for all biologic studies. Biologic studies are becoming increasingly important for diagnosis and in the future may lead to tailored therapeutic approaches. A minimum of 1 cm^3 of tissue is required for cytogenetic, molecular, and immunohistochemistry studies. This is in addition to the fresh tissue needed for diagnosis. Bone tumors can usually be diagnosed by biopsying the soft tissue extension avoiding the need for breaching the already weakened bone which would increase the risk of a subsequent pathologic fracture. This risk is further increased if radiotherapy is subsequently required.

Collaboration between the pediatric oncologist, the radiation oncologist and the surgeon for accurate staging before local therapy will optimize the approach to therapy. Patients who undergo unplanned surgical excision of a "mass" prior to referral to a cancer center for definitive treatment are at increased risk for local recurrence and loss of function (Davis et al. 2002).

4.2.2.2 Surgical Margins

Enneking et al. (2003) described a schema for classifying surgical margins. The surgical margin classification options are: radical, wide, marginal and intralesional. A radical margin is the en bloc excision of an entire tumor bearing muscle compartment. Currently this is rarely done for sarcoma. A wide margin is achieved when the tumor is removed en bloc with the plane of dissection encompassing a rim of normal tissue surrounding the pseudocapsule and reactive zone of the enclosed tumor. In a marginal excision, the tumor is removed en bloc but the plane of dissection runs through the tumor pseudocapsule or reactive area surrounding the tumor. Therefore, microscopic residual disease is likely as satellite tumor lesions are left behind. For an intralesional margin, the tumor is exposed during surgery, thereby contaminating the operating field and leaving gross macroscopic tumor behind. This is a debulking procedure and should rarely be done for any sarcoma.

The surgical margin required for local control of sarcomas is a wide margin. The adequacy of the margin is dependent on the type of tissue near the border of the tumor and the presence of other vital structures. Thick fascial connective tissue is a better barrier to tumor extension than fat or muscle and thus may be an adequate margin even if it is very close to the tumor. Usually the closest margins are near neurovascular structures and while certain major nerves, such as the femoral, can be sacrificed with good functional results, other nerves, such as the median, are essential for hand function. Given the proximity of vital structures to the tumor, the surgeon may have trouble obtaining wide margins in certain anatomic regions such as the pelvis, spine, head and neck, axilla, antecubital fossa, groin, popliteal fossa, forearm, and retroperitoneum. At some sites, if it seems likely that a wide surgical margin will not be achieved, neoadjuvant chemotherapy may be given to chemotherapy sensitive tumors to decrease the size of the tumor or the reactive zone. In some patients, radiotherapy will be required before or after surgery to achieve local control.

4.2.3 Radiation Therapy

Radiotherapy is a valuable tool in the treatment of sarcomas. It can be used preoperatively in an attempt to transform an inoperable tumor into one that can be resected or in the postoperative setting when the margins are inadequate and reexcision is not appropriate. Additionally, radiotherapy can be utilized as an alternative to surgery in cases where surgical resection would prove functionally or cosmetically unacceptable, or where the tumor cannot be completely excised with acceptable margins.

Patients should be evaluated by a radiation oncologist, in conjunction with a surgeon and medical oncologist, prior to the initiation of any therapy. This allows the appropriate integration of radiotherapy into the local control strategy. Additionally, modern radiotherapy depends heavily upon three-dimensional imaging of the tumor for defining target volumes. Therefore, appropriate imaging for radiotherapy planning must often be obtained prior to resection or beginning other treatment.

Radiation affects both tumor and normal tissues through ionization of intracellular organic molecules, which directly and indirectly produce irreparable DNA damage. Biologically, radiotherapy takes advantage of the differences in radiation sensitivity and repair capability between tumor and normal tissue, while not exceeding normal tissue tolerance levels. This is usually accomplished by delivering radiation in multiple daily "fractions" which cause cumulative tumor death while allowing ongoing daily repair of normal tissue. In addition, radiotherapy techniques are used which accurately target tumor while maximally sparing surrounding normal tissues.

4.2.3.1 Types of Radiation

Most types of radiotherapy use X-rays (photons) as the therapeutic agent. X-rays can be accurately shaped and aimed at targets within the body. Another common type of radiotherapy is electron radiation, which has physical properties allowing control over the depth of tissue penetration. Proton radiation acts identically to X-rays and electrons, but can facilitate protection of nearby normal tissues because of its Bragg peak effect of energy deposition and minimal lateral scatter. However, the use of protons is limited by high cost and limited availability.

4.2.3.2 Techniques of Radiotherapy

External beam radiation therapy (XRT) is the method most commonly used to deliver radiation. XRT uses a linear accelerator to produce ionizing radiation that can be directed at the tumor from outside the body. Advantages of XRT are the non-invasive nature of the treatment and the homogeneous fields of ionizing radiation that are produced. Advances in three-dimensional imaging have facilitated significant improvement in the ability to avoid damage of normal tissue through accurate targeting and shaping of radiation beams. A recent advance, intensity modulated radiation therapy (IMRT), controls not only the geometric shape of the beam, but also the intensity within segments of the beam. Consequently, the radiation dose to normal tissue may be significantly decreased, optimizing the risk-benefit ratio.

Brachytherapy refers to treatment with a radiation-producing isotope that is in direct contact with the tumor. Hollow catheters are placed in the tumor bed at the time of resection and subsequently "loaded" with a radiation-producing isotope. Brachytherapy offers some advantages to selected pediatric patients with soft tissue sarcomas. Because of the rapid fall-off of radiation intensity, nearby normal structures can be protected. Duration of treatment may also be shortened. Disadvantages include the potential for dose inhomogeneity, the need for direct access to tissues for placement of the radiation sources, and concerns for radiation exposure to hospital personnel and other patients while the radioactive sources are in place (Merchant et al. 2000; Pisters et al. 1994).

Intraoperative radiation therapy (IORT) is similar to brachytherapy in that the radiation is delivered with direct visualization of the targeted tissues. However, rather than using a radioactive isotope as the source of radiation, a linear accelerator is used, with the treatment given as a single radiation dose at the time of surgical resection or exploration. This allows for direct visualization of the tumor, and organs at risk can be temporarily moved out of the radiation field. However, these benefits are offset by the adverse biological consequences of large radiation doses given in a single fraction and the burdensome technical and logistic issues of delivering XRT to an anesthetized patient in a sterile environment (Merchant et al. 1998).

4.2.3.3 Treatment Morbidity

Both surgery and radiotherapy can cause morbidity, which, in some instances, can be significant. Surgical morbidity is usually related to removal or damage of adjacent tissue or organs during removal of the tumor. The morbidity of radiation therapy can be divided into acute and late effects. Acute side effects relate primarily to rapidly dividing epithelial tissues within the treatment field. Skin can become erythematous or hyperpigmented. Mucous membranes may ulcerate, making intake of adequate nutrition difficult. Alopecia occurs at approximately 3–4 weeks into therapy, but nearly always returns within 4 months of completion when doses do not exceed 50 Gy. Nausea, vomiting, and small bowel enteritis can occur with abdominal radiation. In addition, pelvic irradiation can cause urinary frequency and diarrhea. Most acute side effects resolve after completion of radiotherapy, and are treated symptomatically.

Late treatment effects are defined as occurring several months to years after treatment, and may be permanent in nature. Radiation-induced malignancies can occur in the field of treatment following radiation therapy, usually after a time lapse of several years. Radiation to bone may result in a decrease in bone strength, fatty replacement of bone marrow, and inhibition of future growth. Doses to the testes as low as 4–6 Gy, or doses to the ovaries of 8–10 Gy, may cause permanent sterility. Irradiation of the head and neck region can result in permanent xerostomia, damage to teeth, trismus, and facial abnormalities. Soft tissue fibrosis can occur in any organ such as the lungs, liver or kidneys, and result in diminished function.

4.2.4 Combined Surgery and Radiotherapy for Local Control

When radiation is given alone, the majority of local failures arise from the hypoxic center of the tumor. Surgery is least effective at the periphery where margins may be inadequate but the central necrotic radioresistant part of the tumor is readily removed. Therefore radiotherapy and surgery are well suited for a combined approach to local control. When planned beforehand as part of a comprehensive therapeutic approach, less surgery and a lower dose of radiotherapy may be possible. Combined surgery and radiation therapy are often employed in areas where the morbidity of each modality alone is thought to be worse than their combined effects. If it is difficult to predict that surgery alone will result in a wide margin of normal tissue around the lesion, consideration should be given to neoadjuvant radiotherapy (Davis et al. 2002; Habrand et al. 1991; O'Sullivan et al. 2002; Suit et al. 1981). If surgery alone is planned, but an inadequate margin is achieved, the patient will require a higher dose of postoperative radiation with its associated increased morbidity.

4.2.5 Chemotherapy for Local Control

It is well established that multiagent chemotherapy improves both survival and local control for RMS (Kinsella et al. 1988; Ruymann 1987; Tefft et al. 1981). Not only does chemotherapy work to eradicate microscopic foci of disease, in addition neoadjuvant therapy helps reduce the primary tumor size thereby aiding resection. Chemotherapy must be combined with surgery and XRT to provide a comprehensive local control strategy.

On the other hand the results of chemotherapy for local control in NRSTS are far from clear. Single institution studies have had a difficult time demonstrating any effect of chemotherapy on local control given the small numbers of patients, though the Sarcoma Meta-analysis Collaboration (2000) did show a 10% improvement in local recurrence free interval when chemotherapy was used. In adults, doxorubicin has also been used as a radiosensitizer and when combined with neoadjuvant XRT has been well tolerated with local control rates >90% (Pisters et al. 2002). Studies looking at the use of neoadjuvant chemotherapy have suggested that those patients who have a clinical or pathologic response are more likely to have negative margin resection, improved local control and a decreased incidence of metastatic spread (Eilber et al. 1995; Meric et al. 2002).

4.3 Ewing's Sarcoma

4.3.1 Surgery for Ewing's Sarcoma

The survival of patients with Ewing's sarcoma before the advent of the chemotherapy era in the 1970s was about 10%. Amputation of the limb did not influence survival rates so radiation therapy became the mainstay of local treatment. Advances in surgical techniques, the use of neoadjuvant chemotherapy and improved oncologic training of surgeons resulted in a shift back to surgery for local control of Ewing's sarcoma.

There are two main benefits to surgical excision of these tumors. First, a number of retrospective studies have shown both lower local failure rates and/or a survival advantage for surgical therapy (Craft et al. 1998; Evans et al. 1991; Holt et al. 2002; Kuttesch et al. 1996; Noria et al. 1996; Parsons et al. 2001; Rosito et al. 1999). The second benefit is the opportunity to study the tumoricidal effects of neoadjuvant chemotherapy. The pathologic response of these tumors to chemotherapy has been shown to have prognostic value (Wunder et al. 1998). For these reasons, surgery has become the predominant modality for local control for Ewing's sarcoma in accessible sites.

Criteria which favor surgery as a method for local control include: a small initial tumor volume, location in an expendable bone, tumors in the diaphysis which allow joint and growth plate sparing reconstructions, and tumors which have a good response to chemotherapy making the achievement of a wide surgical margin more likely. The best functional results of surgery are in diaphyseal resections of long bones where the joints can be spared. Limb sparing surgical procedures are no longer contraindicated in patients with pathologic fractures. The fractured limb may be stabilized in traction or a cast during induction chemotherapy following which surgical options or radiotherapy may become feasible. In young children there are added challenges. Local control of long bones leads to diminished future limb growth and a resulting limb length discrepancy that may be very difficult to manage. In some cases achieving a wide surgical margin will necessitate removal of part of a joint surface. This will limit the reconstructive options in a young child. Reconstructive options are more limited in patients less than 10 years of age due to the small size of their joints and the decreased future growth resulting from the loss of growth from the resected end of bone.

4.3.2 Radiation Therapy for Ewing's Sarcoma

Ewing's sarcoma is a radiosensitive tumor, and radiotherapy has historically played a major role in its treatment. The role of radiotherapy has evolved since the first Intergroup Ewing's Sarcoma Study was undertaken in 1973 (IESS-1). In IESS-1 radiotherapy was given to the entire involved bone using an age-dependent dose of 45–55 Gy plus a boost of 5–10 Gy to gross disease. Overall, local control was achieved in 85% of cases (Nesbit et al. 1990). In IESS-II (1978–1982) surgical treatment of the primary tumor was encouraged, with radiotherapy given for residual or inoperable disease. Radiotherapy treatment parameters were similar to those used in IESS-1. Local control was achieved in 91% of patients (Burgert et al. 1990). Local control modality (surgery vs. radiotherapy vs. radiotherapy/surgery) did not appear to impact 5-year overall survival.

A third Intergroup Ewing's Study was completed in 1992 (Grier et al. 2003). The method of local control was at the discretion of the treating physician and included surgery, radiotherapy, or both for patients with gross or suspected residual postoperatively. A detailed analysis of local control from this study is pending, but preliminary results show improved outcome for patients treated with surgery alone compared to radiotherapy or surgery plus radiotherapy. However, a negative selection bias for patients treated with radiotherapy was noted and may have influenced these results.

Schuck et al. (2003) reviewed factors affecting local control of 1,058 patients treated in CESS 81, CESS 86, and a third recently completed European trial, EICESS 92. For this combined population, local failure was greatest (23%) in patients receiving primary radiotherapy, even when patients treated on CESS 81 with suboptimal radiotherapy were excluded. Again, this result was somewhat confounded by the negative selection bias for patients treated with primary radiotherapy (71% had centrally located tumors). Local failure for surgically treated patients was approximately 7%. Of note, local control for patients with intralesional resections followed by radiotherapy was comparable to definitive radiotherapy alone. Therefore, there is no value to "debulking" surgery in these patients.

Radiotherapy alone may be preferred for patients with bulky, primary lesions in surgically difficult sites such as the spine, skull, facial bones, and periacetabular pelvis; and those patients with a poor response to induction chemotherapy, in whom surgery would result in an unacceptable functional outcome. Predictors for favorable local control with radiotherapy vary among studies, but consistently include peripheral tumors and tumors smaller than 8 cm or 100 cc in size. Other factors identified with favorable outcome include radiotherapy doses above 50 Gy and good histologic response of tumor to induction chemotherapy (Arai et al. 1991; Gasparini et al. 1981; Razek et al. 1980; Sauer et al. 1987; Shankar et al. 1999).

4.3.2.1 Radiotherapy Treatment Factors

The appropriate radiotherapy treatment volume has evolved to include less normal tissue with smaller treatment margins around radiographically identifiable tumor. Current guidelines specify inclusion of radiographically identified tumor in bone and soft tissue prior to chemotherapy and surgery plus a 2-cm margin. Additional radiation ("cone-down boost") is then delivered to the volume of initial osseous disease plus any remaining soft-tissue component after chemotherapy and surgery. Lymph nodes are not intentionally included in the treatment volume unless they are known to be involved with tumor. For primary thoracic tumors where pleural effusion, infiltration, or intraoperative contamination occurs, inclusion of the ipsilateral hemithorax in the radiotherapy fields for 15–20 Gy has been shown to improve event-free survival.

Although there has been some success in treating microscopic Ewing's sarcoma with doses as low as 30 Gy (Merchant et al. 1999), the majority of the centers have opted to treat the volume at risk for microscopic disease to a dose of 45 Gy. Unresected or gross residual disease should receive boost radiotherapy to a total of approximately 55 Gy with doses as high as 64 Gy for large tumors, though normal tissue tolerance to radiation may limit the dose that can be used, particularly for vertebral primaries and large, centrally located tumors (Arai et al. 1991; Ozaki et al. 1996).

Radiotherapy is usually given between 8 and 12 weeks following initiation of chemotherapy. If used postoperatively, treatment begins as soon as surgical healing allows. A retrospective review of CESS 86 and EICESS 92 revealed a trend toward increased local failures when postoperative radiotherapy was delayed more than 60 days after surgery.

4.4 Rhabdomyosarcoma

The use of multimodality therapy, including chemotherapy, surgery, and radiotherapy, results in local control rates of 80–90% (Donaldson et al. 2001). However, local failure remains a significant problem in RMS, and for the majority of patients who are unable to undergo complete surgical resection of their tumor, it is the primary mode of failure. Because the approach for local control often plays a major role in determining future quality of life, attention now is directed at minimizing the long-term impact of therapy in survivors, with emphasis on both function and cosmesis.

The diversity of anatomic locations in which RMS occur makes generic algorithms or recommendations for local control management difficult. In addition, the incidence of lymph node and hematogenous metastases as well as the overall prognosis of the patient is also location specific (Table 4.1), further increasing the complexity of local control. In a review of Group III patients on the IRS-III study, lymph node status was found to be the most important factor predictive of local failure. Patients with lymph node involvement had a local failure rate of 32% compared to 16% for those with negative or unknown nodal status (Wharam et al. 2004). Age <10 years and smaller tumor size have also been identified as favorable predictors for local control.

Table 4.1. Rhabdomyosarcoma local failure by site (compiled from Wharam et al. 2004; Raney et al. 2002; Wharam et al. 1997; Donaldson et al. 2001)

Site	Local failure (%)
Parameningeal	15–19
Orbit	2–16
Head & neck	12–29
Extremity	7–25
Bladder/prostate	14–19
Chest	50
Intra-abdominal	22
Pelvis	30
Trunk	32

4.4.1 Surgery for Rhabdomyosarcoma

Surgical excision was originally the mainstay of treatment for RMS, and the only children with a chance of surviving were those who had a complete resection of their tumor (Grosfeld et al. 1983). With the advent of multimodal treatment, surgery continues to play a prominent role in local control of RMS. Local control is improved for many patients who are able to undergo initial complete resection (Table 4.2), and IRS (now COG STS) studies have consistently revealed a survival advantage for initial (prior to adjuvant therapy) complete tumor extirpation (Wiener 1993). Another example for the importance of complete surgical resection is illustrated by the results of a retrospective study from IRS-I and -II which showed that patients with RMS of the trunk or extremities with

Table 4.2. Rhabdomyosarcoma local failure by group (compiled from Michalski et al. 2004; Smith et al. 2001; Wharam et al. 2004; Wharam et al. 1997; Koscielnak et al. 1999; Wolden et al. 1999)

Clinical group	Local failure rate (%)
I	3–6
II	8–20
III	12–20

clinical group IIa disease (microscopic residual tumor without nodal metastases) who underwent a primary site reexcision (PRE) had a significant survival benefit when compared to those not receiving additional surgery (Hays et al. 1995). In fact, patients who underwent PRE had a better survival than patients originally staged as clinical group I (no residual microscopic tumor). This suggests that the pathologic evaluation of the resected specimen in group patients may not be completely accurate in some patients, especially if the original operation was not designed as a "cancer operation."

Surgical guidelines for RMS are site-specific. There are, however, some general principles applicable: (1) biopsy incisions should be oriented in an axial direction that allows for later wide tumor excision without violating tissue planes; (2) initial complete gross and microscopic excision is preferable, although extensive primary resections which will negatively impact form and function should be avoided; (3) debulking has little if any value; delayed complete secondary excisions after initial biopsy and neoadjuvant therapy have a better outcome; (4) primary resection should assure complete excision of the tumor outside of any evident pseudocapsule; the principle of never visualizing tumor tissue during the resection applies; (5) surgical margins should be at least 0.5 cm; (6) certain sites have a high likelihood of regional node involvement, (extremity and paratesticular), while at other sites node involvement is uncommon (head and neck and GU sites); (7) patients who are found to have clinically suspicious lymph nodes as determined by physical examination or pretreatment imaging should have these biopsied at the time of initial surgery or should be managed as if nodes are positive with nodal irradiation; (8) all extremity patients should have pathologic evaluation of node involvement whether or not noted on clinical evaluation. Sentinel node techniques may be employed.

Second-look operations (SLO) may play a role in improving local control for patients who are initially unresectable, but have a significant response to induction chemotherapy and/or radiotherapy. An analysis of 257 group III patients from IRS-III demonstrated that SLO significantly changed the response status in a large number of patients. Twelve percent of presumed CR patients were found to have residual viable tumor (pathologically partial response, or pPR), while 74% of both PR and NR patients were found to have either no viable tumor (pCR) or were able to be converted to CR by a secondary resection. The 3-year survival of PR and NR patients converted to CR after surgical resection was similar to those patients confirmed to be CR at the time of secondary exploration (73% vs. 80%) (Wiener et al. 1991).

4.4.2 Radiotherapy for Rhabdomyosarcoma

With the exception of group I (completely excised) tumors of embryonal histology, the standard of care in North America mandates the use of radiotherapy for RMS. Indeed, in European studies in which RT is less frequently used, local control and failure-free survival rates appear to be inferior for comparable patient groups, despite the use of aggressive chemotherapy regimens (Flamant et al. 1998; Koscielniak et al. 1999).

As in Ewing's sarcoma, the use of radiotherapy for RMS has evolved over the last several decades. The IRS studies have played a major role in defining the indications and techniques for local control with radiation. The first IRS study showed that children with group tumors do not require radiotherapy. However, subsequent meta-analysis of IRS data demonstrated increased local failures in the subset of Group I patients with alveolar histology, and current recommendations include radiotherapy for these children. Radiotherapy is always indicated in patients with microscopic or gross residual tumor after initial resection, and for those patients with spread to regional lymph nodes (Smith et al. 2001).

In general, radiotherapy is begun 3–12 weeks after initiation of chemotherapy, although some studies have suggested improved outcomes when radiotherapy is introduced earlier in the treatment regimen (Crist et al. 1995; Koscielniak et al. 1999; Michalski et al. 2004). Treatment is given to an anatomic volume that encompasses the entire tumor at the time of initial diagnosis, plus a margin of 2 cm. A dose of 36–41.4 Gy is delivered, followed by a "cone-down" reduction of the RT field size for gross residual disease to a total dose of 50.4 Gy. Lymph nodes chains are treated only if involved with tumor, and require a minimum of 41.4 Gy.

Some have based radiotherapy treatment parameters on response to induction chemotherapy, although chemotherapy alone does not provide adequate local control for many patients (Crist et al. 1995; Flamant et al. 1998; Koscielniak et al. 1999). The current IRS study allows reduction of radiotherapy dose to 36–41.4 Gy for patients with gross total resection at the time of second-look operations following induction chemotherapy, and the German CWS-86 study used 32 Gy after a good response to chemotherapy. Though these approaches show promise, their efficacy has not yet been firmly established. Hyperfractionated radiotherapy has been used successfully in the treatment of RMS (Koscielniak et al. 1999). However, when it was studied in a prospective randomized trial in IRS-IV it did not result in improved outcomes compared to conventional schedules using 1.8 Gy/day (Donaldson et al. 2001).

4.4.3 Site Specific Approaches to Local Control

4.4.3.1 Orbit and Head & Neck

About one-third of RMS originate in the head and neck region. Orbital RMS rarely requires surgical treatment beyond biopsy, and is treated with chemoradiotherapy. Careful planning of radiotherapy fields to exclude brain tissue and the contralateral eye can minimize treatment-related morbidity. Sophisticated treatment planning techniques such as IMRT or proton beam therapy may help to achieve these objectives. Orbital primaries have a favorable prognosis, with local control achieved in 95% of patient treated on IRS IV (Donaldson et al. 2001).

The remainder of head and neck tumors are classified as parameningeal (nasopharynx/nasal cavity, paranasal sinuses, pterygopalatine, infratemporal fossa, middle ear/mastoid) or non-parameningeal (face, scalp, oral cavity/oropharynx, larynx).

For non-parameningeal tumors, surgery is often the primary local control modality with radiotherapy given after resection for microscopic residual. Locally advanced tumors are treated primarily with radiotherapy, though in cases of major response to induction chemotherapy a second look operation may be performed and lower radiation doses used postoperatively. A local control rate of 88% was achieved in IRS-IV for these tumors (Donaldson et al. 2001).

Local control of parameningeal RMS is generally achieved with radiotherapy, though there may be a limited role for specialized skull base techniques and reconstructive surgery when such experienced teams are available (Blatt et al. 1997). These tumors may invade the base of skull and involve adjacent meninges, and often present with cranial nerve dysfunction. Radiotherapy treatment fields must include the adjacent meninges, but whole brain therapy as used in early IRS studies is unnecessary (Raney et al. 2002). Initiation of radiotherapy within 2 weeks of diagnosis for tumors with intracranial extension is associated with lower rates of local failure. Five-year local control for these patients is approximately 80% (Michalski et al. 2004).

4.4.3.2 Genitourinary: Bladder/Prostate

Tumors arising in the bladder or prostate are frequently so large that determination of the specific site of primary tumor origin may not be possible. Historically, most RMS of the bladder/prostate were treated by anterior or total pelvic exenterative procedures followed by adjuvant chemoradiotherapy (Hays 1980). Significant clinical effort has shifted toward designing treatment regimens that preserve bladder function in these patients while preserving overall survival. In the third IRS study, treatment began with intensive chemotherapy followed by radiotherapy 6 weeks after the start of CT and supplemented by surgery when necessary. With this approach, 60% of children maintained functional bladders 4 years after diagnosis, compared to 22% of children in the second IRS study treated with less intensive chemotherapy and delayed radiation and surgery (Hays et al. 1995). However, improvements are still needed. In IRS IV, bladder function was preserved in 55% (36/66) of event-free survivors, but of all patients entered on study only 40% (36/88) survive event-free with normal functioning bladders (Arndt et al. 2004). Overall, approximately 80% of these patients achieve local control of their tumors.

Complete response to initial chemo-/radiotherapy may not be rapid, but as long as there is some response, radical or exenterative procedures should be delayed. Even for patients who continue to have viable tumor (other than rhabdomyoblasts) or who suffer early failure or progression of disease after completion of therapy, urethral preservation procedures are still usually possible with good outcome. Patients with prostate RMS will sometimes have an adequate tumor response which allows for prostatectomy with urethral and/or bladder neck reconstruction. Children who are not candidates for bladder salvage can usually be treated with anterior exenteration, which spares the rectum. Reconstruction is best achieved using a non-refluxing colon or ileal conduit.

Partial cystectomy may not be practical in the majority of these tumors due to their location in the area of the trigone. However, approximately 10% of bladder RMS will arise from the dome of the bladder, allowing for a primary partial cystectomy.

4.4.3.3 Vagina and Uterine Sites

Tumors arising in the vulva, vagina, cervix, or uterus are uncommon and are considered as a group, though there are differences in natural history, treatment, and outcome. Girls with vaginal RMS have an excellent prognosis, and can often be cured without the need for radical surgery or radiotherapy (Arndt et al. 2001). These tumors are almost always botryoid and are very responsive to chemotherapy. In IRS III, 83% of girls with vaginal RMS had uterine preservation with chemotherapy alone. There were no relapses and no deaths. In those patients who underwent resection based upon suspicion of incomplete response, there was no residual tumor in the resected specimens (Lawrence et al. 1987; Wiener et al. 1991).

Likewise, uterine RMS, which often occurs in older children, usually does not require aggressive resections, although it may be somewhat less chemoresponsive than vaginal RMS (Corpron et al. 1995; Hays et al. 1985). Vulvar RMS is very uncommon, and can usually be treated with wide local excision and adjuvant chemoradiotherapy.

When radiation therapy is required, brachytherapy can be a valuable technique for delivering radiotherapy for these patients, offering the capability of localized radiation to the tumor with sparing of nearby sensitive organs.

4.4.3.4 Paratestes

Paratesticular RMS should be treated with radical inguinal orchiectomy and resection of any scrotal tissue that is invaded by tumor. Biopsy should be avoided since spillage of the tumor frequently leads to local inguinal recurrence. Transscrotal biopsy or resection with spillage should be treated with an ipsilateral hemiscrotectomy. If there is still residual tumor, scrotal radiotherapy should be used. Retroperitoneal lymph node dissection is not necessary for younger boys with clinically negative nodes as determined by preoperative imaging studies. However, children >10 years of age have a 50% likelihood of node involvement which may often be missed on imaging studies. If involved lymph nodes are not detected and treated appropriately with radiotherapy and more aggressive chemotherapy, there is a high risk of regional and systemic relapse. Therefore, lymph node dissection should be performed in children >10 years, as well as those patients with clinically positive nodes unless there is residual disease elsewhere. All children with positive nodes should receive radiotherapy to the para-aortic and ipsilateral internal iliac nodes (Wiener et al. 1994, 2001).

4.4.3.5 Extremity

RMS arising in the extremities is more amenable to primary resection compared to other sites, with 28% of patients classified as group I and 35% as group II after initial surgery. Complete tumor removal should be attempted in all patients unless this would entail an amputation or disabling surgery. In IRS-III, all patients in clinical group IIa who underwent conversion to group I by PRE survived, while only 60% who did not undergo PRE survived. This has led to a recommendation of performing PRE for all extremity RMS, regardless of clinical group, where the original resection was not designed as a "cancer operation" (Hays et al. 1989). Many of these tumors have alveolar histology, and should receive radiotherapy, even when completely resected. Brachytherapy may be a valuable adjunct to treatment for these patients. Lymph node involvement is demonstrated by imaging studies in 12% of patients with extremity RMS, although when regional nodal sampling is performed the rate of involvement approaches 50%. This emphasizes the need for pathologic evaluation of regional nodes in all children with tumors at these sites so that appropriate regional radiotherapy can be delivered if lymphatic metastasis is found (Hays et al. 1989; Lawrence et al. 1997). Though there has been limited experience with lymph node mapping with sentinel node biopsy for RMS, this technique is being studied in current protocols and may result in increased sensitivity and decreased morbidity of lymph node sampling (Guiliano et al. 1994; Morton et al. 1992).

4.4.3.6 Trunk

RMS of the trunk includes tumors of the chest wall, paraspinal regions, lung/pleura, and heart. These tumors are frequently alveolar, and the majority arise from the chest wall. Wide infiltration of the surrounding tissues is common, and only one-third of tumors are initially resectable. As in extremity tumors, all patients with alveolar histology should receive adjuvant radiotherapy, even if the tumor is felt to be completely resected. Hemithorax or whole abdominal irradiation may be necessary when tumor has disseminated into these body cavities, though treatment is limited by the tolerance of surrounding sensitive organs such as lung, liver, kidneys, and bowel.

4.5 Non-Rhabdomyosarcomatous Soft Tissue Sarcomas

The survival of these patients is dependent on histology, histologic grade, tumor size, invasiveness, and surgical margins (Spunt et al. 2002). Unfortunately the survival for patients with localized disease has not changed significantly over the last 20 years (Weitz et al. 2003).

4.5.1 Surgery for Non-Rhabdo Soft Tissue Sarcomas

Local control is strongly related to the completeness of surgical resection. If surgery is used as the sole local control modality, marginal or lesional excision of the tumor results in a 60–90% local recurrence rate. This data initially led to the use of amputations as the treatment of choice and was associated with recurrence rates of 7–18% (Dinges et al. 1994; Yang et al. 1989). With the addition of radiotherapy, limb sparing operations have become feasible with local recurrence rates as low as 5% (Wilson et al. 1994). Given the efficacy of combined surgical and radiotherapies the current surgical recommendation is that a wide local excision (en bloc resection) be the gold standard for local surgical control in children with NRSTS.

Therefore the main goal of surgical therapy should be the complete eradication of the primary tumor (negative microscopic margins) without resection of vital structures that would seriously compromise subsequent function. These resections are possible in 58–85% of patients (Rao et al. 1989; Skene et al. 1993); however, the success rates at some sites (head and neck, retroperitoneal or mediastinal) are much lower, explaining their higher recurrence rates (Lawrence et al. 1989). The importance of negative margins is best illustrated in synovial sarcoma where patients with positive microscopic margins have a survival of 0% vs. 43% for patients with negative margins (Singer et al. 1996). Similar to the other tumors discussed when definitive resection of a previously biopsied sarcoma is performed the biopsy tract and scar should be removed en bloc with the tumor specimen.

The higher success of extremity local control does not mean that amputation will never be required. In pediatric patients a 21–27% amputation rate has been reported (Philippe et al. 1992; Rao 1993). Amputation is recommended when resection of the primary tumor would result in complete loss of function for the limb. These amputation rates are higher than that recorded for adults (5–15%) (Rao 1993) and may be related to a larger tumor to patient size ratio and the proximity of vital structures to each other in a smaller patient.

Local control is very important for NRSTS since the failure of local resection (positive microscopic margins) has been directly associated with local recurrence, distant disease recurrence and overall survival (Herbert et al. 1993). Pretreatment reexcision (PRE) in this setting has been shown to find residual tumor in 36–45% of patients (Rao 1993; Zornig et al. 1995). Therefore, (PRE) of tumors with unknown or positive microscopic margins is advocated, though a study by the Italian Cooperative suggested that PRE plus chemotherapy did not provide any additional benefit beyond that obtained by radiotherapy and chemotherapy (Cecchetto et al. 2000).

Some exceptions to these guidelines include fibrosarcoma in children <1 year old. In these patients, tumors may spontaneously regress and may respond to chemotherapy (LaQuaglia 1997). In addition, patients with PNET act much like Ewing sarcoma and so may benefit from neoadjuvant chemotherapy after diagnosis has been confirmed by incisional biopsy. Desmoplastic small round cell tumor is a diffuse serosal malignancy and may also benefit from neoadjuvant chemotherapy. Subsequent resection of all gross disease followed by radiotherapy and chemotherapy is the suggested therapy. Leiomyosarcoma should undergo complete surgical resection even if this results in amputation since this tumor is often unresponsive to radiotherapy and chemotherapy. Most infantile hemangiopericytomas can be treated with wide local excision and require no further therapy.

Dissemination of tumor to regional lymph nodes is rare (6–9% of patients) (Dillon et al. 1992; Rao et al. 1991). Therefore, there is no indication for routine lymph node resection unless there is clinical or pathologic evidence of nodal involvement. However, some histologic types such as epithelioid sarcoma, synovial cell sarcoma, clear cell sarcoma and angiosarcoma have a higher incidence of nodal involvement and the treatment strategies for these tumors may be modified to use techniques described for rhabdomyosarcoma.

4.5.2 Radiotherapy for Non-Rhabdo Soft Tissue Sarcomas

The role of radiotherapy in pediatric NRSTS has not been well studied. Only one prospective multi-institution study of pediatric NRSTS has been published in the English literature, and this study focused primarily on the role of chemotherapy for these tumors (Pratt et al. 1999). Many of the recommendations for the use of radiotherapy are taken from adult data, though it is unknown whether this is a valid extrapolation.

The preferred use for radiotherapy in these tumors is as an adjuvant to surgery. Radiotherapy in the presence of unresectable lesions is associated with a 5-year event-free survival of only 31% (Pratt et al. 1998). When combined with surgery, radiotherapy may be given either preoperatively or postoperatively. Both approaches have advantages and disadvantages. Preoperative radiotherapy often allows smaller radiotherapy volumes, allows treatment planning to a non-disturbed tumor bed, may make subsequent resection easier or more complete, and may decrease the risk of dissemination of viable tumor cells at the time of resection (Lindberg et al. 1981; O'Sullivan et al. 2002; Suit et al. 1981). Alternatively, postoperative radiotherapy allows treatment to be tailored to the extent of residual tumor after maximal resection; patients who have substantial amounts of residual tumor can receive a planned course of higher dose radiation, and some patients who have completely resected tumors may avoid radiotherapy altogether. Additionally, complications of local control may be fewer when radiotherapy is used postoperatively. Results have been reported for brachytherapy (Merchant et al. 2000) though the role of this modality in pediatric NRSTS is still unclear.

In the POG NRSTS study, radiotherapy was used postoperatively for marginal resections or when resection was not feasible. Analysis of local control by treatment received showed no advantage for the use of radiotherapy in children with low grade tumors, even when marginally resected. Children with high grade tumors, however, benefited from radiotherapy when tumor was incompletely resected. Ten of 11 patients in this setting were controlled with radiotherapy versus only one of four when radiotherapy was omitted. The benefit of radiation after wide resection of high grade tumors was less clear in this study, though a randomized trial has shown a benefit in this setting for adults (Yang et al. 1998).

Prescribed radiotherapy doses vary. Preoperatively, many institutions use 45–50 Gy given at 1.8–2.0 Gy daily. Some would give an additional 10–15 Gy postoperatively when resection is incomplete, but the value of this "boost" is questionable. When radiotherapy is given postoperatively, data would suggest that a dose of 50 Gy or more is necessary to control microscopic residual (Brizel et al. 1988; Brown et al. 2003) with doses of 60 Gy or more needed for gross tumor.

Radiotherapy treatment volume also varies, though few continue to treat the entire anatomic compartment encompassing the tumor. With improved imaging techniques, many now use 5-cm margins around visible tumor with subsequent cone-down "boosts" to 2 cm for doses in excess of 45–50 Gy. As with other sarcomas, circumferential irradiation of an extremity is to be avoided.

4.6 Osteosarcoma

4.6.1 Surgery for Osteosarcoma

Surgery is the mainstay of local therapy in osteosarcoma. Neoadjuvant chemotherapy is usually given to treat micrometastatic disease at diagnosis and to decrease the surrounding reactive zone around the tumor, thereby making a wide excision more feasible. There are two components of surgery for osteosarcoma. The first is wide tumor excision to diminish the risk of local relapse. The second component of surgery is the subsequent limb reconstruction. The extent of resection is determined by the tumor location. Patients usually have options to consider, which depend on age, physical activity and emotional demands. Most osteosarcomas are metaphyseal and require removal of part of the joint.

Osteoarticular allografts can provide for future joint mobility with good bone integration, but there are many early complications such as infection, nonunions and fractures. Late results may be satisfying if the patient has a good anatomic size match of the graft and there are sufficient ligamentous structures available for reconstruction (Hornicek et al. 1998).

Reconstruction with tumor endoprostheses allows reliable early mobility with fewer early complications than allografts. The endoprostheses can be cemented into the patient's bone or can be press fit depending on bone strength for future stability. Eventually all implants will fail due to infection, mechanical failures and/or aseptic loosening inevitably requiring prosthetic revision. When used as a knee replacement, the prosthesis violates the growth plate increasing future limb length discrepancies. Complications have been reported in between 12% and 41% (Ham et al. 1998; Jeys et al. 2003; Kaste et al. 2001). Endoprosthesis placement requires a large resection of healthy bone adjacent to the bone being replaced. In order to function efficiently, musculature is required to provide movement. Often much of the muscle surrounding the tumor has to be resected, severely limiting strength and mobility of the reconstructed joint. Cemented endoprostheses have the advantage of early weight bearing but make future revisions extremely difficult compared to uncemented endoprosthesis. Fixation of uncemented endoprosthesis is often delayed due to chemotherapy effects, but future revisions are more successful due to the preservation of bone stock. Expandable prostheses appear to be a good option for the growing child but are subject to more mechanical problems, and often require a greater number of revisions than traditional prostheses (Windhager et al. 1991). Newer prostheses allow non-invasive expansion (Neel et al. 2003).

Joint arthrodeses are good for shoulder reconstruction and are also durable reconstructions for the knee. Knee arthrodesis makes sitting in confined spaces difficult and most patients walk with a limp. The best results for allograft reconstruction are when an intercalary allograft is used such as in an arthrodesis (Wolf et al. 1999). The results of arthrodesis are very site specific with the best results in the shoulder.

Rotationplasty is a good reconstructive technique for very young patients with future growth potential and patients with very large tumors requiring extensive muscle excision. Rotationplasty has been utilized for tumors located in the proximal femur, distal femur or proximal tibia (Gottsauner-Wolf et al. 1991; Kotz et al. 1982). After removal of the tumor the remaining limb is rotated 180 degrees and reattached. Physical activity is unrestricted and there are no problems with durability. In a study comparing patient satisfaction and quality of life in patients with endoprostheses versus rotationplasty, the patients with rotationplasty scored higher (Hillmann et al. 1999).

4.6.2 Radiotherapy for Osteosarcoma

The role of radiotherapy in local control of osteosarcoma is quite limited due to the radioresistance of the disease. Prior to the use of chemotherapy, radiation was sometimes used as a method of delaying surgical amputation for those who survived the first few months after diagnosis without developing metastatic disease. Local control rates were poor and viable tumor was observed in amputation specimens after radiation doses that exceeded 80 Gy (Lee et al. 1964). Radiotherapy may play a role in patients with microscopic or minimal residual tumor after surgery where local control rates of 70–80% have been reported (DeLaney et al. 2003).

References

Arai Y, Kun LE, Brooks MT, Fairclough DL, Fontanesi J, Meyer WH, Hayes FA, Thompson E, Rao BN (1991) Ewing's sarcoma: local tumor control and patterns of failure following limited-volume radiation therapy. Int J Radiat Oncol Biol Phys 21(6):1501–1508

Arndt CA, Donaldson SS, Anderson JR, Andrassy RJ, Laurie F, Link MP, Raney RB, Maurer HM, Crist WM (2001) What constitutes optimal therapy for patients with rhabdomyosarcoma of the female genital tract? Cancer 91(12):2454–2468

Arndt CA, Rodeberg D, Breitfeld P, Raney R, Ullrich F, Donaldson S (2004) Does bladder preservation (as a surgical principle) lead to retaining bladder function in bladder/prostate rhabdomyosarcoma? Results from IRS IV. J Urol 171:2396–2403

Blatt J, Snyderman C, Wollman MR, Mirro J Jr, Janecka IP, Albo VC, Deutsch M, Janosky JE, Wiener ES (1997) Delayed resection in the management of non-orbital rhabdomyosarcoma of the head and neck in childhood. Med Pediatr Oncol 28:294–298

Brizel DM, Weinstein H, Hunt M, Tarbell NJ (1988) Failure patterns and survival in pediatric soft tissue sarcoma. Int J Radiat Oncol Biol Phys 15(1):37–41

Brown LB, Breitfeld PP, Marcus JRB (2003) Use of a multimodal team to optimize local control and function in young patients with bone and soft tissue sarcomas: A practical approach. American Society of Clinical Oncology 39th Annual Meeting, Chicago, IL

Burgert EO Jr, Nesbit ME, Garnsey LA, Gehan EA, Herrmann J, Vietti TJ, Cangir A, Tefft M, Evans R, Thomas P et al. (1990) Multimodal therapy for the management of nonpelvic, localized Ewing's sarcoma of bone: intergroup study IESS-II. J Clin Oncol 8(9):1514–1524

Cecchetto G, Carli M, Sotti G, Bisogno G, Dall'Igna P, Boglino C, Granata C, Antoniello L, Guglielmi M (2000) Importance of local treatment in pediatric soft tissue sarcomas with microscopic residual after primary surgery: results of the Italian Cooperative Study RMS-88. Med Pediatr Oncol 34(2):97–101

Collin C, Godbold J, Hajdu S, Brennan M (1987) Localized extremity soft tissue sarcoma: an analysis of factors affecting survival. J Clin Oncol 5(4):601–612

Corpron CA, Andrassy RJ, Hays DM, Raney RB, Wiener ES, Lawrence W, Lobe TE, Maurer HM (1995) Conservative management of uterine pediatric rhabdomyosarcoma: a report from the Intergroup Rhabdomyosarcoma Study III and IV pilot. J Pediatr Surg 30(7):942–944

Craft A, Cotterill S, Malcolm A, Spooner D, Grimer R, Souhami R, Imeson J, Lewis I (1998) Ifosfamide-containing chemotherapy in Ewing's sarcoma: The Second United Kingdom Children's Cancer Study Group and the Medical Research Council Ewing's Tumor Study. J Clin Oncol 16(11):3628–3633

Crist W, Gehan EA, Ragab AH, Dickman PS, Donaldson SS, Fryer C, Hammond D, Hays DM, Herrmann J, Heyn R et al. (1995) The Third Intergroup Rhabdomyosarcoma Study. J Clin Oncol 13(3):610–630

Davis AM, O'Sullivan B, Bell RS, Turcotte R, Catton CN, Wunder JS, Chabot P, Hammond A, Benk V, Isler M, Freeman C, Goddard K, Bezjak A, Kandel RA, Sadura A, Day A, James K, Tu D, Pater J, Zee B (2002) Function and health status outcomes in a randomized trial comparing preoperative and postoperative radiotherapy in extremity soft tissue sarcoma. J Clin Oncol 20(22):4472–4477

DeLaney TF, Park L, Goldberg SI, Hug EB, Liebsh NJ, Munzenrider JD, Suit HD (2003) Radiation therapy for local control of osteosarcoma. Int J Radiat Oncol Biol Phys 57(2 Suppl 0):S449

Dillon P, Maurer H, Jenkins J, Krummel T, Parham D, Webber B, Salzberg A (1992) A prospective study of nonrhabdomyosarcoma soft tissue sarcomas in the pediatric age group. J Pediatr Surg 27(2):241–244; discussion 244–245

Dinges S, Budach V, Budach W, Feldmann HJ, Stuschke M, Sack H (1994) Local recurrences of soft tissue sarcomas in adults: a retrospective analysis of prognostic factors in 102 cases after surgery and radiation therapy. Eur J Cancer 30A(11):1636–1642

Donaldson SS, Meza J, Breneman JC, Crist WM, Laurie F, Qualman SJ, Wharam M (2001) Results from the IRS-IV randomized trial of hyperfractionated radiotherapy in children with rhabdomyosarcoma – a report from the IRSG. Int J Radiat Oncol Biol Phys 51(3):718–728

Eilber F, Eckardt J, Rosen G, Forscher C, Selch M, Fu YS (1995) Preoperative therapy for soft tissue sarcoma. Hematol Oncol Clin North Am 9(4):817–823

Enneking WF, Spanier SS, Goodman MA (2003) A system for the surgical staging of musculoskeletal sarcoma. 1980. Clin Orthop(415):4–18

Evans RG, Nesbit ME, Gehan EA, Garnsey LA, Burgert O Jr, Vietti TJ, Cangir A, Tefft M, Thomas P, Askin FB et al. (1991) Multimodal therapy for the management of localized Ewing's sarcoma of pelvic and sacral bones: a report from the second intergroup study. J Clin Oncol 9(7):1173–1180

Flamant F, Rodary C, Rey A, Praquin MT, Sommelet D, Quintana E, Theobald S, Brunat-Mentigny M, Otten J, Voute PA, Habrand JL, Martelli H, Barrett A, Terrier-Lacombe MJ, Oberlin O (1998) Treatment of non-metastatic rhabdomyosarcomas in childhood and adolescence. Results of the second study of the International Society of Paediatric Oncology: MMT84. Eur J Cancer 34(7):1050–1062

Gasparini M, Lombardi F, Gianni C, Fossati-Bellani F (1981) Localized Ewing sarcoma: results of integrated therapy and analysis of failures. Eur J Cancer Clin Oncol 17(11):1205–1209

Gottsauner-Wolf F, Kotz R, Knahr K, Kristen H, Ritschl P, Salzer M (1991) Rotationplasty for limb salvage in the treatment of malignant tumors at the knee. A follow-up study of seventy patients. J Bone Joint Surg Am 73(9):1365–1375

Grier HE, Krailo MD, Tarbell NJ, Link MP, Fryer CJ, Pritchard DJ, Gebhardt MC, Dickman PS, Perlman EJ, Meyers PA, Donaldson SS, Moore S, Rausen AR, Vietti TJ, Miser JS (2003) Addition of ifosfamide and etoposide to standard chemotherapy for Ewing's sarcoma and primitive neuroectodermal tumor of bone. N Engl J Med 348(8):694–701

Grosfeld JL, Weber TR, Weetman RM, Baehner RL (1983) Rhabdomyosarcoma in childhood: analysis of survival in 98 cases. J Pediatr Surg 18(2):141–146

Guiliano AE, Kirgan JM, Guenther DM, Morton DL (1994) Lymphatic mapping and sentinel lymphadenectomy for breast cancer. Ann Surg 220(3):391–401; discussion 398–401

Habrand JL, Gerbaulet A, Pejovic MH, Contesso G, Durand S, Haie C, Genin J, Schwaab G, Flamant F, Albano M et al. (1991) Twenty years experience of interstitial iridium brachytherapy in the management of soft tissue sarcomas. Int J Radiat Oncol Biol Phys 20(3):405–411

Ham SJ, Schraffordt Koops H, Veth RP, van Horn JR, Molenaar WM, Hoekstra HJ (1998) Limb salvage surgery for primary bone sarcoma of the lower extremities: long-term consequences of endoprosthetic reconstructions. Ann Surg Oncol 5(5):423–436

Hays D (1980) The management of rhabdomyosarcoma in children and young adults. World J Surg 4:15–28

Hays DM, Shimada H, Raney RB Jr, Tefft M, Newton W, Crist WM, Lawrence W Jr, Ragab A, Maurer HM (1985) Sarcomas of the vagina and uterus: the Intergroup Rhabdomyosarcoma Study. J Pediatr Surg 20(6):718–724

Hays D, Lawrence W, Wharam M, Newton W Jr, Ruymann FB, Beltangady M, Maurer H (1989) Primary re-excision for patients with microscopic residual tumor following initial excision of sarcomas of trunk and extremity sites. J Pediatr Surg 24(1):5–10

Hays DM, Raney RB, Wharam MD, Wiener E, Lobe TE, Andrassy RJ, Lawrence W Jr, Johnston J, Webber B, Maurer HM (1995) Children with vesical rhabdomyosarcoma (RMS) treated by partial cystectomy with neoadjuvant or adjuvant chemotherapy, with or without radiotherapy. A report from the Intergroup Rhabdomyosarcoma Study (IRS) Committee. J Pediatr Hematol Oncol 17(1):46–52

Herbert SH, Corn BW, Solin LJ, Lanciano RM, Schultz DJ, McKenna WG, Coia LR (1993) Limb-preserving treatment for soft tissue sarcomas of the extremities. The significance of surgical margins. Cancer 72(4):1230–1238

Hillmann A, Hoffmann C, Gosheger G, Krakau H, Winkelmann W (1999) Malignant tumor of the distal part of the femur or the proximal part of the tibia: endoprosthetic replacement or rotationplasty. Functional outcome and quality-of-life measurements. J Bone Joint Surg Am 81(4):462–468

Holt GE, Wunder JS, Griffin AM (2002) Fractures following radiation therapy and limb salvage surgery for soft tissue sarcomas: High versus low dose radiotherapy. Proceedings of the Musculoskeletal Tumor Society 41, Toronto, Canada

Hornicek FJ Jr, Mnaymneh W, Lackman RD, Exner GU, Malinin TI (1998) Limb salvage with osteoarticular allografts after resection of proximal tibia bone tumors. Clin Orthop 352:179–186

Jeys LM, Grimer RJ, Carter SR, Tillman RM (2003) Risk of amputation following limb salvage surgery with endoprosthetic replacement, in a consecutive series of 1261 patients. Int Orthop 27(3):160–163

Kaste SC, Neel MN, Rao BN, Thompson VF, Pratt CB (2001) Complications of limb-sparing procedures using endoprosthetic replacements about the knee for pediatric skeletal sarcomas. Pediatr Radiol 31(2):62–71

Kinsella TJ, Miser JS, Triche TJ, Horvath K, Glatstein E (1988) Treatment of high-risk sarcomas in children and young adults: analysis of local control using intensive combined modality therapy. NCI Monogr 6:291–296

Koscielniak E, Harms D, Henze G, Jurgens H, Gadner H, Herbst M, Klingebiel T, Schmidt BF, Morgan M, Knietig R, Treuner J (1999) Results of treatment for soft tissue sarcoma in childhood and adolescence: a final report of the German Cooperative Soft Tissue Sarcoma Study CWS-86. J Clin Oncol 17(12):3706–3719

Kotz R, Salzer M (1982) Rotation-plasty for childhood osteosarcoma of the distal part of the femur. J Bone Joint Surg Am 64(7):959–969

Kuttesch JF Jr, Wexler LH, Marcus RB, Fairclough D, Weaver-McClure L, White M, Mao L, Delaney TF, Pratt CB, Horowitz ME, Kun LE (1996) Second malignancies after Ewing's sarcoma: radiation dose-dependency of secondary sarcomas. J Clin Oncol 14(10):2818–2825

LaQuaglia M (1997) Rhabdomyosarcoma and nonrhabdomyomatous sarcomas. Surgery of Infants and Children. In: Oldham KT, Colombani PM, Foglia RP (eds) Scientific principles and practice. Lippincott-Raven, Philadelphia, pp 614–631

Lawrence W Jr, Neifeld J (1989) Soft tissue sarcomas. In: Wells S (ed) Current problems in surgery, vol XXVI. Year Book Medical Publishers, Chicago, pp 753–827

Lawrence W, Gehan E, Hays D, Beltangady M, Maurer H (1987) Prognostic significance of staging factors of the UICC staging system in childhood rhabdomyosarcoma: A report from the Intergroup Rhabdomyosarcoma Study (IRS II). J Clin Oncol 5(1):46–54

Lawrence W, Hays D, Heyn R (1997) Lymphatic metastasis with childhood rhabdomyosarcoma. Cancer 39:556–550

Lee ES, Mackenzie DH (1964) Osteosarcoma: A study of the value of preoperative megavoltage radiotherapy. Br J Surg 51:252–274

Lindberg RD, Martin RG, Romsdahl MM, Barkley HT Jr (1981) Conservative surgery and postoperative radiotherapy in 300 adults with soft-tissue sarcomas. Cancer 47(10):2391–2397

Link MP, Goorin AM, Horowitz M, Meyer WH, Belasco J, Baker A, Ayala A, Shuster J (1991) Adjuvant chemotherapy of high-grade osteosarcoma of the extremity. Updated results of the Multi-Institutional Osteosarcoma Study. Clin Orthop (270):8–14

Link MP, Goorin AM, Miser AW, Green AA, Pratt CB, Belasco JB, Pritchard J, Malpas JS, Baker AR, Kirkpatrick JA et al. (1986) The effect of adjuvant chemotherapy on relapse-free survival in patients with osteosarcoma of the extremity. N Engl J Med 314(25):1600–1606

Merchant TE, Zelefsky MJ, Sheldon JM, LaQuaglia MB, Harrison LB (1998) High-dose rate intraoperative radiation therapy for pediatric solid tumors. Med Pediatr Oncol 30(1): 34–39

Merchant TE, Kushner BH, Sheldon JM, LaQuaglia M, Healey JH (1999) Effect of low-dose radiation therapy when combined with surgical resection for Ewing sarcoma. Med Pediatr Oncol 33(2):65–70

Merchant TE, Parsh N, del Valle PL, Coffey DH, Galindo CR, Jenkins JJ, Pappo A, Neel MD, Rao BN (2000) Brachytherapy for pediatric soft-tissue sarcoma. Int J Radiat Oncol Biol Phys 46(2):427–432

Meric F, Hess KR, Varma DG, Hunt KK, Pisters PW, Milas KM, Patel SR, Benjamin RS, Plager C, Papadopoulos NE, Burgess MA, Pollock RE, Feig BW (2002) Radiographic response to neoadjuvant chemotherapy is a predictor of local control and survival in soft tissue sarcomas. Cancer 95(5):1120–1126

Michalski JM, Meza J, Breneman JC, Wolden SL, Laurie F, Jodoin M, Raney R, Wharam M, Donaldson S (2004) Influence of radiation therapy parameters on outcome in children treated with radiation therapy for localized parameningeal rhabdomyosarcoma in Intergroup Rhabdomyosarcoma Study Group trials II through IV. Int J Radiat Oncol Biol Phys (in press)

Morton DL, Wen DR, Wong JH, Economou JS, Cagle LA, Storm FK, Foshag LJ, Cochran AJ (1992) Technical details of intraoperative lymphatic mapping for early stage melanoma. Arch Surg 127(4):392–399

Neel MD, Wilkins RM, Rao BN, Kelly CM (2003) Early multicenter experience with a noninvasive expandable prosthesis. Clin Orthop(415):72–81

Nesbit ME Jr, Gehan EA, Burgert EO Jr, Vietti TJ, Cangir A, Tefft M, Evans R, Thomas P, Askin FB, Kissane JM et al. (1990) Multimodal therapy for the management of primary, nonmetastatic Ewing's sarcoma of bone: a long-term follow-up of the First Intergroup study. J Clin Oncol 8(10):1664–1674

Noria S, Davis A, Kandel R, Levesque J, O'Sullivan B, Wunder J, Bell R (1996) Residual disease following unplanned excision of soft-tissue sarcoma of an extremity. J Bone Joint Surg Am 78(5):650–655

O'Sullivan B, Davis AM, Turcotte R, Bell R, Catton C, Chabot P, Wunder J, Kandel R, Goddard K, Sadura A, Pater J, Zee B (2002) Preoperative versus postoperative radiotherapy in soft-tissue sarcoma of the limbs: a randomised trial. Lancet 359(9325):2235–2241

Ozaki T, Hillmann A, Hoffmann C, Rube C, Blasius S, Dunst J, Jurgens H, Winkelmann W (1996) Significance of surgical margin on the prognosis of patients with Ewing's sarcoma. A report from the Cooperative Ewing's Sarcoma Study. Cancer 78(4):892–900

Parsons JT, Zlotecki RA, Reddy KA, Mitchell TP, Marcus RB Jr, Scarborough MT (2001) The role of radiotherapy and limb-conserving surgery in the management of soft-tissue sarcomas in adults. Hematol Oncol Clin North Am 15(2):377–388, vii

Philippe PG, Rao BN, Rogers DA, Fontanesi J, Bowman L, Parham D, Shapiro D, Lobe TE, Fleming I (1992) Sarcomas of the flexor fossae in children: is amputation necessary? J Pediatr Surg 27(8):964–967

Pisters PW, Harrison LB, Woodruff JM, Gaynor JJ, Brennan MF (1994) A prospective randomized trial of adjuvant brachytherapy in the management of low-grade soft tissue sarcomas of the extremity and superficial trunk. J Clin Oncol 12(6):1150–1155

Pisters PW, Ballo MT, Patel SR (2002) Preoperative chemoradiation treatment strategies for localized sarcoma. Ann Surg Oncol 9(6):535–542

Pratt CB, Maurer HM, Gieser P, Salzberg A, Rao BN, Parham D, Thomas PR, Marcus RB, Cantor A, Pick T, Green D, Neff J, Jenkins JJ (1998) Treatment of unresectable or metastatic pediatric soft tissue sarcomas with surgery, irradiation, and chemotherapy: a Pediatric Oncology Group study. Med Pediatr Oncol 30(4):201–209

Pratt CB, Pappo AS, Gieser P, Jenkins JJ, Salzbergdagger A, Neff J, Rao B, Green D, Thomas P, Marcus R, Parham D, Maurer H (1999) Role of adjuvant chemotherapy in the treatment of surgically resected pediatric nonrhabdomyosarcomatous soft tissue sarcomas: A Pediatric Oncology Group Study. J Clin Oncol 17(4):1219

Raney RB, Meza J, Anderson JR, Fryer CJ, Donaldson SS, Breneman JC, Fitzgerald TJ, Gehan EA, Michalski JM, Ortega JA, Qualman SJ, Sandler E, Wharam MD, Wiener ES, Maurer HM, Crist WM (2002) Treatment of children and adolescents with localized parameningeal sarcoma: experience of the Intergroup Rhabdomyosarcoma Study Group protocols IRS-II through -IV, 1978–1997. Med Pediatr Oncol 38(1):22–32

Rao BN (1993) Nonrhabdomyosarcoma in children: prognostic factors influencing survival. Semin Surg Oncol 9(6):524–531

Rao BN, Etcubanas EE, Green AA (1989) Present-day concepts in the management of sarcomas in children. Cancer Invest 7(4):349–356

Rao BN, Santana VM, Parham D, Pratt CB, Fleming ID, Hudson M, Fontanesi J, Philippe P, Schell MJ (1991) Pediatric nonrhabdomyosarcomas of the extremities. Influence of size, invasiveness, and grade on outcome. Arch Surg 126(12): 1490–1495

Razek A, Perez CA, Tefft M, Nesbit M, Vietti T, Burgert EO Jr, Kissane J, Pritchard DJ, Gehan EA (1980) Intergroup Ewing's Sarcoma Study: local control related to radiation dose, volume, and site of primary lesion in Ewing's sarcoma. Cancer 46(3):516–521

Rosito P, Mancini AF, Rondelli R, Abate ME, Pession A, Bedei L, Bacci G, Picci P, Mercuri M, Ruggieri P, Frezza G, Campanacci M, Paolucci G (1999) Italian Cooperative Study for the treatment of children and young adults with localized Ewing sarcoma of bone: a preliminary report of 6 years of experience. Cancer 86(3):421–428

Ruymann FB (1987) Rhabdomyosarcoma in children and adolescents. A review. Hematol Oncol Clin North Am 1(4):621–654

Sarcoma Meta-analysis Collaboration (SMAC) (2000) Adjuvant chemotherapy for localised resectable soft tissue sarcoma in adults. Cochrane Database Syst Rev (2):CD001419

Sauer R, Jurgens H, Burgers JM, Dunst J, Hawlicek R, Michaelis J (1987) Prognostic factors in the treatment of Ewing's sarcoma. The Ewing's Sarcoma Study Group of the German Society of Paediatric Oncology CESS 81. Radiother Oncol 10(2):101–110

Schuck A, Ahrens S, Paulussen M, Kuhlen M, Konemann S, Rube C, Winkelmann W, Kotz R, Dunst J, Willich N, Jurgens H (2003) Local therapy in localized Ewing tumors: results of 1058 patients treated in the CESS 81, CESS 86, and EICESS 92 trials. Int J Radiat Oncol Biol Phys 55(1):168–177

Shankar AG, Pinkerton CR, Atra A, Ashley S, Lewis I, Spooner D, Cannon S, Grimer R, Cotterill SJ, Craft AW (1999) Local therapy and other factors influencing site of relapse in patients with localised Ewing's sarcoma. United Kingdom Children's Cancer Study Group (UKCCSG). Eur J Cancer 35(12):1698–1704

Singer S, Baldini EH, Demetri GD, Fletcher JA, Corson JM (1996) Synovial sarcoma: prognostic significance of tumor size, margin of resection, and mitotic activity for survival. J Clin Oncol 14(4):1201–1208

Skene AI, Barr L, Robinson M, Fisher C, Thomas JM (1993) Adult type (nonembryonal) soft tissue sarcomas in childhood. Med Pediatr Oncol 21(9):645–648

Smith LM, Anderson JR, Qualman SJ, Crist WM, Paidas CN, Teot LA, Pappo AS, Link MP, Grier HE, Wiener ES, Breneman JC, Raney RB, Maurer HM, Donaldson SS (2001) Which patients with microscopic disease and rhabdomyosarcoma experience relapse after therapy? A report from the Soft Tissue Sarcoma Committee of the Children's Oncology Group. J Clin Oncol 19(20):4058–4064

Spunt SL, Hill DA, Motosue AM, Billups CA, Cain AM, Rao BN, Pratt CB, Merchant TE, Pappo AS (2002) Clinical features and outcome of initially unresected nonmetastatic pediatric nonrhabdomyosarcoma soft tissue sarcoma. J Clin Oncol 20(15):3225–3235

Suit HD, Proppe KH, Mankin HJ, Wood WC (1981) Preoperative radiation therapy for sarcoma of soft tissue. Cancer 47(9):2269–2274

Tefft M, Lindberg RD, Gehan EA (1981) Radiation therapy combined with systemic chemotherapy of rhabdomyosarcoma in children: local control in patients enrolled in the Intergroup Rhabdomyosarcoma Study. Natl Cancer Inst Monogr(56):75–81

Weitz J, Antonescu CR, Brennan MF (2003) Localized extremity soft tissue sarcoma: improved knowledge with unchanged survival over time. J Clin Oncol 21(14):2719–2725

Wharam MD, Hanfelt JJ, Tefft MC, Johnston J, Ensign LG, Breneman J, Donaldson SS, Fryer C, Gehan EA, Raney RB, Maurer HM (1997) Radiation therapy for rhabdomyosarcoma: local failure risk for Clinical Group III patients on Intergroup Rhabdomyosarcoma Study II. Int J Radiat Oncol Biol Phys 38(4):797–804

Wharam M, Meza J, Anderson JR, Breneman JC, Donaldson S, Fitzgerald TJ, Michalski JM, Teot LA, Wiener E, Meyer WH (2004) Failure pattern and factors predictive of local failure in rhabdomyosarcoma: A report of group III patients on the third Intergroup Rhabdomyosarcoma Study. J Clin Oncol (in press)

Wiener ES (1993) Rhabdomyosarcoma: New dimensions in management. Semin Pediatr Surg 2:47–58

Wiener E, Lawrence W, Hays D (1991) Survival is improved in clinical Group III children with complete response established by second-look operations in the Intergroup Rhabdomyosarcoma Study (IRS III). Med Pediatr Oncol 19:399 (abstr. 228)

Wiener ES, Lawrence W, Hays D, Lobe TE, Andrassy R, Donaldson S, Crist W, Newton W, Johnson J, Gehan E et al. (1994) Retroperitoneal node biopsy in paratesticular rhabdomyosarcoma. J Pediatr Surg 29(2):171–177; discussion 178

Wiener E, Anderson JR, Ojima J (2001) Controversies in the management of paratesticular rhabdomyosarcoma: Is staging retroperitoneal lymph node dissection necessary for adolescents with resected paratesticular rhabdomyosarcoma? Sem Pediatr Surg 10(3):146–152

Wilson AN, Davis A, Bell RS, O'Sullivan B, Catton C, Madadi F, Kandel R, Fornasier VL (1994) Local control of soft tissue sarcoma of the extremity: the experience of a multidisciplinary sarcoma group with definitive surgery and radiotherapy. Eur J Cancer 30A(6):746–751

Windhager R, Schiller C, Giesinger B, Kotz R (1991) Complications and problems with expandable prostheses in children: treatment and prophylaxis. In: Brown KLB (ed) Complications of limb salvage: prevention, management and outcome. ISOLS, Montreal, pp 511–513

Wolden SL, Anderson JR, Crist WM, Breneman JC, Wharam MD Jr, Wiener ES, Qualman SJ, Donaldson SS (1999) Indications for radiotherapy and chemotherapy after complete resection in rhabdomyosarcoma: A report from the Intergroup Rhabdomyosarcoma Studies I to III. J Clin Oncol 17(11):3468–3475

Wolf RE, Scarborough MT, Enneking WF (1999) Long-term followup of patients with autogenous resection arthrodesis of the knee. Clin Orthop 358:36–40

Wunder JS, Paulian G, Huvos AG, Heller G, Meyers PA, Healey JH (1998) The histological response to chemotherapy as a predictor of the oncological outcome of operative treatment of Ewing sarcoma. J Bone Joint Surg Am 80(7):1020–1033

Yang JC, Rosenberg SA (1989) Surgery for adult patients with soft tissue sarcomas. Semin Oncol 16(4):289–296

Yang JC, Chang AE, Baker AR, Sindelar WF, Danforth DN, Topalian SL, DeLaney T, Glatstein E, Steinberg SM, Merino MJ, Rosenberg SA (1998) Randomized prospective study of the benefit of adjuvant radiation therapy in the treatment of soft tissue sarcomas of the extremity. J Clin Oncol 16(1): 197–203

Zornig C, Peiper M, Schroder S (1995) Re-excision of soft tissue sarcoma after inadequate initial operation. Br J Surg 82(2):278–279

Drug Discovery in Pediatric Bone and Soft Tissue Sarcomas Using In Vivo Models

Jennifer K. Peterson, Peter J. Houghton

Contents

5.1 Introduction

In the United States there are approximately 8,500 new cases of cancer diagnosed annually in children under the age of 15 and 12,000 cases annually in patients under 21 years of age. Current multimodality therapies including surgery, radiation therapy and chemotherapy cure over 70% of patients. For those patients that ultimately succumb to their disease current therapies may induce significant remissions. Hence, the number of children eligible for phase I or phase II clinical trials is small. Further, as shown in early studies, a phase II population may not be optimal for identifying agents that may have significant clinical activity against disease at diagnosis (Horowitz et al. 1988). Thus, with an increasing number of new agents under development for treating cancer it is imperative that a mechanism is developed that can accurately identify those agents having the greatest potential to impact children that have poor outcome with current therapies. Work over the past 2 decades suggests that when used intelligently, xenograft models (human cancers grown in mice) may accurately identify drugs that have significant activity against childhood cancer.

Over the past 35 years, cure rates for children with solid tumors have risen dramatically, with one-half to two-thirds of children with neuroblastoma, rhabdomyosarcoma, or osteosarcoma surviving disease-free for prolonged periods after aggressive treatment with surgery, radiation and multiagent chemotherapy (Crist and Kun 1991). For the remaining patients, it has been possible to slow or stop the progression of disease with use of intensified therapy, but cure has remained elusive. The apparent plateau in survival

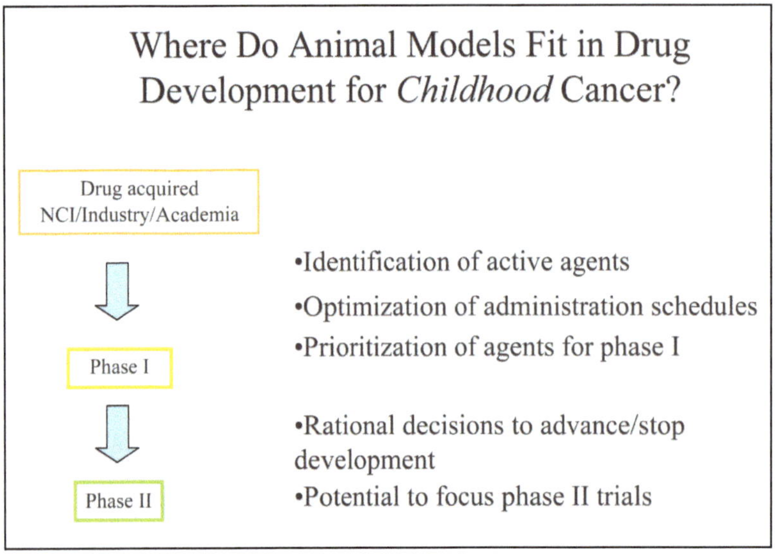

Figure 5.1

Schematic representation of clinical drug development and where animal tumor models may have some impact

rates may reflect the lack of major improvements in our therapeutic armamentarium. The overriding problem is treatment failure due to the development of drug resistance by clonogenic tumor cells, presumably because of mutations or epigenetic silencing. A second major problem is the limited repertoire of active antineoplastic agents, making it difficult to develop effective therapy for resistant tumor subtypes, even when they are identified early in the clinical course. Clearly, the avenue to more successful treatment of childhood solid tumors lies in understanding the biologic characteristics that confer the malignant phenotype, and through this the potential to identify both new targets and novel effective agents, and in the optimization of cytotoxic therapy.

For relatively rare diseases, such as pediatric cancers in general, and rhabdomyosarcoma and osteosarcoma as the focus of this article, one can view models and their potential uses in the context of the clinical development paradigm outlined in Fig. 5.1. It is probably realistic to assume that the majority of agents identified by the pharmaceutical industry, or through the NCI screening program (which does not use cell lines derived from pediatric cancers), will not have been developed with the intent to treat childhood cancer per se. As more academic laboratories become involved in therapeutics, it is possible that new chemical entities will be developed that target molecular changes in such cancers. Listed in Fig. 5.1 are some of the areas in which animal models may be useful during the preclinical and clinical development of new agents. Here we will use examples to illustrate such uses of currently available animal models.

5.2 Pediatric Tumor Models

Available models of rhabdomyosarcoma, osteosarcoma and other pediatric malignancies have been summarized recently (Houghton et al. 2002). In addition to multiple well characterized cell lines there are syngeneic models of metastatic osteosarcoma (Khanna et al. 2000; Yu et al. 2004), and genetically engineered models of both rhabdomyosarcoma (Fleischmann et al. 2003; Sharp et al. 2002) and certain bone tumors (Jensen et al. 1993). For a complete list see http://emice.nci.nih.gov/emice/communication/index.html. The advent of genetically engineered mouse models of human cancer has raised great excitement, and clearly these models have become critical in understanding the etiology and biology of certain childhood cancers. Less clear is their role in drug discovery and development. One concern is whether the genetic alterations that give rise to particular cancers in mice accurately recapitulate the human disease. For example, orbital rhabdomyosarcomas develop with high frequency in $p53^{-/-}$ $fos^{-/-}$ double knockout mice, whereas the incidence of p53 mutations in childhood rhabdomyosarcoma is low (~5%) (Fleischmann et al. 2003). Of concern also is that fos is detected in cell lines derived from human embryonal rhabdomyosarcomas; consequently the model may not be representative of embryonal RMS. This is particularly problematic considering the role of p53 in determining the cellular response to anticancer agents. At present there is no tumor model of translocation-driven t(2;13) alveolar rhabdomyosarcoma, although the PAX3-FKHR knock-in mice have developmental abnormalities (Lagutina et al. 2002). The multifocal rhabdomyosarcoma model (INK4a/ARF/HGF transgenic) developed at NCI was originally engineered to create a model of melanoma, but resulted in myogenic tumors. It will be important to determine whether these tumors indeed represent the human disease with respect to gene expression profiles, pathway activation, and chemosensitivity. This model may be valuable in identifying novel molecular targets (Yu et al. 2004); for example, overexpression of ezrin in metastatic variants of the transgenic RMS model was found, and hence is similar to metastatic variants of murine osteosarcoma (Khanna et al. 2004). It will be important to relate such data to the human disease to determine its relevance. Thus, while such models are of particular interest, and may be valuable in context, their relevance to drug development remains to be determined. To date there are no published studies using these models as drug discovery tools; hence this article will focus on available models where such data are published.

It is clear that tumors that arise in children have characteristics quite distinct from adult carcinomas. Childhood tumors are characterized by unique molecular events, and in many instances are exquisitely sensitive to available cytotoxic agents. Cytogenetic abnormalities such as the t(2;13) chromosomal rearrangement found in xenografts derived from alveolar rhabdomyosarcoma were subsequently determined in ~80% of these tumors in clinical samples (Douglass et al. 1987; Hazelton et al. 1987). Importantly, these models identified agents known to be active against clinical disease (vincristine, actinomycin D, cyclophosphamide), and were valuable in prospectively identifying new effective agents and drug combinations.

5.3 General Criteria for Selecting Appropriate Models

It is essential that the model systems reflect accurately biological and metabolic characteristics of the same tumor type in children. Substantial data supports maintenance of certain characteristics when tumors are heterografted into mice. These characteristics include gene amplification, chromosomal translocations and antigen expression. Information derived from the Pediatric Oncology Preclinical Protein Array Project (POPP-TAP), an NCI-supported initiative to characterize expression profiles at the RNA and protein levels, may be valuable for establishing criteria for preclinical models using more global profiling than has been done so far. Expression profiling will determine the similarity or divergence in gene expression patterns between patient samples and specific tumor types (i.e., do neuroblastoma xenografts show similar expression patterns to clinical neuroblastoma by clustering analysis). Although not possible in the POPP-TAP study it would be beneficial if xenograft tumors could be directly compared to the tumor sample taken from the same patient.

5.4 Expression Profiles

It will become potentially more important to establish that signaling pathways or gene expression in the models closely mimics that in patient tumors. That is, signaling pathways, or expression of potential drug targets, are not changed when a tumor is heterografted into mice. We have started to characterize expression profiles in early passage tumor xenografts, and have compared these to the same primary tumor resected from the patient at the time the sample for heterografting was obtained. The high correlation in ex-

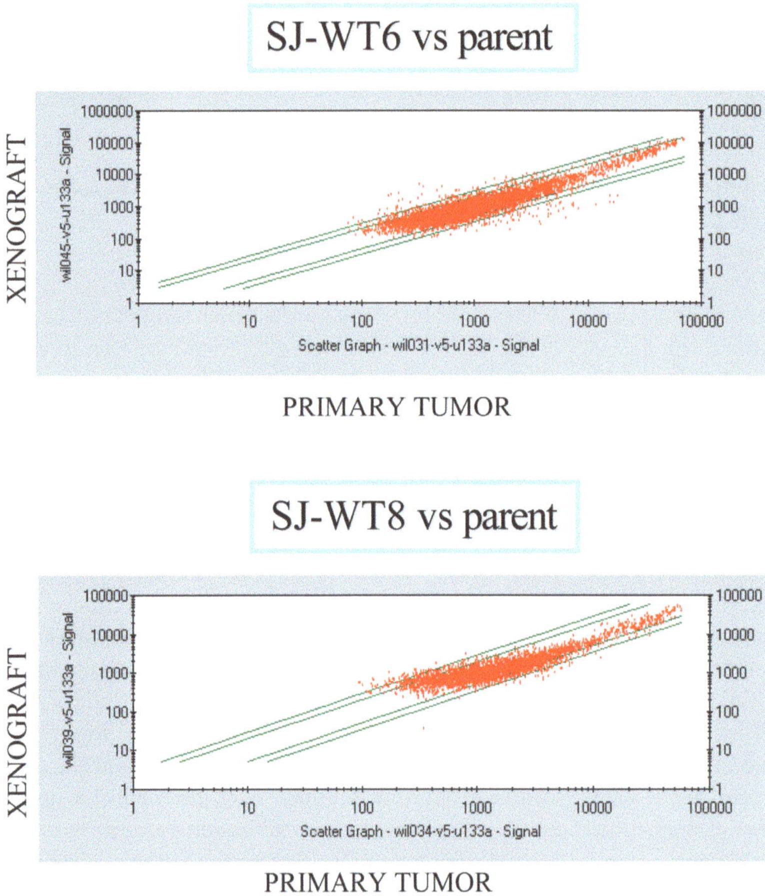

Figure 5.2

Comparison of expression profiles for primary Wilms' tumors and the respective xenografts (SJ-WT6, SJ-WT8) growing in scid mice. Results demonstrate correlation between expression in patient tumor and respective xenograft using Affymetrix U133A arrays (J. Dome, P. Houghton, unpublished results)

pression between primary tumor and the xenografts suggest the models may accurately recapitulate the human condition. An example of an expression profile comparison between patient tumor and early passage xenograft is shown for a Wilms' tumor, SJ-WT6 (Fig. 5.2). These results demonstrate that expression profiles (at least for genes expressed at adequate levels for accurate detection) found in primary tumor are retained in early passage xenograft models. The data attest to the stability of expression, and suggest that "molecular signatures" may prove informative as to drug action and biological response of tumors. Obviously, to be of value the expression profiles for a given tumor line should be consistent, in which case it may be possible to establish drug-induced molecular signatures that can be clearly analyzed and related to biological responses. Expression profiling should permit also an objective assessment of tumor to model fidelity, and if the model is representative of the original tumor, such studies should allow criteria to be established to determine the validity of the model as it is passaged in mice (i.e., genetic drift of the tumor with serial transplantation in mice).

5.5 Criteria for Selecting RMS Xenografts for Drug Evaluation

As a panel, tumors established from rhabdomyosarcoma samples taken at diagnosis are very sensitive to vincristine, cyclophosphamide, and to a lesser extent

Table 5.1. Response rates to standard chemotherapeutics in RMS models

Agent	Xenografts (%)	Clinical (%)
Vincristine	78	59
Cytoxan	44	54
Dactinomycin	11	24
Adriamycin	19	31
Melphalan	83	81
Topotecan	86	46
Irinotecan	88	45

Table 5.2. Relative systemic exposures and therapeutic dose range for cytotoxic agents

Drug	Relative systemic exposures @ MTD (mouse: human)	Effective dose range in mice[a]
Carzelesin	~80	<2
DMP840	15–20	~2–3
Sulofenur	~8	~3
Melphalan	1	~3–4
Topotecan	~3	>10
Irinotecan (SN-38)	~16	>100
Irofulven (MGI-114)	>10	~2–3

[a] The therapeutic range is the lowest drug dose causing tumor regressions (≥50% volume reduction) relative to the MTD dose

actinomycin D and doxorubicin (Houghton et al. 1982, 1984). Xenografts established from relapsed patients are far less sensitive to these agents. We have extensively characterized tumors established from patients prior to therapy with respect to chemosensitivity to agents known to have activity against clinical RMS, and in a prospective manner to identify agents that may have clinical utility (Table 5.1). These tumors demonstrate the histology of the patient tumors, and express appropriate myogenic markers (MyoD1, myogenin), and t(2;13) chromosomal translocation in alveolar RMS. Tumors have high take-rates in mice, have consistent growth rates, and have consistent responses when re-tested to the same agents. Four were diagnosed as embryonal histology and three are alveolar. This panel of RMS xenografts was used to identify camptothecin analogs as active agents.

5.5.1 In Vivo Models in Drug Discovery

As discussed above, there is a critical need to develop models that accurately identify new agents that will have significant biological activity in clinical trials. The limitations of current models have been reviewed quite recently (Peterson and Houghton 2004). Clearly, a major problem in extrapolating rodent tumor data to the clinic lies in species differences in drug metabolism and tolerance between man and mice. Thus, there are examples where a drug has dramatic activity against human cancers in mice, but has limited utility in the clinic. This may be a consequence of mice tolerating much greater systemic drug exposures than can be achieved in patients without excessive toxicity. Such examples are shown in Table 5.2. The drug systemic exposure achieved in patients at the MTD is contrasted to that in the mouse at its MTD. For example, mice tolerate high systemic exposures to carzelesin compared to humans (~80-fold), although the useful therapeutic dose range is narrow (~2-fold). Consequently, human cancers in mice are exposed to far greater drug levels than are achieved clinically; hence the model over-predicts true clinical activity. In contrast, although the systemic exposure to topotecan is greater in mice at the MTD, this agent has a broad dose range for activity in the animal models. Consequently, one would anticipate clinical activity at tolerated drug systemic exposures. On the other hand, if the mouse is more sensitive to a drug than human, the model may un-

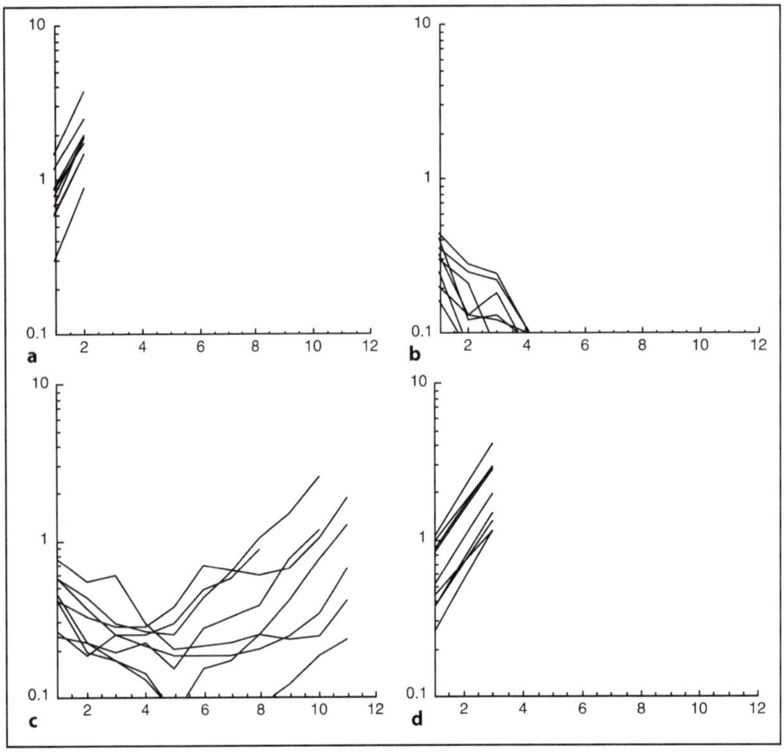

Figure 5.3 a–d

Evaluation of platinum analogs against OS33 osteosarcoma xenografts. a Controls; b carboplatin 75 mg/kg every 21 days ×3; c cisplatin 7 mg/kg every 21 days ×3; d oxaliplatin 15 mg/kg. Each curve represents the growth of an individual tumor and mice were observed for up to 12 weeks. Note: oxaliplatin treated tumors progressed and the experiment was terminated after one cycle of therapy

derestimate the true utility of the drug. Despite these limitations, xenograft models seem to have utility in being able to identify agents of known utility in a particular disease and in distinguishing between analogues. For example, whereas cisplatin and carboplatin cause regressions of several osteosarcoma xenografts, oxaliplatin demonstrates less activity at equitoxic dose levels (Fig. 5.3). The models also have value in prospectively identifying active agents. Examples are the camptothecin analogues topotecan and irinotecan (CPT-11) that exhibit broad-spectrum activity against rhabdomyosarcoma, neuroblastoma and several other tumors (Houghton et al. 1992, 1993; Thompson et al. 1997), although osteosarcoma xenografts are less sensitive than other sarcomas examined (unpublished data).

In the context of the drug development schema depicted in Fig. 5.1, such studies as described have two uses. First, they have value in identifying a subset of new agents that are in development and may allow these to be prioritized for pediatric trials. The second is that upon establishment of the drug systemic exposure at the maximum tolerated dose level in adult patients which usually precedes pediatric testing, it should be possible to determine whether such exposure is consistent with tumor regressions in the preclinical model(s). Where the human exposure is consistent with significant activity in preclinical models one would anticipate the agent would demonstrate clinical utility, whereas in the instances where responses of model tumors occurs at systemic exposures to drug that far exceed those achieved in adults one may de-emphasize further development prior to starting phase II trials.

5.5.2 Models for Optimizing Therapy

The models are of value, also, in identifying schedules of drug administration that may be optimal, and may potentially focus clinical studies on schedules that

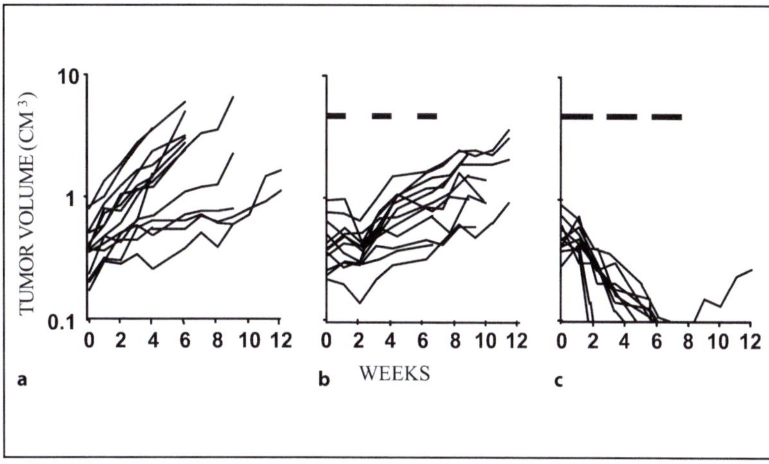

Figure 5.4 a–c

Schedule-dependent antitumor activity of topotecan. a Control; b topotecan 1.5 mg/kg administered daily for 5 days per 21-day cycle; c topotecan administered at 0.75 mg/kg for 5 days on two consecutive weeks [(dx5)2] per 21-day cycle. The cumulative dose in b and c was 22.5 mg/kg over three cycles of treatment. Each curve shows the growth of an individual tumor and mice were observed for up to 12 weeks. *Horizontal bars* indicate treatment periods

may be most effective. The antitumor activity of camptothecins, agents that target DNA topoisomerase I, is highly schedule-dependent with protracted courses of treatment being most effective in the models examined (Fig. 5.4). This is consistent with the mechanism of action as topoisomerase I poisons are S-phase toxins and require ongoing DNA replication to exert cytotoxic effects (Fiorani and Bjornsti 2000). Published phase I results suggest a relatively high response rate to protracted courses of irinotecan (Furman et al. 1999; Cosetti et al. 2002). Whether protracted cycles of irinotecan therapy do indeed induce higher response rates is currently being tested in relapsed RMS comparing daily for 5 days [(dx5)1] versus daily for 5 days for two consecutive weeks [(dx5)2 (COG ARST 0121 Trial).

5.6 Combination Therapy

Although identifying new active agents is important, understanding how best to combine them perhaps presents a greater dilemma. Binary drug combinations, at least, can be screened with relative ease in xenograft models, and may identify interesting combinations worthy of clinical evaluation. One such combination was topotecan with vincristine (Thompson et al. 1999) that demonstrated marked synergy against many tumor models including rhabdomyosarcoma. Both in the mouse and in patients the limiting toxicity was thrombocytopenia, although significant antitumor activity was observed in the phase I trials. Similar synergy was observed when the less myelosuppressive camptothecin, irinotecan, was combined with vincristine in xenograft models of neuroblastoma and other tumors, and this is illustrated for Rh28 alveolar RMS xenografts in Fig. 5.5. This combination is currently being evaluated in newly diagnosed advanced rhabdomyosarcoma (COG Protocol D9802). Similarly, the combination of temozolomide, a DNA methylating agent, demonstrated synergistic activity when combined with irinotecan in various pediatric solid tumor models (Fig. 5.6), and this combination has recently completed phase I evaluation with objective responses in Ewing sarcoma (Houghton et al. 2000; Wagner et al. 2004). These results suggest that effective antitumor combinations can be identified using currently available animal models. Less clear, however, is the value of these studies for predicting toxicity that will be encountered in patients.

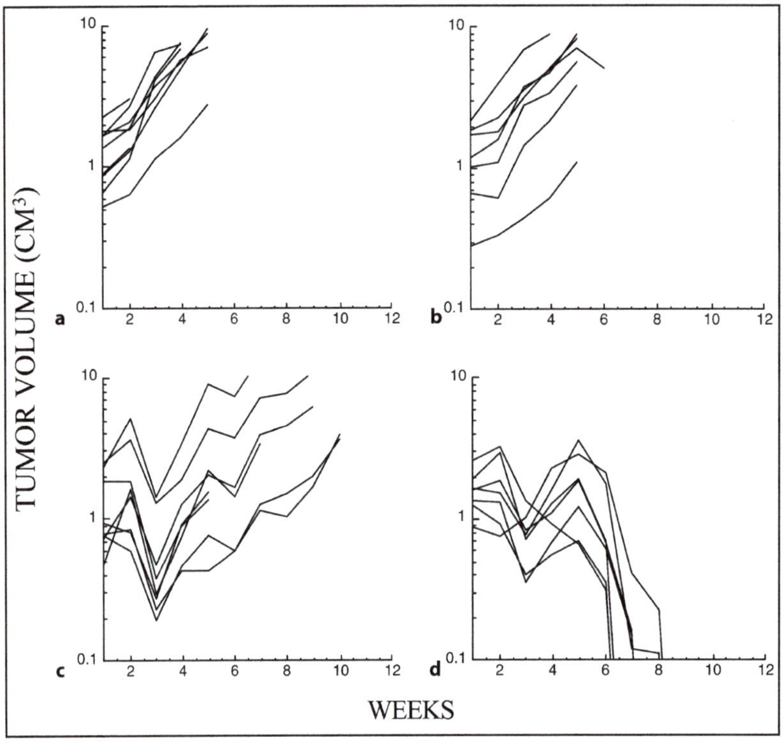

Figure 5.5 a–d

Synergistic activity of irinotecan (CPT-11) and vincristine in Rh28 rhabdomyosarcoma xenografts. **a** Control; **b** vincristine 0.14 mg/kg administered every 7 days; **c** irinotecan given at 0.06 mg/kg using the [(dx5)2] schedule; **d** combination of vincristine and irinotecan at the same doses and schedule. Vincristine was administered on the first day of each irinotecan course. Each curve represents the growth of an individual tumor, and mice were observed for up to 12 weeks

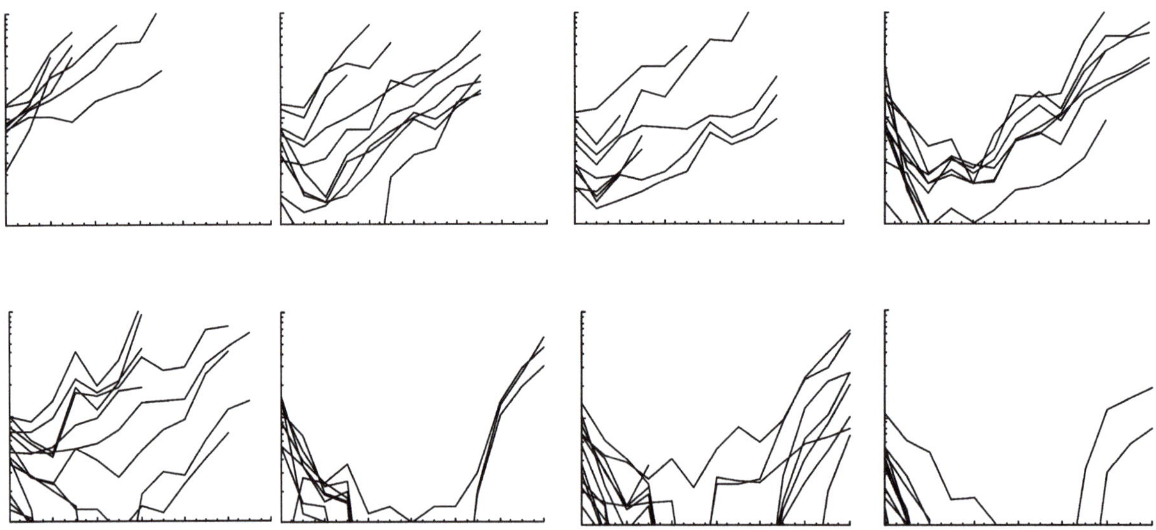

Figure 5.6

Antitumor activity of temozolomide (TMZ) and irinotecan (CPT-11) as single agents and in combination against Rh18 rhabdomyosarcoma xenografts deficient in mismatch repair and expressing high methylguanine DNA methyltransferase (MGMT) levels. Each curve represents growth of an individual tumor, and mice were observed for up to 12 weeks (Houghton et al. 2000)

5.7 Molecular Targeted Agents

Drug development in cancer is moving from the classical cytotoxic agents to development of small molecules or antibodies targeted to signaling pathways that may be altered in specific tumor types. As in the past, however, such development is aimed at targets that may be altered frequently in adult carcinomas, and which may not be relevant to treatment of pediatric sarcomas. For childhood solid tumors limited information is only now becoming available to demonstrate pathways altered in transformation that may be legitimate targets for drug development. Of critical importance is that such alterations in pathways are recapitulated in the models, and raises the question of whether the site of tumor growth will significantly impact phenotypic characteristics. That is, will orthotopic or disseminated models be a requirement to identify active agents? At present there is inadequate information to make such decisions; however, approaches such as comparative gene expression profiling of tumors growing either at the subcutaneous site or as orthotopic or disseminated sites may be informative.

On the other hand, new agents may themselves prove to be useful tools in elucidating biological properties of tumors. Thus, screening may identify specific tumor traits that predispose to being highly sensitive to inhibitors of specific signaling pathways. For example, it has been proposed that activation of the Akt/mTOR pathway through mutations or inactivation of the dual phosphatase PTEN sensitizes tumors to rapamycin analogues that specifically block mTOR signaling (Neshat et al. 2001). Determination of activation of the Akt/mTOR pathway in pediatric solid tumors has not been consistently studied, but could potentially assist in selection of patients or tumor subtypes that would benefit from rapamycin therapy. In this context the relationship between pathway activation, target inhibition (pharmacodynamic endpoints) and biological effect (tumor response) can most readily be examined in model systems (Boulay et al. 2004; Dudkin et al. 2001). Thus, a concerted effort to identify altered signaling pathways, one of the objectives of the POPP-TAP initiative, could be rewarding in that it will characterize and identify specific preclinical models against which targeted therapies can be evaluated.

5.8 Combining Signal Transduction Inhibitors

The conventional approach to developing signaling inhibitors, both preclinically and clinically, has been to combine them with cytotoxic agents that are standard of care for a particular tumor type. For example, gefitinib (Iressa), an inhibitor of the epidermal growth factor receptor (ErbB1), demonstrated single agent activity in refractory non-small cell lung carcinoma, and was subsequently combined with standard platinum-based therapy for non-small cell lung cancer in a large randomized phase III trial (the so-called INTACT trial). Similarly, imatinib (Gleevec) is being combined with cytotoxic agents for treatment of several cancer types. In part the combination trials in NSCLC were based on promising preclinical results that indicated greater than additive activity when gefitinib was combined with taxanes, anthracyclines, and platinum-based agents (Sirotnak et al. 2000). However, the mechanism of this interaction is unclear, as synergy was not associated with expression of ErbB1 in these model tumors. Gefitinib, like another anilinoquinazoline ErbB1 inhibitor, CI-1030 (Boulay et al. 2004), and the 2-phenylamino pyrimidine imatinib (Gleevec), are potent inhibitors of the ABCG2 (BCRP) drug transporter (Erlichman et al. 2001; Houghton et al. 2004). As shown in Fig. 5.7a, combination of gefitinib with irinotecan (the active metabolite of which is a substrate for the ABCG2 transporter), gives greater than additive activity that may be through gefitinib inhibiting ABCG2 expressed in OS17 xenografts (Fig. 5.7b). Thus, unexpected results in animal tumor models, combined with appropriate biochemical studies to elucidate mechanisms of action, provide important models for developing effective drug combinations. These results suggest that tyrosine kinase inhibitors such as imatinib and gefitinib may have potent activities not related to their primary molecular target that should be considered in design and interpretation of clinical trials. One obvious extension of these results is to

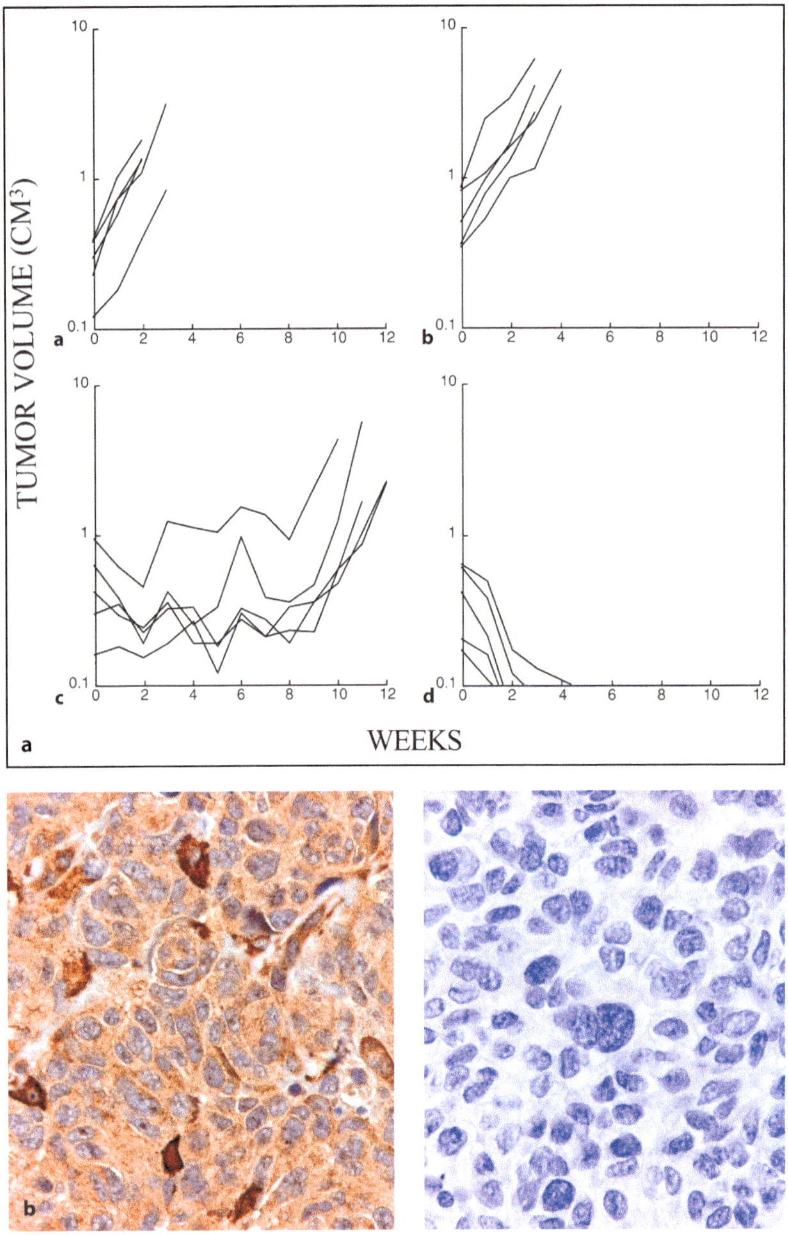

Figure 5.7 a,b

a Potentiation of irinotecan by the ErbB1 inhibitor gefitinib in OS17 osteosarcoma xenografts. *A* Control; *B* gefitinib 100 mg/kg twice daily 5 days/week by oral gavage; *C* irinotecan 2.5 mg/kg [(dx5)2] intravenously; *D* gefitinib combined with irinotecan at the same dose levels. Cycles of irinotecan were repeated twice at 21-day intervals. Each curve represents growth of an individual tumor, and mice were observed for up to 12 weeks (Stewart et al. 2004). b Detection of ABCG2 transporter in OS17 xenograft tissue by immunohistochemistry. *Left panel* demonstrates diffuse staining with anti-ABCG2, whereas the negative isotype matched control shows no staining (*right panel*) (J. Jenkins, P. Houghton, unpublished results)

evaluate gefitinib (or imatinib) as modulators of oral bioavailability of camptothecin analogs or other drugs that have poor absorption due to expression of ABCG2 in the upper intestine. In mice gefitinib dramatically increases the oral bioavailability of irinotecan (Stewart et al. 2004). Whether this can be translated to children is the focus of an ongoing phase I clinical trial. One concern is that both gefitinib and irinotecan have overlapping gastrointestinal toxicity that may limit tolerance of this combination.

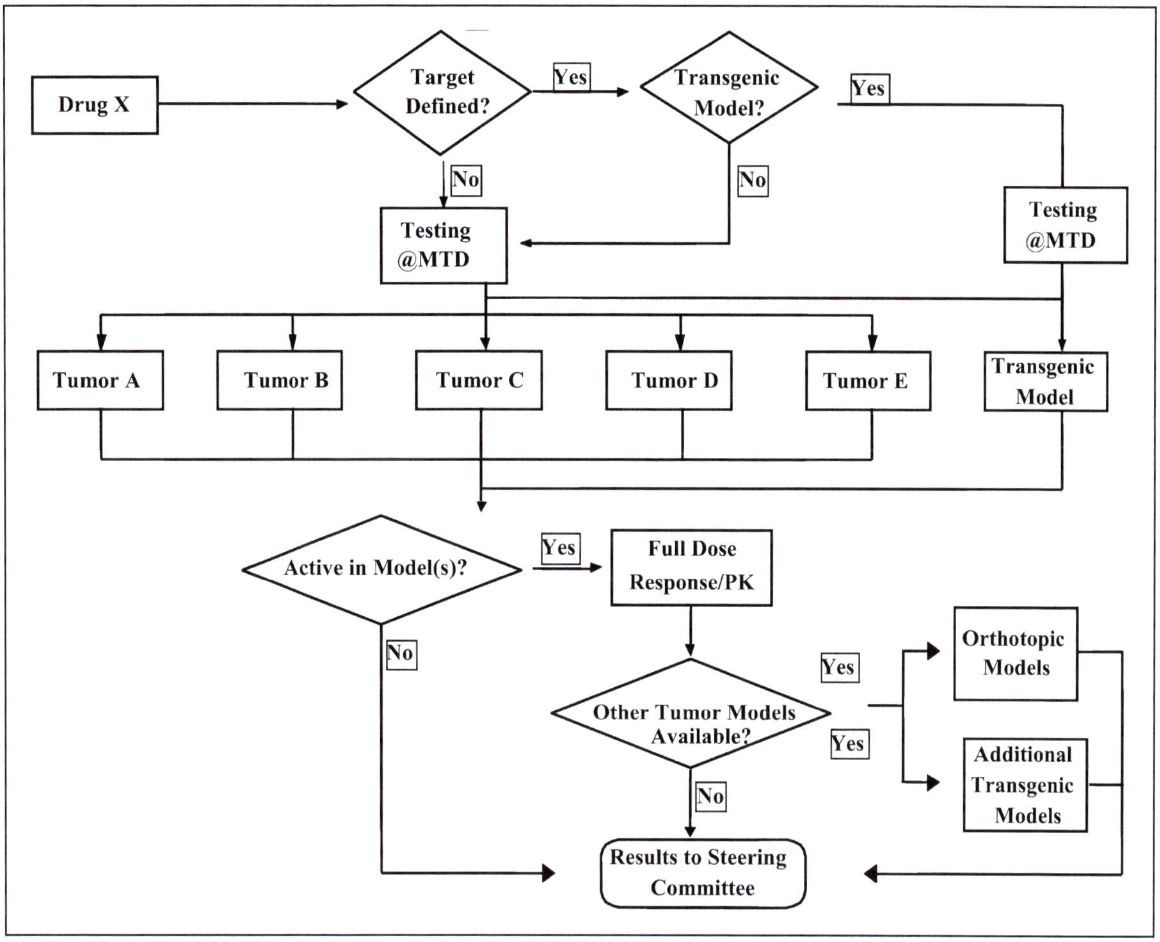

Figure 5.8

Schema for the Pediatric Preclinical Testing Program to evaluate new agents in panels of pediatric preclinical models (Houghton et al. 2002)

5.9 Future Directions

The studies presented serve to illustrate several uses that animal tumor models may serve particularly in the context of developing drugs for treating childhood tumors. As relevant genetic models of pediatric cancers are developed, one can foresee focused attempts to develop drugs specifically targeted against those molecular changes associated with malignant transformation. In addition, these and currently available models can be used in a systematic way to evaluate new agents as they enter clinical trials in adults with the anticipation that activity in models of childhood cancer can be used to prioritize which agents are tested in pediatric trials. A recent NCI initiative, the Pediatric Preclinical Testing Program (PPTP), seeks to establish a comprehensive testing program using pediatric cancer models. The process is diagrammed in Fig. 5.8, and was the product of several NCI sponsored workshops on pediatric drug development (Houghton et al. 2002). The overall idea is to access new agents from pharmaceutical or academic sources, and to screen them against panels of tumors representative of pediatric cancers (Tumor A, for example, may be a panel of six to ten osteosarcomas). In addition, where transgenic models and orthotopic models are available these will be incorporated into the screen. Further, pharmacokinetics studies will be undertaken to determine whether model tumor responses are observed at clinically achieved drug exposures. While the PPTP is an ambitious undertaking, and its success far from assured, the program may potentially serve as a paradigm for drug development in childhood cancer and be a relevant model for other rare cancers in adults.

Acknowledgements. We thank Jeff Dome for making available unpublished results, and the many members of this laboratory who have contributed to the work reviewed here. Work reported from this laboratory was supported through USPHS grants CA23099, CA77776 and CA96696 and CA21675 (Cancer Center Support Grant), and by American, Lebanese, Syrian Associated Charities (ALSAC).

References

Boulay A, Zumstein-Mecker S, Stephan C, Beuvink I, Zilbermann F, Haller R, Tobler S, Heusser C, O'Reilly T, Stolz B, Marti A, Thomas G, Lane HA (2004) Antitumor efficacy of intermittent treatment schedules with the rapamycin derivative RAD001 correlates with prolonged inactivation of ribosomal protein S6 kinase 1 in peripheral blood mononuclear cells. Cancer Res 64:252–261

Cosetti M, Wexler LH, Calleja E, Trippett T, LaQuaglia M, Huvos AG, Gerald W, Healey JH, Meyers PA, Gorlick R (2002) Irinotecan for pediatric solid tumors: the Memorial Sloan-Kettering experience. J Pediatr Hematol Oncol 24:101–105

Crist WM, Kun LE (1991) Common solid tumors of childhood. N Engl J Med 324:461–471

Douglass EC, Valentine M, Etcubanas E, Parham D, Webber BL, Houghton PJ, Houghton JA, Green AA (1987) A specific chromosomal abnormality in rhabdomyosarcoma. Cytogenet Cell Genet 45:148–155

Dudkin L, Dilling MB, Cheshire PJ, Harwood FC, Hollingshead M, Arbuck SG, Travis R, Sausville EA, Houghton PJ (2001) Biochemical correlates of mTOR inhibition by the rapamycin ester CCI-779 and tumor growth inhibition. Clin Cancer Res 7:1758–1764

Erlichman C, Boerner SA, Hallgren CG, Spieker R, Wang XY, James CD, Scheffer GL, Maliepaard M, Ross DD, Bible KC, Kaufmann SH (2001) The HER tyrosine kinase inhibitor CI1033 enhances cytotoxicity of 7-ethyl-10-hydroxycamptothecin and topotecan by inhibiting breast cancer resistance protein-mediated drug efflux. Cancer Res 61:739–748

Fiorani P, Bjornsti MA (2000) Mechanisms of DNA topoisomerase I-induced cell killing in the yeast *Saccharomyces cerevisiae*. Ann N Y Acad Sci 922:65–75

Fleischmann A, Jochum W, Eferl R, Witowsky J, Wagner EF (2003) Rhabdomyosarcoma development in mice lacking Trp53 and Fos: tumor suppression by the Fos protooncogene. Cancer Cell 4:477–482

Furman WL, Stewart CF, Poquette CA, Pratt CB, Santana VM, Zamboni WC, Bowman LC, Ma MK, Hoffer FA, Meyer WH, Pappo AS, Walter AW, Houghton PJ (1999) Direct translation of a protracted irinotecan schedule from a xenograft model to a phase I trial in children. J Clin Oncol 17:1815–1824

Hazelton BJ, Houghton JA, Parham DM, Douglass EC, Torrance PM, Holt H, Houghton PJ (1987) Characterization of cell lines derived from xenografts of childhood rhabdomyosarcoma. Cancer Res 47:4501–4507

Horowitz ME, Etcubanas E, Christensen ML, Houghton JA, George SL, Green AA, Houghton PJ (1988) Phase II testing of melphalan in children with newly diagnosed rhabdomyosarcoma: a model for anticancer drug development. J Clin Oncol 6:308–314

Houghton JA, Houghton PJ, Green AA (1982) Chemotherapy of childhood rhabdomyosarcomas growing as xenografts in immune-deprived mice. Cancer Res 42:535–539

Houghton JA, Cook RL, Lutz PJ, Houghton PJ (1984) Childhood rhabdomyosarcoma xenografts: responses to DNA-interacting agents and agents used in current clinical therapy. Eur J Cancer Clin Oncol 20:955–960

Houghton PJ, Cheshire PJ, Myers L, Stewart CF, Synold TW, Houghton JA (1992) Evaluation of 9-dimethylaminomethyl-10-hydroxycamptothecin against xenografts derived from adult and childhood solid tumors. Cancer Chemother Pharmacol 31:229–239

Houghton PJ, Cheshire PJ, Hallman JC, Bissery MC, Mathieu-Boue A, Houghton JA (1993) Therapeutic efficacy of the topoisomerase I inhibitor 7-ethyl-10-(4-[1-piperidino]-1-piperidino)-carbonyloxy-camptothecin against human tumor xenografts: lack of cross-resistance in vivo in tumors with acquired resistance to the topoisomerase I inhibitor 9-dimethylaminomethyl-10-hydroxycamptothecin. Cancer Res 53:2823–2829

Houghton PJ, Stewart CF, Cheshire PJ, Richmond LB, Kirstein MN, Poquette CA, Tan M, Friedman HS, Brent TP (2000) Antitumor activity of temozolomide combined with irinotecan is partly independent of O6-methylguanine-DNA methyltransferase and mismatch repair phenotypes in xenograft models. Clin Cancer Res 6:4110–4118

Houghton PJ, Adamson PC, Blaney S, Fine HA, Gorlick R, Haber M, Helman L, Hirschfeld S, Hollingshead MG, Israel MA, Lock RB, Maris JM, Merlino G, Patterson W, Reynolds CP, Shannon K, Yu A, Yu J, Smith MA (2002) Testing of new agents in childhood cancer preclinical models: meeting summary. Clin Cancer Res 8:3646–3657

Houghton PJ, Germain GS, Harwood FC, Schuetz JD, Stewart CF, Buchdunger E, Traxler P (2004) Imatinib mesylate is a potent inhibitor of the ABCG2 (BCRP) transporter and reverses resistance to topotecan and SN-38 in vitro. Cancer Res 64:2333–2337

Jensen NA, Rodriguez ML, Garvey JS, Miller CA, Hood L (1993) Transgenic mouse model for neurocristopathy: Schwannomas and facial bone tumors. Proc Natl Acad Sci USA 90: 3192–3196

Khanna C, Prehn J, Yeung C, Caylor J, Tsokos M, Helman L (2000) An orthotopic model of murine osteosarcoma with clonally related variants differing in pulmonary metastatic potential. Clin Exp Metastasis 18:261–271

Khanna C, Wan X, Bose S, Cassaday R, Olomu O, Mendoza A, Yeung C, Gorlick R, Hewitt SM, Helman LJ (2004)The membrane-cytoskeleton linker ezrin is necessary for osteosarcoma metastasis. Nat Med 10:182–186

Lagutina I, Conway SJ, Sublett J, Grosveld GC (2002) Pax3-FKHR knock-in mice show developmental aberrations but do not develop tumors. Mol Cell Biol 22:7204–7216

Neshat MS, Mellinghoff IK, Tran C, Stiles B, Thomas G, Petersen R, Frost P, Gibbons JJ, Wu H, Sawyers CL (2001) Enhanced sensitivity of PTEN-deficient tumors to inhibition of FRAP/mTOR. Proc Natl Acad Sci USA 98:10314–10319

Peterson JK, Houghton PJ (2004) Integrating pharmacology and in vivo cancer models in pre-clinical and clinical drug development. Eur J Cancer (in press)

Ries LAG, Miller BA, Guerney JG, Linet M, Tamra T, Young JL, Bunin GR (eds) SEER Program, 1975–1995. Res 42:535–539

Sharp R, Recio JA, Jhappan C, Otsuka T, Liu S, Yu Y, Liu W, Anver M, Navid F, Helman LJ, DePinho RA, Merlino G (2002) Synergism between INK4a/ARF inactivation and aberrant HGF/SF signaling in rhabdomyosarcomagenesis. Nat Med 8:1276–1280

Sirotnak FM, Zakowski MF, Miller VA, Scher HI, Kris MG (2000) Efficacy of cytotoxic agents against human tumor xenografts is markedly enhanced by coadministration of ZD1839 (Iressa), an inhibitor of EGFR tyrosine kinase. Clin Cancer Res 6:4885–4892

Stewart CF, Leggas M, Schuetz JD, Panetta JC, Cheshire PJ, Peterson JK, Daw NC, Jenkins JJ III, Gilbertson R, Germain GS, Harwood FC, Houghton PJ (2004) Gefitinib enhances the antitumor activity and oral bioavailability of irinotecan in mice. Cancer Res 64:7491–7499

Thompson J, Zamboni WC, Cheshire PJ, Lutz L, Luo X, Li Y, Houghton JA, Stewart CF, Houghton PJ (1997) Efficacy of systemic administration of irinotecan against neuroblastoma xenografts. Clin Cancer Res 3:423–431

Thompson J, George EO, Poquette CA, Cheshire PJ, Richmond LB, de Graaf SS, Ma M, Stewart CF, Houghton PJ (1999) Synergy of topotecan in combination with vincristine for treatment of pediatric solid tumor xenografts. Clin Cancer Res 5:3617–3631

Wagner LM, Crews KR, Iacono LC, Houghton PJ, Fuller CE, McCarville MB, Goldsby RE, Albritton K, Stewart CF, Santana VM (2004) Phase I trial of temozolomide and protracted irinotecan in pediatric patients with refractory solid tumors. Clin Cancer Res 10:840–848

Yu Y, Khan J, Khanna C, Helman L, Meltzer PS, Merlino G (2004) Expression profiling identifies the cytoskeletal organizer ezrin and the developmental homeoprotein Six-1 as key metastatic regulators. Nat Med 10:175–181

Pediatric Rhabdomyosarcoma: Biology and Results of the North American Intergroup Rhabdomyosarcoma Trials

Alberto Pappo, Fred G. Barr, Suzanne L. Wolden

Contents

Rhabdomyosarcoma, a primitive malignant mesenchymal tumor of the soft tissue which recapitulates the phenotypic and biological features of developing skeletal muscle, is the most common soft tissue sarcoma in children (Ries et al. 1999). Advances in the understanding and treatment of this disease have equaled or surpassed the progress seen in other childhood tumors and can, in part, be attributed to the establishment of multi-institutional trials which integrate a coordinated approach to treatment using risk-directed multimodal therapies. Furthermore, improved knowledge of the genetic features of this disease will likely improve our ability to identify the factors responsible for treatment failure and facilitate the discovery of novel targets for therapy.

6.1 Epidemiology

Rhabdomyosarcoma accounts for approximately 40% of all soft tissue sarcomas in patients younger than 20 years of age, with an estimated 350 new cases diagnosed each year in the United States (Ries et al. 1999). It is the third most common extracranial tumor, accounting for 3% of all childhood neoplasms. There is a slight male predominance, with a peak incidence during the first 5 years of life. The incidence for black females is about half that of white females, whereas the rate for males is similar for races.

Although most rhabdomyosarcomas are sporadic, this tumor has been described in association with a variety of syndromes and environmental factors as described below. In addition, in a large autopsy series of 115 children and adolescents with rhabdomyosarcoma who were registered in the first and second Intergroup Rhabdomyosarcoma Studies (IRSG), 32% were noted to have at least one congenital anomaly that most commonly affected the central nervous system or the genitourinary tract (Ruymann et al. 1988).

Costello Syndrome. This syndrome is characterized by mental retardation, low birth weight, neonatal feeding problems, coarse facies, nasal papillomata, curly hair with hirsutism, and loose soft skin with deep palmar and plantar creases (DeBaun 2002; Gripp et al. 2002). There have been 10 cases of rhabdomysarcoma reported among 103 patients with this syndrome (Hennekam 2003). The age of affected individuals ranged from 6 months to 6 years. Most of the cases reported are of embryonal histology and originated in the abdomen, pelvis and urogenital area (Gripp et al. 2002). Some investigators have suggested that the high incidence of rhabdomyosarcoma and other tumors in patients with Costello syndrome justifies tumor screening for this patient population (DeBaun 2002; Gripp et al. 2002).

Beckwith-Wiedemann Syndrome. This syndrome is an overgrowth syndrome characterized by macroglossia, macrosomia, omphalocele, organomegaly, and hemihypertrophy. Seven cases of rhabdomyosarcoma have been reported in association with this syndrome, with both alveolar and embryonal histologies being represented. Imprinting defects involving the *KCNQ1OT1* gene in the telomeric domain of 11p15 have been implicated as a possible pathogenic mechanism in these patients (Smith et al. 2001a; Weksberg et al. 2003).

Li-Fraumeni Syndrome and p53. Rhabdomyosarcoma is the most frequently observed childhood cancer in classic Li-Fraumeni cancer syndrome families, in whom germ-line mutations of the *p53* gene have consistently been detected (Malkin et al. 1990). An excess of breast carcinomas and other tumors has also been reported in young mothers with germ-line *p53* mutations whose children have been diagnosed with rhabdomyosarcoma (Moutou et al. 1996; Olivier et al. 2003). Furthermore, in a study of 33 patients with sporadic rhabdomyosarcoma, germ-line mutations of the *p53* gene were detected in 3 of 13 patients, all of whom were under the age of 3 years (Diller et al. 1995). In a study of 1,770 patients enrolled in the first and second IRSG, Heyn identified 22 children who developed a second malignant neoplasm. Twelve of 13 families for whom adequate family history was available had a pattern of malignancies suggestive of the Li-Fraumeni syndrome (Heyn et al. 1993). In another study by Hartley, genetic predisposition to the development of cancer was noted in up to 33% of families of children younger than 15 years who were diagnosed with a soft tissue sarcoma (most of which were rhabdomyosarcoma) and who were registered at the Manchester Children's Tumor Registry among others (Hartley et al. 1993). These findings indicate that germline *p53* mutations predispose individuals to a wide spectrum of cancer development at an early age and should alert physicians to closely assess cancer risk among family members of such patients.

Neurofibromatosis Type 1. The prevalence of NF1 among patients with rhabdomyosarcoma who were enrolled in IRS-IV was 0.5%, which is about 20 times greater than that reported for the general population. Three of the five children in this series were younger than 3 years of age and the majority of patients had large embryonal tumors that originated in the prostate or bladder (Sung et al. 2004a).

Environmental Factors. In a case controlled study of 351 children who were enrolled in the second and third IRSG trials, parental use of recreational drugs such as cocaine and marijuana during the year before the child's birth was associated with an increased risk of rhabdomyosarcoma in the offspring (Grufferman et al. 1993). In utero X-ray exposure has also been associated with an increased risk of rhabdomyosarcoma (Ruymann 1991).

6.2 Pathology and Biology of Rhabdomyosarcoma

6.2.1 Pathologic Classification of Rhabdomyosarcoma

Rhabdomyosarcoma comprises a heterogeneous family of tumors related to the skeletal muscle lineage. Though histopathologic classification has evolved over time, a classification system has been established with subtypes that contribute to the assessment of a patient's prognosis (Table 6.1) (Newton et al. 1995). The current system that is termed the International Classification of Rhabdomyosarcoma provides a strong relationship between pathologic subtype and patient outcome according to the following categories: superior prognosis (botryoid and spindle cell variants of embryonal rhabdomyosarcoma), intermediate prognosis (embryonal rhabdomyosarcoma, not otherwise specified), and poor prognosis (alveolar rhabdomycosarcoma and undifferentiated sarcoma). Within this classification system, the two largest categories

Table 6.1. Pathologic subtypes of RMS (Newton et al. 1995)

Category	Prognosis	Site	Age (years)	Pathologic features
Botryoid	Superior	Head and neck, genitourinary tract	<10	Condensed layer of tumor cells (cambial layer) underlying intact epithelium
Spindle cell	Superior	Paratesticular		Spindle-shaped cells forming tumors of low cellularity – within either collagen-rich or collagen-poor stroma
ERMS, NOS	Intermediate	Head and neck, genitourinary tract	<10	Usually moderately cellular in a loose myxoid stroma with characteristic strap-shaped cells with elongated nuclei; may show considerable variation in cytology, ranging from primitive to highly differentiated muscle cells
ARMS	Poor	Extremities, trunk	>10	Anastomosing fibrovascular connective tissue septa lined by tumor cells – usually monotonous small round cells with coarse chromatin
Undifferentiated sarcoma	Poor	Extremities	>5	Primitive non-committed mesenchymal cells with no discernible architecture – generally diagnosis of exclusion – no expression of common immunohistochemical markers

are embryonal and alveolar rhabdomyosarcoma. As the criteria for distinguishing these two categories have been refined over time, comparison of clinical features between patients with these two types of RMS demonstrated distinct ages of onset, primary sites, and prognoses. These clinical and pathologic differences between alveolar and embryonal rhabdomyosarcomas are hypothesized to be the result of different molecular alterations and differences in the resulting biological mechanisms of tumorigenesis.

In addition to the complexities of the categorization within the rhabdomyosarcoma family of tumors, the diagnosis in general is often complicated by a paucity of features of striated muscle differentiation. The problem is compounded by the fact that a variety of pediatric solid tumors including rhabdomyosarcoma, neuroblastoma, Ewing's sarcoma, and non-Hodgkin's lymphoma can present as collections of poorly differentiated cells. To detect more subtle evidence of myogenic differentiation, a variety of immunohistochemical reagents have been used to identify muscle-specific proteins such as desmin, myoglobin, or muscle-specific actin (Qualman et al. 1998). More recently, antibodies to the muscle-specific transcription factors MyoD and myogenin have also been shown to be useful immunohistochemical tools for these differential diagnostic purposes (Sebire and Malone 2003). In addition, further evidence of the myogenic phenotype can be gathered by the detection of myofilaments in electron microscopic examination (Peydro-Olaya et al. 2003). However, it should be emphasized that there is no well-established ultrastructural or immunohistochemical marker that will distinguish among the RMS subtypes, and particularly between alveolar and embryonal rhabdomyosarcoma.

6.2.2 Chromosomal Translocations in Alveolar Rhabdomyosarcoma

In studies of chromosomal changes in rhabdomyosarcoma, recurrent chromosomal translocations have been specifically identified in the alveolar subtype. The most characteristic translocation involves chromosomes 2 and 13, t(2;13)(q35;q14) (Turc-Carel et al. 1986). In addition, a t(1;13) (p36;q14) variant translocation was identified in a smaller fraction of cases (Biegel et al. 1991). The loci on chromosomes 2 and 1 rearranged by the t(2;13) and t(1;13) are *PAX3* and *PAX7*, respectively (Fig. 6.1) (Barr et al. 1993; Davis et al. 1994). These two genes encode highly related

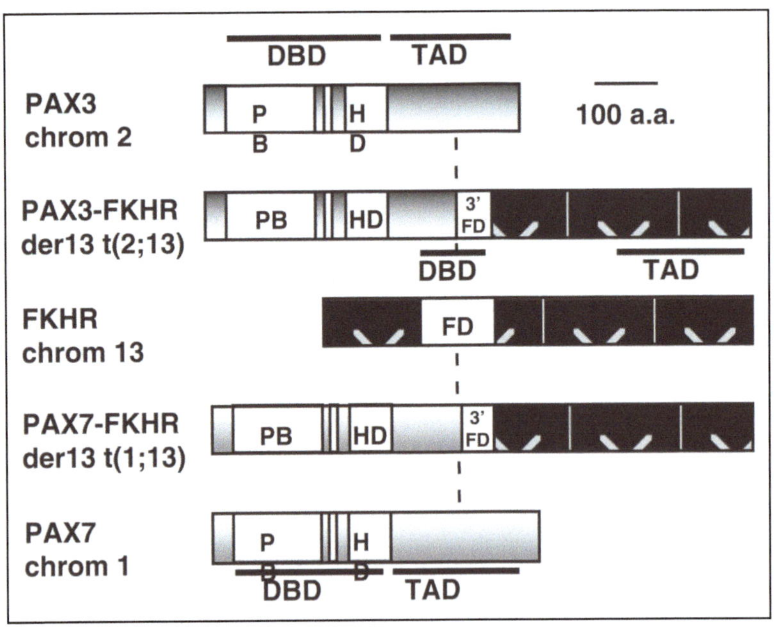

Figure 6.1

Comparison of wild-type and fusion products associated with the 2;13 and 1;13 translocations. The paired box, octapeptide, homeobox and fork head domain are indicated as *open boxes*, and transcriptional domains (*DBD* DNA binding domain, *TAD* transcriptional activation domain) are shown as *solid bars*. The *vertical dashed line* indicates the translocation fusion point

members of the paired box transcription factor family, which contain N-terminal DNA binding domains consisting of paired box and homeobox motifs and C-terminal transcriptional activation domains. The chromosome 13 locus involved in these translocations is *FKHR (FOX01A)*, which encodes a member of the fork head transcription factor family with an N-terminal fork head DNA binding domain and a C-terminal transcriptional activation domain (Galili et al. 1993). The translocations break within *PAX3* or *PAX7* and *FKHR* to create two chimeric genes on the derivative chromosomes. The *PAX3-FKHR* and *PAX7-FKHR* chimeric genes on each derivative chromosome 13 are more consistently and highly expressed as chimeric transcripts that encode fusion proteins containing the PAX3 or PAX7 DNA binding domain and the C-terminal FKHR transcriptional activation domain. These fusion proteins function as transcription factors that activate transcription from PAX-binding sites but are 10- to 100-fold more potent as transcriptional activators than the wild-type PAX3 and PAX7 proteins (Bennicelli et al. 1996, 1999).

In addition to showing a gain of function, the PAX3-FKHR and PAX7-FKHR fusion products are expressed at higher levels in alveolar rhabdomyosarcoma tumors than the corresponding wild-type PAX3 and PAX7 products (Davis and Barr 1997). Though both fusion genes are consistently overexpressed in the two fusion subtypes, there is a striking difference in the mechanism of fusion gene overexpression between these subtypes. In PAX7-FKHR-expressing tumors, the fusion gene is overexpressed secondary to in vivo amplification of the genomic region containing the fusion gene whereas the *PAX3-FKHR* fusion gene is overexpressed due to a copy number-independent increase in transcriptional rate (Barr et al. 1996; Davis and Barr 1997). By combining changes in protein function and changes in gene expression, the combined effect of these alterations in alveolar rhabdomyosarcoma is to produce high levels of potent activators of transcription from PAX3/PAX7 DNA binding sites. The end result is inappropriate activation of PAX3/PAX7 target genes, which is hypothesized to contribute to tumorigenic behavior by alterations in growth, differentiation, and apoptosis control.

Gene transfer studies in cultured cells provide support for an oncogenic role of the PAX3-FKHR protein. Under conditions in which PAX3 is not transforming, introduction of PAX3-FKHR into chicken embryo fibroblasts and NIH 3T3 murine fibroblasts produced evidence of cellular transformation, including morphological changes, focus formation, and anchorage-independent growth (Scheidler et al. 1996; Lam et al. 1999). A role in protecting cells from apoptosis was indicated by the induction of cell death when PAX3-FKHR expression was downregulated with antisense oligonucleotides (Bernasconi et al. 1996). Gene transfer studies with C2C12 myoblasts and MyoD-transfected C3H 10T1/2 fibroblasts, which undergo myogenic differentiation under low serum conditions, showed that PAX3-FKHR is more effective than PAX3 in inhibiting terminal differentiation (Epstein et al. 1995). However, microarray analyses showed that PAX3-FKHR transduction into NIH 3T3 fibroblasts induced expression of genes involved in myogenesis (Khan et al. 1999). The apparent contrast of these findings and those of the preceding study may be explained by the hypothesis that these fusion proteins facilitate entry into the myogenic pathway but inhibit its final steps. The findings of these phenotypic studies indicate that PAX3-FKHR can influence growth, differentiation, and apoptosis, and may exert an oncogenic effect through multiple pathways that exaggerate the normal developmental role of wild-type PAX3.

The PAX3-FKHR and PAX7-FKHR chimeric transcripts can be readily detected with reverse transcription-polymerase chain reaction (RT-PCR) methodology, facilitating molecular diagnostic detection of this molecular hallmark of the alveolar rhabdomyosarcoma subtype (Barr et al. 1995). Using RT-PCR assays for the PAX3-FKHR and PAX7-FKHR transcripts, studies were conducted to analyze RMS tumors and determine the frequency of gene fusions in the alveolar and embryonal categories. In tumor panels of varying size, ~80% of ARMS cases expressed one of the two fusions, with the frequency of PAX3-FKHR being severalfold higher than that of PAX7-FKHR (Sorensen et al. 2002). In contrast, the vast majority of embryonal tumors (>95%) are negative for the PAX3- and PAX7-FKHR fusions.

6.2.3 Allelic Loss of 11p15.5 in Embryonal Rhabdomyosarcoma

Although no recurrent chromosomal rearrangements were found in embryonal rhabdomyosarcoma, frequent allelic loss was found on chromosome 11, with the smallest region of consistent allelic loss in cases localized to chromosomal region 11p15.5 (Koufos et al. 1985; Scrable et al. 1987). Allelic loss results from a genetic event such as chromosome loss, deletion, or mitotic recombination that effectively eliminates the allelic contribution of all or part of one of the two chromosomes from a patient's tumor cells. In cancer genetics, the finding of a consistent region of allelic loss often indicates that a tumor suppressor gene has been inactivated in the tumor under investigation. In the case of embryonal rhabdomyosarcoma, the presence of a putative tumor suppressor in chromosomal region 11p15 has been further supported by chromosome transfer studies in which normal human chromosome 11 or fragments containing the 11p15 region suppress proliferation of the RD embryonal rhabdomyosarcoma cell line (Loh et al. 1992; Koi et al. 1993). Furthermore, the mechanism for tumor suppressor gene inactivation is generally postulated to be a two step process in which both gene copies are sequentially inactivated. To date, specific genetic alteration of genes in this region have not been identified in embryonal rhabdomyosarcoma. However, in studies of these tumors, analysis of the parental derivation of the two alleles with respect to the allelic loss pattern in the tumors revealed that the tumors preferentially maintain the paternal allele and lose the maternal allele (Scrable et al. 1989). This preferential involvement of parental alleles suggests the existence of genomic imprinting, an epigenetic developmental process that specifically inactivates expression of alleles in a gamete-of-origin-dependent process. In other studies of the human 11p15 chromosomal region and the corresponding mouse region, imprinting of several genes has been demonstrated; *H19* and *IGF2* are imprinted in opposite directions so that *H19* is preferentially expressed from the maternally inherited alleles and *IGF2* is preferentially expressed from paternally inherited alleles. Another gene preferentially expressed from the maternal allele is *CDKN1C* (*p57/KIP2*) gene, which encodes a cyclin-dependent kinase inhibitor that negatively regulates cell-cycle progression. These combined studies suggest that embryonal rhabdomyosarcoma tumorigenesis often involves inactivation of these and other imprinted tumor suppressor genes by allelic loss of the active maternal allele and retention of the inactive paternal allele.

6.2.4 Other Genetic Changes in Rhabdomyosarcoma

Additional genetic alterations have been demonstrated in rhabdomyosarcoma tumors using the technology of comparative genomic hybridization (CGH), which identifies copy number gains and losses in tumor DNA relative to a normal DNA control. These findings point to additional differences between the alveolar and embryonal categories and provide further support for the premise that distinct molecular pathways are involved in the development of these two rhabdomyosarcoma subtypes. CGH studies of embryonal tumors identified whole chromosome gains such as 2, 7, 8, 12, and 13 and whole chromosome losses of chromosomes such as 14 (Weber-Hall et al. 1996; Bridge et al. 2000). In contrast, CGH analyses of alveolar cases identified genomic amplification of the chromosomal regions 12q13–15 and 2p24, each occurring in ~30% of cases. Less common amplicons were found by CGH at 2q34-qter, 15q24–26, 1p36 (corresponding to amplification of the *PAX7-FKHR* fusion), 13q31, 1q21, and 8q13–21 (Gordon et al. 2000; Bridge et al. 2002). Though genomic amplification is an infrequent event in most cases of embryonal rhabdomyosarcoma (1 of 10 and 1 of 16 cases in two independent studies), CGH analysis detected evidence of genomic amplification in 4 of 6 cases of embryonal tumors with evidence of anaplasia (Bridge et al. 2002), a subset of ERMS associated with a poor clinical outcome (Kodet et al. 1993).

Mutations of p53, amplification of MDM2 (in 12q13–15 amplicon), and deletions of the CDKN2A locus affecting the ARF product have been demonstrated in various cases of rhabdomyosarcoma and lead to effective loss of p53 protein function by one of a variety of mechanisms (Iolascon et al. 1996; Taylor

Table 6.2. Mouse models of rhabdomyosarcoma

Mouse model	Genetic alteration	Genetic background	Predominant tumor	RMS incidence	
				% mice	% tumors
NBCCS (Goodrich et al. 1997)	*Ptch* +/–, deletion of exons 1–2	129SV	Medulloblastoma	2/27 (7%)	2/8 (25%)
NBCCS (Hahn et al. 1998)	*Ptch* +/–, deletion of exons 6–7	CD1	RMS	10/117 (9%)	10/10 (100%)
Li-Fraumeni (Lavigueur et al. 1989)	Mutant *Trp53* transgenic	C57BL/6	Lung CA	2/112 (2%)	2/27 (7%)
Li-Fraumeni (Jacks et al. 1994)	*Trp53* +/–, deletion of exon 2 to intron 6	C57BL/6	Sarcomas	1/232 (0.4%)	1/44 (2%)
	Trp53 –/–		Lymphoma	3/70 (4%)	3/56 (5%)
Neu/Li-Fraumeni (Nanni et al. 2003)	*Trp53* +/–, Neu transgenic	BALB/c	GU RMS (males), salivary gland tumors	100%	N/A
HGF (Takayama et al. 1997)	*Hgf* transgenic	FVB/N	Mammary gland CA	3/69 (4%)	N/A
HGF/CDKN2A (Sharp et al. 2002)	*Hgf* transgenic Ink4a/Arf –/–	FVB/ C57BL/6	RMS	35/36 (97%)	~90%
	Hgf transgenic Ink4a/Arf +/–		RMS, melanoma	20/57 (35%)	~53%

et al. 2000). Similarly amplification of CDK4 (in 12q13–15 amplicon) or deletion of the CDKN2A locus that affect the p16 product lead to an effective loss of RB1 protein function (Khatib et al. 1993; Iolascon et al. 1996). Amplification of MYCN in the 2p24 amplicon and RAS mutations has also been reported in rhabdomyosarcoma cases (Stratton et al. 1989; Driman et al. 1994). The finding of these additional genetic changes indicates that alveolar and embryonal tumors arise and evolve by a multistep process. The specific changes are found at variable frequencies and constitute a repertoire of possible collaborative events that may occur during RMS tumor progression.

Mouse models of rhabdomyosarcoma development have arisen as part of an attempt to recapitulate critical steps in multistep tumorigenesis, both with rhabdomyosarcoma as a specific goal and with rhabdomyosarcoma as a fortuitous outcome of the system (Table 6.2). Some of these models involve use of homologous recombination technology to inactivate tumor suppressor genes which, in the models shown here, occur in a non-specific cell type-independent pattern. Other models use transgenic technology to express oncogenes from exogenous expression constructs in a cell type-dependent pattern. In earlier models, such as the Tp53 and the Ptch gene knockouts and the HGF transgenic, the incidence of rhabdomyosarcoma was quite low and thus the utility of these models as a system for analysis was limited. However, in more recent models combining a transgene and a knockout (Neu transgenic Tp53 knockout and the Hgf transgenic Cdkn2A knockout), the incidence of rhabdomyosarcoma has increased substantially, and these systems now present interesting opportunities for analysis of the multistep process of rhabdomyosarcoma development and developmental therapeutics. However, it should be pointed out that the correspondence of these tumors to human embryonal and alveolar rhabdomyosarcoma is unclear and requires further investigation.

6.3 Clinical Presentation and Evaluation of Extent of Disease

Rhabdomyosarcoma is a clinically heterogeneous tumor which can arise anywhere in the body where mesenchymal tissue is found. The initial symptoms of rhabdomyosarcoma are closely related to the extent of tumor involvement and the location of the primary tumor.

6.3.1 Head and Neck Region (Flamant 1991)

Approximately one-third of all rhabdomyosarcomas arise in the head and neck region. The three major anatomic areas where rhabdomyosarcoma can arise in the head and neck region include the orbit, the parameningeal area (nasopharynx, paranasal sinuses, middle ear, mastoid, nasal cavity, pterygoid fossa, and orbital tumors with intracranial tumor or bone destruction) and non-parameningeal head and neck sites which include the parotid gland, oropharynx, oral cavity, larynx and soft tissues of the head and neck. Orbital tumors characteristically present with proptosis and occasionally ophthalmoplegia. Tumors in this location tend to be localized and have a very low incidence of distant or nodal spread. Parameningeal tumors more commonly arise within the nasopharynx and middle ear. Presenting symptoms are insidious and include persistent nasal discharge, nasal obstruction, noisy breathing, epistaxis, recurrent episodes of otitis media, swelling around the cheek, and gingival ulceration. Headache and cranial nerve palsies should alert the physician about the presence of meningeal extension. Tumors arising in other areas of the head and neck region can present with dysphonia, dysphagia, and palpable adenopathy.

6.3.2 Genitourinary Tumors (Flamant 1991)

Approximately 25% of rhabdomyosarcomas arise in the genitourinary tract and the majority of these tumors are located in the bladder and prostate. Signs and symptoms in this location include dysuria, polyuria, hematuria, and urinary retention. A palpable mass may be evident and hydronephrosis and renal insufficiency are occasionally seen in advanced cases. Vaginal tumors, which are commonly of botryoid histology and affect young children, often present with vaginal inflammation, an extruding mass, and bloody vaginal discharge. Uterine tumors occur in older patients and may present as a pelvic mass. Tumors located in the paratesticular area usually manifest as a non-transilluminant painless mass that can have an associated hydrocele.

6.3.3 Extremity Tumors (Flamant 1991)

The extremities are affected in approximately 18% of patients with rhabdomyosarcoma. Signs and symptoms often include swelling and pain after trauma and the lower extremities are involved more frequently than the upper extremities. Lymphatic involvement is common and the tumor can extend along the fascial planes.

6.3.4 Trunk (Flamant 1991)

This designation includes breast tumors located in the chest wall, paraspinal area, and abdominal wall. Patients can present with dyspnea, thoracic pain, evidence of nerve root compression, and pericardial disease.

6.3.5 Other Sites (Flamant 1991)

Intra-abdominal and pelvic tumors usually present with a palpable abdominal mass and can occasionally produce ascites. Tumors in the perineal and perianal region often present with compression of the rectum and difficulty in defecation, and can be confused with an abscess (Hill et al. 2002). Biliary tract tumors are extremely rare and can produce obstructive jaundice, cholestasis, and a picture similar to that seen in acute cholecystitis.

The initial evaluation of a child with rhabdomyosarcoma must include a detailed physical examination, a complete blood count with differential, serum electrolytes, serum calcium (hypercalcemia has been reported to occur in 0.4–6% of patients with metastatic rhabdomyosarcoma), liver function tests, uric acid (hyperuricemia was reported to occur in 5% of patients in IRSG-III), renal function tests, and coagulation studies including fibrinogen (disseminated intravascular coagulation was reported in 10% of patients with bone marrow metastases in IRSG-I). Bilateral bone marrow aspirates and biopsies should be performed routinely in all patients at the time of diagnosis even in the presence of normal hematologic values, and cerebrospinal fluid examination should be reserved for patients with cranial parameningeal tumors. Radiographic evaluation should include imaging of the primary tumor site with either magnetic resonance imaging (MRI) or computed tomography (CT) and a thorough search for metastases in the lung (CT of chest) and bone (bone scintigraphy). Patients with paratesticular tumors should have thin cut double contrast CT of abdomen and pelvis to accurately identify nodal disease; patients with abdominal, pelvic, and genitourinary tumors should have complete imaging of the abdomen and pelvis to search for occult metastases. It is recommended that a baseline CT scan of the head be performed at diagnosis in asymptomatic patients with metastatic paraspinal tumors (Spunt et al. 2001a). Routine lymph node sampling is routinely indicated for patients with extremity lesions whereas lymph node dissection (ipsilateral nerve sparing resection of spermatic vessels and nodes) is required for patients ≥10 years of age with paratesticular tumors (Neville et al. 2000; Wiener et al. 2001).

6.4 Staging

The development of an accurate and reproducible staging system for rhabdomyosarcoma is essential in order to interpret and compare treatment results of various multi-institutional trials and to help refine risk-directed treatment strategies aimed at maximizing the potential for cure while minimizing the potential side effects of therapy. The IRSG grouping system (Table 6.3) was developed in 1972 and categorizes patients into four distinct risk groups based on the postoperative extent of disease (Maurer et al. 1988). Briefly, patients with clinical Group I have complete excision of all tumor, Group II disease includes patients with microscopic residual tumor (IIa), patients with negative margins and resected positive nodes (IIb), and patients with microscopic residual disease and positive margins (IIc). Patients with clinical Group III have evidence of macroscopic residual disease after initial biopsy and clinical

Table 6.3. Surgicopathologic staging system for rhabdomyosarcoma (Maurer et al. 1988)

Group I	Localized disease, completely resected
Group II	Total gross resection with evidence of regional spread (a) Grossly resected tumor with microscopic residual disease (b) Regional disease with involved nodes, completely resected with no microscopic residual (c) Regional disease with involved nodes, grossly resected, but with evidence of microscopic residual and/or histologic involvement of the most distal regional node (from the primary site) in the dissection
Group III	Incomplete resection with gross residual disease
Group IV	Distant metastatic disease present at onset

Table 6.4. Pretreatment TNM staging system for rhabdomyosarcoma (Lawrence et al. 1987). Staging prior to treatment requires thorough clinical examination, laboratory and imaging examinations. Biopsy is required to establish the histologic diagnosis

Stage	Sites	T	Size	N	M
1	Orbit, head and neck (excluding parameningeal), GU non-bladder/non-prostate, biliary tract	T_1 or T_2	a or b	N_0 or N_1 or N_x	M_0
2	Bladder/prostate, extremity, cranial, parameningeal, other (includes trunk, retroperitoneum, etc.)	T_1 or T_2	a	N_0 or N_x	M_0
3	Bladder/prostate	T_1 or T_2	a	N_1	M_0
	Extremity, cranial, parameningeal, other (includes trunk, retroperitoneum, etc.)		b	N_0 or N_1 or N_x	M_0
4	All	T_1 or T_2	a or b	N_0 or N_1	M_1

Definitions			
	Tumor	T(site)$_1$	Confirmed to anatomic site of origin (a) ≤5 cm in diameter in size (b) >5 cm in diameter in size
		T(site)$_2$	Extension and/or fixative to surrounding tissue (a) ≤5 cm in diameter in size (b) >5 cm in diameter in size
	Regional nodes	N_0	Regional nodes not clinically involved
		N_1	Regional nodes clinically involved by neoplasm
		N_x	Clinical status of regional nodes unknown (especially sites that preclude lymph node evaluation)
	Metastasis	M_0	No distant metastasis
		M_1	Metastasis present

Group IV patients have evidence of distal metastasis at the time of diagnosis. Despite the fact that the surgicopathologic staging system is a robust tool that accurately identifies distinct risk groups of patients with rhabdomyosarcoma, its validity has been criticized by various clinical investigators since clinical grouping does not account for the pre-treatment characteristics of the tumor or the patient. Thus, using data from IRSG-II, a pre-treatment staging system was developed and prospectively tested in IRSG-III (Table 6.4) (Lawrence et al. 1987, 1997). This system takes into consideration the size and the site of the primary tumor as well as the degree of invasion of adjacent structures, the presence or absence of nodal involvement, and the presence or absence of distant metastases. The combination of group and stage was used for treatment assignment for the first time in IRSG-IV and is currently being used to identify risk categories and allocate therapies in IRSG-V (see Table 6.5).

Table 6.5. Risk assignment and therapy for patients enrolled in IRS-V (Raney et al. 2001). *Favorable* orbit/eyelid, head and neck (excluding parameningeal), genitourinary (not bladder or prostate), and biliary tract. *Unfavorable* bladder, prostate, extremity, parameningeal, trunk, retroperitoneal, pelvis, other. *a* tumor size ≤5 cm in diameter; *b* tumor size >5 cm in diameter; *EMB* embryonal botryoid, or spindle-cell rhabdomyosarcomas or ectomesenchymomas with embryonal RMS; *ALV* alveolar rhabdomyosarcomas or ectomesenchymomas with alveolar RMS; *UDS* undifferentiated sarcomas; *NO* regional nodes clinically not involved; *N1* regional nodes clinically involved; *NX* node status unknown; *VAC* vincristine, actinomycin D, cyclophosphamide; *XRT* radiotherapy; *TOPO* topotecan; *CPT-11* irinotecan

Risk (protocol)	Stage	Group	Site	Size	Age	Histology	Metastasis	Nodes	Treatment
Low, subgroup A	1	1	Favorable	a or b	<21	EMB	MO	NO	VA
(D9602)	1	II	Favorable	a or b	<21	EMB	MO	NO	VA+XRT
	1	III	Orbit only	a or b	<21	EMB	MO	NO	VA+XRT
	2	I	Unfavorable	a	<21	EMB	MO	NO or NX	VA
Low, subgroup B	1	II	Favorable	a or b	<21	EMB	MO	N1	VAC+XRT
(D9602)	1	III	Orbit only	a or b	<21	EMB	MO	N1	VAC+XRT
	1	III	Favorable (excluding orbit)	a or b	<21	EMB	MO	NO or N1 or NX	VAC+XRT
	2	II	Unfavorable	a	<21	EMB	MO	NO or NX	VAC+XRT
	3	I or II	Unfavorable	a	<21	EMB	MO	N1	VAC (+XRT, Gp II)
	3	I or II	Unfavorable	b	<21	EMB	MO	NO or N1 or NX	VAC (+XRT, Gp II)
Intermediate	2	III	Unfavorable	a	<21	EMB	MO	NO or NX	VAC±Topo+XRT
(D9803)	3	III	Unfavorable	a	<21	EMB	MO	N1	VAC±Topo+XRT
	3	III	Unfavorable	b	<21	EMB	MO	NO or N1 or NX	VAC±Topo+XRT
	1 or 2 or 3	I or II or III	Favorable or unfavorable	a or b	<21	ALV/UDS	MO	NO or N1 or NX	VAC±Topo+XRT
	4	I or II or III or IV	Favorable or unfavorable	a or b	<10	EMB	M1	NO or N1 or NX	VAC±Topo+XRT
High (D9802)	4	IV	Favorable or unfavorable	a or b	≥10	EMB	M1	NO or N1 or NX	CPT-11, VAC+XRT
	4	IV	Favorable or unfavorable	a or b	<21	ALV/UDS	M1	NO or N1 or NX	CPT-11, VAC+XRT

6.5 Prognostic Factors

Identification of prognostic factors is of pivotal importance in planning and developing risk-directed therapies for patients with rhabdomyosarcoma. The patient and tumor characteristics that have consistently been associated with survival in patients with rhabdomyosarcoma include clinical group, primary tumor site, histology, age, and treatment era (Pappo et al. 1995). These attributes have been used to identify distinct subsets of patients who are at different risk of treatment failure and to tailor therapy accordingly. Clinical Group has been shown to accurately predict clinical outcome in all of the published IRSG studies (Maurer et al. 1988, 1993; Crist et al. 1995). Among patients with clinical Group I disease, an inferior outcome was documented in those with alveolar histology tumors and in those who, in addition to having alveolar histology, were spared radiotherapy (Maurer et al. 1988, 1993; Crist et al. 1990; Wolden et al. 1999). Among patients with Group II tumors, those with microscopic residual tumor or resected nodal disease with negative margins (IIa and IIb) fare significantly better than those who present with both features (Group IIc) (5-year failure-free survival 75% vs. 74% vs. 58% $p=0.003$) (Smith et al. 2001). For patients with clinical Group III, those with embryonal histology and orbital or head and neck sites have an excellent survival and in patients with metastatic disease, the combination of embryonal histology, limited number of metastatic sites and age less than 10 years has been associated with a superior clinical outcome (survival of 47%) (Breneman et al. 2003).

In a study of over 2,300 patients enrolled in IRSG-III, IV pilot and IV, patients <1 year and those >10 year had a significantly poorer clinical outcome compared to patients who were 1–9 years of age. In this study, age emerged as an independent risk factor for failure even when adjusted for other unfavorable features such as alveolar and undifferentiated histology advanced group and stage (Joshi et al. 2004). Similarly, an Italian study has also demonstrated that patients younger than 1 year of age have a poor clinical outcome (Ferrari et al. 2003). The overriding prognostic importance of treatment is illustrated in Fig. 6.2. The subgroups of patients who have benefited the most from the therapeutic approaches pioneered by the IRSG include patients with Group I and II alveolar tumors, those with Group III tumors, and children with stage 1 Group II N1 and stage 2, 3 Group I, II disease (Crist et al. 1995; Baker et al. 2000). Other prognostic factors that have been identified as potential predictors of outcome in patients with rhabdomyosarcoma include lymphocyte count, tumor cell DNA content (ploidy), nodal status, tumor size, and for alveolar tumors, the subtype of fusion transcript (Maurer et al. 1988; Pappo et al. 1993; Lawrence et al. 1997; Neville et al. 2000; Sorensen et al. 2002).

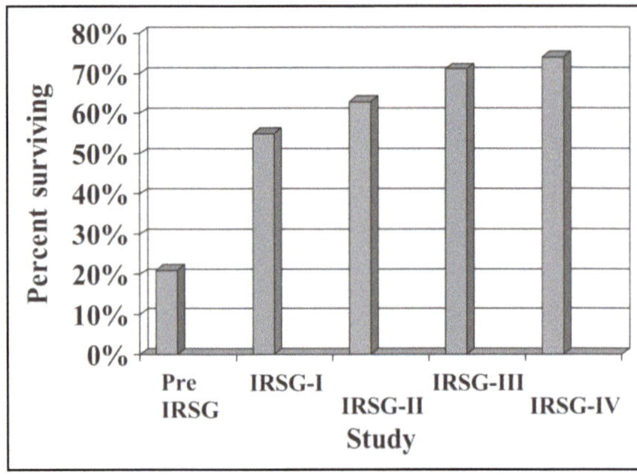

Figure 6.2

Treatment outcome according to treatment era

6.6 Treatment

The cure of patients with rhabdomyosarcoma has dramatically improved over the past 40 years. Prior to the use of multimodal therapy, less than 30% of children who were treated with local therapies alone (radiotherapy or surgery) survived (Pinkel 1961; Porterfield 1962; Lawrence 1964; Soule 1968; Grosfeld 1969) (Fig. 6.2). Single agent activity with drugs such as vincristine (V), actinomycin D (A), and cyclophosphamide (C) was documented in the early 1960s, and in 1969 combination chemotherapy with VAC was reported to be active in advanced stage disease (Pinkel 1961; Sutow 1966; Pratt 1969). In the early 1970s the use of combination chemotherapy with radiation therapy and/or surgery, pioneered by Pratt and Wilbur (Pratt 1972; Wilbur 1974), was shown to increase the response rate and resectability of large tumors and to improve the survival of patients who had completely resected disease. In 1974, Heyn et al. conclusively demonstrated that the administration of adjuvant chemotherapy improves the survival of children with surgically resected rhabdomyosarcoma (Heyn 1974). In an effort to further the understanding of treatment of this disease and to accrue significant numbers of patients to be able to ask clinically significant randomized questions, the first national trial (IRSG-I) was initiated in 1972.

6.7 Role of Local Therapies

Radiation therapy is an important component for the success of multi-modality therapy for rhabdomyosarcoma. The role of radiation has been studied extensively by the IRSG as well as the European cooperative groups and single institutions. The indications and delivery of radiation therapy depend upon a variety of factors including disease stage, clinical group, site, and histology. It is useful to review the basic radiation related findings of IRSG-I–IV, to better understand current recommendations and investigational directions.

In IRSG-I, all patients with clinical Group I disease were randomized to receive or not radiotherapy (RT). Overall, there was no benefit for RT in this group of patients. All other patients were intended to receive RT. Patients who received RT to the tumor plus a margin were compared to those who had treatment to the whole muscle bundle. No difference in control was noted, so a field that includes the tumor and a 2-cm margin became the standard treatment volume. Radiation doses in IRSG-I and II ranged from 40 to 60 Gy, depending upon patient age and tumor size (Maurer et al. 1988).

There were no randomized RT questions in IRSG-II. During this study, the practice of using prophylactic craniospinal or whole brain RT along with intrathecal chemotherapy for parameningeal tumors was abandoned. This was associated with considerable toxicity with no significant improvement in outcome (Maurer et al. 1993).

In IRSG-III, doses were standardized so that patients with residual gross disease (Group III) received 50.4 Gy while those with microscopic disease (Group II) received 41.4 Gy, irrespective of patient age and tumor size (Crist et al. 1995). Radiotherapy was added back for patients with Group I disease who had alveolar or undifferentiated histology because of their inferior outcome in previous studies. This was later validated in a larger review (Wolden et al. 1999).

IRSG-IV featured a randomization for clinical Group III patients to standard RT using 50.4 Gy in once daily fractions of 1.8 Gy compared to hyperfractionated RT to 59.4 Gy in twice daily fractions of 1.1 Gy. In theory, the higher dose should have produced higher rates of local control with equivalent late effects. Unfortunately, local control was not improved and 50.4 Gy in once daily fractions remains the standard treatment for children with gross residual disease (Donaldson et al. 2001).

The radiation questions in IRSG-V are non-randomized reductions in dose and treatment volumes in selected clinical scenarios where control rates have been excellent. For example, Group I alveolar and undifferentiated tumors as well as all Group II node negative patients receive 36 Gy instead of 41.4 Gy and Group III embryonal orbit tumors receive 45 Gy rather than 50.4 Gy. Patients who undergo delayed resection, or "second look surgery," may also receive reduced doses of 36 or 41.4 Gy depending upon margin status. Also, the target volume for Group III patients may be reduced from a margin of 2 cm, to 0.5 cm after 36 (if node negative) or 41.4 Gy (if node positive) (IRSG-V protocols). The results of IRSG-V will need to be compared to historical data to know whether these reductions in RT dose and volume are to become the standard of care.

Currently, patients with clinical Group I disease only require postoperative radiation therapy if they are alveolar or undifferentiated subtypes. All clinical Group II patients should have postoperative radiation therapy. This recommendation has been validated not only in the United States but also in Europe (Schuck et al. 2004). Group III patients should receive 50.4 Gy unless they are enrolled in a study allowing dose reduction for special circumstances. Group IV patients receive radiotherapy to the primary site and also to sites of metastasis, to the extent this is feasible. Bone marrow obviously cannot be irradiated but cortical bone lesions should be treated. Whole lung RT to 14.4 Gy is recommended for parenchymal lung metastases and hemithorax RT can be used for unilateral pleural contamination. In the very rare instance that a patient presents with positive CSF cytology or other evidence of leptomeningeal spread, craniospinal radiation therapy should be considered.

The standard RT field should target the initial (pre-chemotherapy, pre-surgery) extent of disease plus a 2-cm margin. As previously mentioned, IRSG-V is investigating a "cone-down" to a smaller margin during RT. Favorable results with this technique or the use of smaller margins from the beginning of therapy have been reported at single institutions (Wolden, personal communication). Margins may be customized to the extent that it is necessary to limit doses to critical normal tissues, provided that the tumor is not being underdosed.

Radiation therapy is generally integrated into chemotherapy between weeks 3 and 15. This has varied in different protocols because of different chemotherapy schedules. Actinomycin D and doxorubicin are potent radiosensitizers and are contraindicated during RT. Typically patients continue to receive vincristine and cyclophosphamide during radiotherapy. In the past, it was recommended that patients with parameningeal tumors with skull base erosion, intracranial extension or cranial nerve palsies begin RT immediately. In IRSG-V, only those with intracranial extension are required to start RT at the beginning of chemotherapy. Analyses are ongoing to determine the optimal timing of RT for high risk parameningeal tumors.

There has been an explosion of new technology in imaging and radiation therapy in the past several decades. The use of CT, MRI and now PET imaging has revolutionized the way tumors are targeted for radiotherapy. Furthermore, advancements in radiation delivery include three-dimensional conformal and now intensity modulated radiation therapy (IMRT) as well as proton beams. These techniques allow improved coverage and dosing of the target (tumor) with decreased exposure of surrounding tissues. Preliminary clinical results with these high-technology approaches are very promising (Michalski et al. 1995; Hug et al. 2002; Wolden et al. 2003). Brachytherapy, although not a new technology, is now being actively considered for certain rhabdomyosarcoma patients. Examples include interstitial afterloading catheters for treatment of a tongue or extremity tumor. For infants with vaginal tumors, an intracavitary cylinder is an ideal way to treat the vaginal mucosa while preserving fertility and bone growth. Intraoperative radiation therapy has also been used at the time of second-look or salvage surgery, as an adjunct to external beam RT (Goodman et al. 2003).

Acute side-effects during RT depend upon the site being treated and vary significantly from patient to patient. The most common problem for patients with head and neck tumors is severe mucositis. Some patients require narcotic analgesia and tube feeding. Breaks in treatment are discouraged since tumor cells will repopulate and local control will decrease when there are significant treatment interruptions. Patients with orbital tumors may have conjunctival irritation. Radiotherapy for sites in the thorax may result in esophagitis and, very rarely, pneumonitis or pericarditis. Abdominal radiation can cause nausea and emesis as well as diarrhea and cramping. Treatment of the pelvis may be associated with proctitis, cystitis and, when the perineum is included, severe pain from perineal desquamation in females. Extremity radiotherapy is generally well tolerated except for a potentially severe skin reaction. Bone marrow suppression from radiation therapy is proportional to the amount of bone in the treatment field.

Long-term complications of radiation therapy depend upon the age of the patient, the site treated, and the dose and technique used. There may also be interactions with surgery and chemotherapy as well as patient related factors. A common concern is that bone growth arrest may occur above doses of approximately 20–25 Gy in pre-pubertal children. This could lead to cosmetic or functional deformity. This outcome must be weighed against the morbidity of a wide surgical resection to determine which form of local control will be less damaging to a child. Organ dysfunction is also a major consideration. Each organ or structure has a unique radiation dose-response relationship and all structures within a radiation field must be carefully considered by the radiation oncologist for a determination of risk. Potential problems include but are not limited to hormone deficiency, cataract, xerostomia, cardiopulmonary dysfunction, liver abnormalities, and infertility.

Secondary solid tumors are another significant risk for children receiving radiation therapy. Such tumors tend to occur after a latency of at least 15–20 years, but the risk appears to continue throughout life. There is a dose-response relationship so that tumors are most common in tissues that receive very high doses (Kuttesch et al. 1996). Some tissues are more susceptible to carcinogenesis than others; these include thyroid, breast, salivary glands, and brain. Life-long screening for second malignancies and behavior education (i.e., avoidance of smoking, excessive sun exposure) is important for survivors.

Radiation therapy is perhaps the most effective “single agent” in the treatment of rhabdomyosarcoma. Its use continues to be carefully refined through academic investigation and development of new technologies with the goal of maximizing cure and long-term quality of life for children with rhabdomyosarcoma.

6.8 Multi-institutional Trials

The majority of children treated in North America are enrolled in trials conducted by the IRSG (now known as the soft Tissue Sarcoma Committee of the Children’s Oncology Group). This group has conducted, analyzed, and reported four consecutive trials which have accrued over 3,700 patients (Maurer et al. 1988; Maurer et al. 1993; Crist et al. 1995; Crist et al. 2001; Breneman et al. 2003): IRSG-I: 1972–1978, n=686; IRSG-II: 1978–1984, n=999; IRSG-III: 1984–1991, n=1,062; and IRSG-IV: 1991–1997, n=1,010. These studies have provided significant and useful insights into the natural history, biology, and response to therapy of this heterogeneous tumor. The median age at diagnosis for all patients is approximately 5 years and two-thirds of the patients were less than 10 years of age. The most common primary tumor sites included the head and neck region (36%), the genitourinary tract (25%), and the extremities (18%). Detailed results by group and site of the four consecutive IRSG trials and the current approach for these children is depicted in Tables 6.5, and 6.6. As shown in Table 6.6 and Figure 6.2, the survival of patients with rhabdomyosarcoma has progressively increased from 55% in IRSG-I to 72% in IRSG-IV.

6.8.1 Clinical Group I (Maurer et al. 1988, 1993; Crist et al. 1995, 2001; Raney et al. 2001)

Over 90% of patients with completely resected tumors and negative margins are expected to be cured from their disease. In the first IRSG study, patients were randomized to receive vincristine, actinomycin and cyclophosphamide (VAC) for 2 years with or without radiation. The estimated percentage of patients surviving at 5 years was similar; therefore, radiotherapy was avoided in these patients in subsequent trials. Therapy for patients with Group I disease in IRSG-II was stratified according to site and histology. All patients excluding those with extremity alveolar tumors were randomized to receive VAC chemotherapy or vincristine and actinomycin D (VA) for 2 years. The survival and disease-free survival at 5 years was similar for both groups demonstrating that cyclophosphamide can be safely omitted in the majority of children with Group I disease, IRSG-III used an intensified VA regimen for all patients with favorable histology tumors, resulting in a 5-year survival of 93%. Two-drug VA therapy was only given to patients with orbital and testicular tumors in IRSG-IV with excellent results (3-year S ≥90%), whereas all other Group I patients were randomized to receive VAC vs. vincristine, actinomycin, ifosfamide (VAI) or vincristine, ifosfamide and etoposide (VIE). Although no differences were noted between randomized arms, the use of three drugs in patients with Group I embryonal stage 2 and 3 tumors significantly improved the failure-free survival of these patients when compared to IRSG-III (Baker

Table 6.6. Summary of clinical groups, treatment and outcome in four major Intergroup Rhabdomyosarcoma Study (IRSG) studies (detailed descriptions of treatment may be found in references) (*VAC* vincristine, actinomycin, cyclophosphamide; *RT* radiation therapy; *ADR* Adriamycin (doxorubicin); *VADRC* vincristine-Adriamycin, cyclophosphamide; *CDDP* cisplatin; *VP-16* etoposide; *DTIC* dacarbazine; *M* melphalan; *I* ifosfamide; 3 drug, VAC, VAF, VFE). (Modified from Pappo et al. 1995: Biology and therapy of pediatric rhabdomyosarcoma. *J Clin Oncol* 13:2123–2139; with permission)

	IRS-1 (1972–1978)		IRS-II (1978–1984)		IRS-III (1984–1991)		IRS-IV (1991–1997)	
Clinical group	Treatment (regimen)	Survival (%)	Treatment (regimen)	Survival (%)	Treatment (regimen)	Survival (%)	Treatment (regimen)	Survival (%)
Group I (favorable histology)	VAC×2y (A)	93	VAC×2y (21)	85	Cyclic-sequential VA for 1y (31)	93	Overall VA 3 drug	90 88 94
	VAC+RT×2y (B)	81	VA×1y (22)	84				
	Amputees, VAC×2y (G)	83						
Group II (favorable histology)	VA+RT×1y (C)	73	VA+RT×1y (23)	88	VA+RT×1y (32)	54	3 drug+RT	96
	VAC+RT×2y (D)	70	Pulsed VAC+RT×1y (24)	79	VA+ADR+RT×1y (33)	89		
Group III (excluding special pelvic[a], orbit, and selected head sites[e])	VAC+RT×2y (E)[b]	53	Pulsed VAC×2y+RT (25)[d]	–	Pulsed VAC+RT×2y (34)[c,d]	70	3 drug+RT	70%
	VAC+ADR +RT×2y (F)[b]	51	Pulsed VADRC-VAC +RT×2y (26)	–	Pulsed VADRC-VAC +CDDP+RT×2y (35)	63	VAC+RT	67
	E+F[b]	52	Regimens 25+26	59[f]	Pulsed VADRC-VAC +CDDP-VP-16 +RT×2y (36)	64	VAI+RT	66
					Regimens 34+35+36	65[f]	VIE+RT	75
Group IV	VAC+RT×2y (E)[b]	14	Pulsed VAC×2y +RT (25)[d]	–	Pulsed VAC+RT×2y (34)[c,d]	27	VIE+RT	33
							VM+RT	19
	VAC+ADR +RT×2y (F)[b]	26	Pulsed VADRC-VAC +RT×2y (26)	–	Pulsed VADRC-VAC+CDDP +VP-16+RT×2y (35)	31	overall	25
	E+F[b]	20	Regimens 25+26	27	Pulsed VADRC-VAC +CDDP+VP-16+RT×2y (36)	29		
					Regimens 34+35+36	30		

Table 6.6. (Continued)

Clinical group	IRS-1 (1972–1978) Treatment (regimen)	IRS-1 (1972–1978) Survival (%)	IRS-II (1978–1984) Treatment (regimen)	IRS-II (1978–1984) Survival (%)	IRS-III (1984–1991) Treatment (regimen)	IRS-III (1984–1991) Survival (%)	IRS-IV (1991–1997) Treatment (regimen)	IRS-IV (1991–1997) Survival (%)
Special pelvic sites[a] (Group III)	–	71	Pulsed VAC±RT ±surgery×2y (27)	72[f]	Pulsed VADRC-VAC +CDDP±AMD±VP16±RT ±surgery ×2y[c] (37) A&B	83[g]	3 drug+RT	86
Unfavorable histology, alveolar (Groups I and II)	–	57[h]	Pulsed VAC ±RT×1y (25)	71	Pulsed VADRC-VAC +CDDP+RT×1y (38)	80	3 drug±RT	86
Orbit and selected head sites[e] (favorable histology)					VA+RT×1y (32)			
Group II	–	–	VA+RT or VAC +RT×1y (23&24)		VA+RT×1y (32)		2 or 3 drug +RT	97
Group III			VAC or VADRC +RT×1y (25&26)	91[f]	VA+RT×1y (32)	91[g]	3 drug+RT	100
			Regimens 23–26 (combined results)		Regimen 32 (combined results)			
Paratesticular sites (Group II, favorable histology)	–	–	VA+RT or VAC +RT×1y (23&24)	81	VA+RT×1y (32)	81	3 drug+RT	94
All sites and groups		55		63		71		72

[a] Bladder, prostate and vagina, uterus
[b] For all sites
[c] Second-look surgery recommended at week 20 for all patients in partial or complete remission. Patients in partial remission were to receive ADR+DTIC (regimen 34) or AMD+VP-16 (regimens 35&37 A&B), or AMD+DTIC (regimen 26)
[d] Differences in outcome between regimens 25 vs. 26 in IRS-II, and 34 vs. 35 vs. 36 in IRS-III were not statistically significant
[e] Oral cavity, cheek, oropharynx, larynx, scalp, parotid gland
[f] Overall 5-year survival for all Group III patients treated in IRS-II is 66%
[g] Overall 5-year survival for all Group III patients treated in IRS-III is 74%
[h] Three-year estimate

et al. 2000). Since these results were not widely available at the time the IRSG-V opened, all Group I patients received two drugs in this trial. However, the next generation trial for low-risk rhabdomyosarcoma will incorporate limited exposure to an alkylating agent. Finally, as previously mentioned, current therapies for Group I patients should include the addition of radiotherapy for patients with alveolar histology since this strategy significantly improves the 10-year survival and failure-free survival (Wolden et al. 1999).

6.8.2 Clinical Group II (Maurer et al. 1988, 1993; Crist et al. 1995, 2001; Raney et al. 2001; Smith et al. 2001)

Nearly 700 patients with clinical Group II disease have been treated in IRSG trials and approximately 90% of these patients are long term survivors. In IRSG-I, the addition of cyclophosphamide to standard VA therapy with radiotherapy failed to improve the survival and progression free survival of these patients. In IRSG-II, patients with clinical Group II tumors (excluding those with extremity alveolar tumors) were randomized to receive radiotherapy and intensive sequential VA or repetitive VAC therapy. The addition of cyclophosphamide did not improve the outcome of these patients. In IRSG III, patients with favorable histology tumors (excluding orbit, head and paratesticular sites) were randomized to receive radiotherapy and either VA or VA with doxorubicin. Although the 5-year progression free survival and survival rates for the doxorubicin treated patients were superior (77% and 89% vs. 56% and 54% respectively), the outcome of VA patients in this trial was inferior when compared to IRSG II and the beneficial effect of doxorubicin became less obvious when the results of VA for IRSG-II and III were combined. In IRSG-IV, all patients except for those with orbital tumors were treated with three drugs including an alkylating agent. Patients with embryonal Group II N1 disease and those with Group II stage 2, 3 disease benefited from this approach (Baker et al. 2000). Therefore, in the current IRSG-V trial (see Table 6.6), these patients are being treated with VAC chemotherapy. The next generation soft tissue sarcoma trial will examine the feasibility of reducing the dose of cyclophosphamide in these patients in an attempt to limit the long-term complications of this agent.

6.8.3 Clinical Group III (Maurer et al. 1988, 1993; Crist et al. 1995, 2001; Baker et al. 2000; Donaldson et al. 2001)

Patients with clinical Group III comprise the largest group of patients enrolled in IRSG studies and are the largest group of children who have benefited the most from intensified therapies. The combined overall 5-year survival for these patients has increased from 52% in IRSG I to 76% in IRSG-IV (Crist et al. 1995, 2001). In the first IRSG, the addition of doxorubicin to a VAC backbone failed to improve the outcome of these patients. In IRSG II, increases in the cumulative doses of actinomycin D, doxorubicin and vincristine and the use of a repetitive pulse VAC regimen improved the response rates and outcome of these patients (5-year survival: 52–66%). The promising results of IRSG II prompted changes in IRSG-III to include a more intense and complex treatment regimen for most Group III patients (excluding those with special pelvic, orbit, and selected head sites). This treatment strategy compared VAC with VAC, doxorubicin and cisplatin and VAC with cisplatin and etoposide. Patients who failed to achieve a complete response by week 20 received alternate pulsed chemotherapy. Although the combined results of these three regimens were similar, producing complete responses of 81%, the progression free survival and survival was superior when compared to the outcomes of patients who were treated in IRSG-II. In IRSG-IV, patients were randomized to receive VAC, VIE, or VAI and either conventional radiotherapy or hyperfractionated radiotherapy. Patients with pre-existing renal abnormalities were treated with VAC chemotherapy. The outcome of patients treated with a cyclophosphamide or an ifosfamide-based regimen were similar, with 3-year failure-free survival rates of approximately 75%. No differences in outcome were evident amongst patients randomized to conventional or hyperfractionated radiotherapy. In IRSG-V patients with embryonal stage 1 Group III, non-orbital tumors received VAC chemotherapy those with Group III orbital disease received VA, and the remainder of patients are being randomized to receive

VAC alone or VAC alternating with topotecan and cyclophosphamide.

6.8.4 Clinical Group IV (Maurer et al. 1988, 1993; Crist et al. 1995, 1995; Breitfeld et al. 2001; Sandler et al. 2001)

The majority of patients with metastatic disease (except for those with embryonal histology tumors and fewer than three metastatic sites) (Breneman et al. 2003) have a dismal outcome, with less than 25% of patients expected to be failure free at 3 years. The addition of a variety of agents including doxorubicin, cisplatin and etoposide to standard VAC therapy have failed to significantly improve the outcome of these patients. In IRSG-IV, 127 patients were treated with a variety of drug pairs, some of them identified through the xenograft model (described in Chap. 5) and using an "up-front" phase II window approach. Sixty-eight patients were treated with vincristine and melphalan followed by VAC, and 59 received ifosfamide and etoposide followed by VAC. Despite similar response rates for both regimens, the 3-year progression-free survival and survival rates were significantly better for patients who received ifosfamide and etoposide (33% vs. 19% and 55% and 27% respectively), likely resulting from the inability to deliver adequate cyclophosphamide doses after initial melphalan administration. Other drugs recently tested by the IRSG have included topotecan, cyclophosphamide in combination with topotecan and ifosfamide in combination with doxorubicin. Although the response rates to these agent (s) have been promising, the survival of responding patients has not been significantly improved (Pappo et al. 2001; Sandler et al. 2001; Walterhouse et al. 2004).

6.9 Management of Specific Tumor Sites

6.9.1 Parameningeal Tumors (Raney 2002, Michalski 2004)

Patients with parameningeal tumors account for approximately 16% of cases of rhabdomyosarcoma. In IRSG-I, 35% of patients with Group III and IV tumors experienced direct meningeal extension either at the time of study entry or within 12 months of diagnosis, and 90% of these patients died of their disease (Tefft et al. 1978). These findings prompted changes in IRSG-II including prompt initiation of radiotherapy after diagnosis for patients who presented with high risk features such as cranial nerve palsy, base of skull erosion or intracranial extension. In addition, these patients received whole spine radiotherapy at week 6 and triple intrathecal medications from weeks 0 to 78. These treatment modifications improved the 5-year survival of these patients from 47% in IRSG-I to 67% in IRSG-II. Unfortunately, the repetitive and extensive use of triple intrathecal medications was associated with a 3.4% risk of developing ascending myelitis (Raney et al. 1992). Evolving therapeutic modifications for these patients have included the elimination of spinal radiotherapy, and intrathecal medications, and limiting whole brain radiotherapy for patients who present with high risk features such as intracranial extension. These changes have not adversely influenced the outcome of these patients (Crist et al. 1995). More recently, in IRSG-IV, elimination of whole brain radiotherapy and intrathecal medications for all patients with parameningeal rhabdomyosarcoma has produced similar excellent results (3 year FFS 72%) and limited central nervous system failure rates (7%) similar to those observed in IRSG-III (Raney et al. 2002). Current treatment recommendations for patients with parameningeal tumors include the use of a three-drug regimen that incorporates and alkylating agent and administration of radiotherapy to the primary tumor. Early radiation therapy (within 2 weeks of diagnosis) is associated with a significant decrease in local failure in patients with meningeal impingement (18% vs. 33%) and intracranial extension (16% vs. 37%). Radiation doses above 47.5 Gy are required for optimal local tumor control in patients with larger tumors (≥5 cm) (Michalski et al. 2004).

6.9.2 Orbital Tumors (Maurer et al. 1988, 1993; Crist et al. 1995, 2001; Oberlin et al. 2001)

The median age of patients with orbital rhabdomyosarcoma is 6.8 years, and embryonal histology accounts for the majority of cases (87%). Patients with primary tumors in the orbit faired well in IRSG-

I and II with 89% and 92% of the patients respectively being long term survivors. For this reason, patients enrolled in IRSG-III were excluded from treatment randomizations and were treated with VA plus radiotherapy for 1 year. The outcome of these patients showed a survival rate of 91%, a similar result to that observed in IRSG-II when patients were treated with more intense therapies. In IRSG-IV, patients with Group I–II disease were also treated with VA therapy with an associated 3-year failure-free survival and survival rate of 89% and 100% respectively. Patients with Group III disease were randomized to receive VAC, VIE or VAI. The failure-free survival rate was slightly improved for these patients when compared to those treated in IRSG-III (92% vs. 81%), but survival remained essentially unchanged (100% vs. 96). Because of similar survival rates, patients in IRSG-V continued to be treated with intensified VA. However, for the upcoming IRSG trial, patients with orbital tumors will receive low dose of cyclophosphamide in combination with VA in an attempt to improve the failure-free survival.

6.9.3 Head and Neck Non-Orbital, Non-Parameningeal Tumors (Pappo et al. 2003)

A review of 164 patients whose primary tumors arose in the non-orbital, non-parameningeal head and neck area and who were envolved in IRSG-III and IV revealed that the median age of these patients was 5 years and that two-thirds were between 1 and 9 years of age. The most common primary tumor sites were the cheek, followed by the neck, the parotid area, and the oral cavity. The majority of patients (76%) had Group II or III disease and most of the tumors were of embryonal histology. Lymphatic involvement was present in 20% of the cases. The estimated 5-year failure-free survival and survival for all patients was 76% and 83% respectively.

The relatively good prognosis of patients with non-parameningeal non-orbital head and neck tumors was first recognized in IRSG-I (5-year survival 74%). In IRSG-II the overall outcome of these patients increased to 81% and, given their relatively good prognosis, patients with Group II/III primary head tumors were excluded from randomization in IRSG-III and were treated with VA therapy. Patients with neck primary tumors were treated more aggressively. In planning for IRSG-IV, the committee determined that the results of the first three trials were similar and therefore opted to incorporate an alkylating agent into the standard VA backbone therapy. In this study, patients with primary tumors of the neck fared as well as other patients. Only the 5-year failure-free survival was significantly improved in IRSG-IV when compared to IRSG-III and this difference was most evident among patients who presented with clinical Group I and II disease. For patients with alveolar and undifferentiated tumors there was no difference in outcome. Failure-free survival was significantly influenced by the age of the patient, with those under the age of 1 faring significantly worse than those aged 1–9 years of age or those older than 10 years of age. The current IRSG trial incorporates VA therapy for Group I/II patients and VAC therapy for those with Group II N1 and III disease (Table 6.5). The upcoming IRSG trial will incorporate low doses of cyclophosphamide for all patients in an attempt to maintain the promising failure-free survival rates observed in IRSG-IV.

6.9.4 Parotid Tumors (Walterhouse et al. 2001)

Rhabdomyosarcoma arising in the parotid gland accounts for 1.5% of all cases of rhabdomyosarcoma. All patients present with a palpable mass in the parotid region and its presence can be confused with an infectious process. The age at diagnosis is usually 6 years and approximately half have parameningeal extension. Over three-fourths of the patients have embryonal histology tumors. The 5-year event-free survival and survival for these patients is approximately 81% and 84% respectively. The outcome is not influenced by the presence or absence of parameningeal extension; however, those with parameningeal extension were treated more intensively with three drugs and therefore this treatment approach is recommended for such patients. Patients with Group III disease may also benefit from the addition of an alkylating agent since most of these patients were cured with a three-drug therapy in a review of patients enrolled in the four IRSG trials.

6.9.5 Extremity Tumors (Neville 2000, Christ 1995)

Approximately 20% of children with rhabdomyosarcoma present with tumors located in the extremities. The lower extremities are more commonly affected, nearly 50% of these patients have Group I and II disease and over two-thirds have alveolar histology (Neville et al. 2000). Among surgically evaluated patients in IRSG-III and IV, nearly 50% had regional nodal involvement. The final report of the IRSG-I trial demonstrated that patients with Group I and II alveolar extremity tumors had a poorer survival when compared to patients with tumors in other sites; therefore, the prescribed therapy for such patients in IRSG-II was more intense and used repetitive pulse VAC chemotherapy for 2 years (Heyn et al. 1989). This change in therapy boosted 3-year survival rates from 57% to 77% (Heyn et al. 1989). Intensification of therapy in IRSG-III with a regimen comprising VADRAC and cisplatin further improved the survival of these patients (5-year survival of 80%) (Crist et al. 1995). In IRSG-IV, patients with Group I–IV extremity tumors were randomized to receive VAC vs. VAI or VIE. Their outcome was similar to that reported in previous trials. The current IRSG trial incorporates a randomization between VAC and VAC alternating with vincristine, topotecan, and cyclophosphamide (VTC) in an attempt to improve the outcome of these patients.

6.9.6 Paratesticular Rhabdomyosarcoma (Raney et al. 1987; Wiener et al. 2001)

Paratesticular rhabdomyosarcoma accounts for approximately 7% of all rhabdomyosarcomas. Over 95% of these patients have embryonal tumors and over half of them have tumors that measure more than 5 cm. The majority of patients present with localized disease (Group I disease). The median age at diagnosis of these patients is approximately 6 years. A relatively good prognosis of patients with this primary site was recognized in IRSG-I and IRSG-II with an estimated survival of 89% at 3 years. Protocol mandated investigations in IRSG-III specified surgical evaluation of retroperitoneal lymph nodes; however, those who were enrolled in IRSG-IV were only required to have clinical evaluation by computed tomography. Among 234 patients enrolled in IRSG-III and IRSG-IV, a significant shift in the staging of Group I and II patients was noted (68% of patients had clinically documented Group I disease in IRSG-III vs. 82% in IRSG-IV). This change in frequency was attributed to a higher rate of nodal involvement in IRSG-III vs. IRSG-IV (23% vs. 7%). Patients 10 years of age or older were more likely to have retroperitoneal lymph node involvement in IRSG-III (14% vs. 47%), but these numbers decreased to 4% and 13% in IRSG-IV due to the fact that routine nodal sampling was not required in this protocol. The outcome between patients enrolled in IRSG-III and IV was similar with 3-year survival estimates for Group I and II disease of 96% vs. 92% in IRSG-III and IV respectively and with failure-free survival rates of 90% and 96% respectively (Wiener et al. 2001). However, a slightly higher regional failure was seen in patients in IRSG-IV, presumably as a consequence of omitting radiation therapy in patients who were missed by clinical staging and were actually node positive. Patients treated in IRSG-IV who were treated with three-drug therapy and who were truly Group II had a superior failure-free survival (100%) when compared to patients who were treated with two drugs in IRSG-III. The results of this analysis suggest that retroperitoneal node dissection should be routinely recommended for patients who are 10 years of age or older and that patients with Group II disease should receive intensified therapy with three drugs.

6.9.7 Female Genital Tract Tumors (Arndt et al. 2001)

Rhabdomyosarcoma of the female genital tract (vulva, vagina, uterus or cervix) is rare, accounting for 3.5% of all rhabdomyosarcomas. The vagina is the most commonly affected site followed by the uterus and cervix, and the majority of patients present with clinical Group III disease (65%). The mean age at diagnosis is 5.2 years, and approximately 52% of patients have tumors of botryoid histology. Most of the patients who present with vaginal or uterine lesions are younger than 10 years of age whereas those that have lesions of the vulva and cervix are usually older. Furthermore, patients with tumors of the vulva and cervix more often have resected tumors when compared to patients who present with tumors in the uterus or vagina. The outcome for these patients is excellent with the estimated 5-year overall survival of 82%. The majority of failures are local or locoregional and most of these are seen in patients with clinical Group III and IV disease. Fortunately, over two-thirds of patients who present with non-metastatic disease and fail therapy can be salvaged with aggressive second line therapies. Patients between the ages of 1 and 9 years had an improved outcome when compared to younger or older children. Those with botryoid tumors have an improved 5-year survival when compared to patients with embryonal tumors. A uterine primary is associated with an inferior outcome when compared to other sites and this finding could be in part explained by the high incidence of reported toxic deaths among this group of patients. Therapy on the most recent protocols (IRSG-III and IV) significantly benefited patients who are less than 1 year of age or over 10 years of age. Furthermore, the use of primary intensive chemotherapy in the most recent trials has produced a significant reduction in the rates of hysterectomies and vaginectomies. However, the use of radiotherapy has also increased in recent trials from approximately 23% in IRSG-II to 43% in IRSG-IV. This finding is a reflection of increased efforts to avoid the use of aggressive surgery. Only 20% of patients in the IRSG trials were cured without the use of local therapies. Current recommendations include the use of VAC chemotherapy for the majority of patients who have clinical Group III disease (Table 6.5). Local therapy should be individualized but early local regional therapy is indicated for patients with uterine, cervical and vulvar tumors. The current approach in IRSG-V is to reserve the use of local therapies such as radiotherapy for vaginal tumors only if tumor persists after 20 weeks of therapy and if residual disease is not completely resected with negative margins. Patients with Group III uterine tumors should be evaluated for resection or hysterectomy at week 12 and the addition of radiotherapy is recommended for those patients with nodal, microscopic, or gross residual disease. Patients with vulvar lesions should receive radiotherapy at week 3 for Group II tumors and at week 12 for Group III tumors.

6.9.8 Bladder and Prostate Rhabdomyosarcoma (Hays et al. 1982; Raney et al. 1990b; Heyn et al. 1997; Arndt et al. 2004a)

These sites account for approximately 10% of all rhabdomyosarcomas. The majority of these patients are between the ages of 1 and 9 years, present with Group III disease, and most have embryonal histology tumors. The bladder is affected more commonly than the prostate. In the past, a significant number of patients were treated with radical surgical procedures such as pelvic exoneration. However, increased awareness of the chemosensitivity of these tumors drastically reduced the rates for this procedure from 44% in IRSG-I to 4% in IRSG-II. The use of conservative delayed surgery and primary chemotherapy was explored in IRSG-II, producing inferior disease-free survival rates but similar survival and bladder preservation rates (about 20%) than those reported in IRSG-I. In IRSG-III, all patients received intensified chemotherapy with VAC/VADRC (doxorubicin) plus cisplatin followed by second look surgery at week 20, and alternate induction chemotherapy for patients with residual tumor improved the complete response to 81% and survival rates to 83%. Furthermore, there was more than a twofold improvement in the bladder salvage rate from 25% to 60%. In IRSG IV, most patients with bladder/prostate tumors fell into the category of Group III disease or in one of three regimens that incorporate an alkylating agent as prescribed before. Radiotherapy was given according to their group; those with stage II disease and Group I disease initially received radiotherapy, with patients with stage III Group I disease and outpatients with residual microscopic disease receiving 41.4 Gy and patients with gross residual tumors receiving 50.4 Gy. In this analysis, only a small percentage of patients underwent an initial partial cystectomy. Among 66 event-free survivors, 55 retained their bladder and 36 had normal bladder function. Among all study patients 40% were event free with normal function in bladders. Current local control recommendations in these patients include an evaluation in week 12 to determine the respectability of these patients with negative margins. All patients who are Group III at diagnosis receive radiotherapy ranging from 36 Gy to 50.4 Gy depending on the margin status. Only those who are biopsied or undergo surgical procedures can have their radiotherapy modified.

6.10 Other Sites

6.10.1 Biliary Tract Tumors

Biliary tract rhabdomyosarcoma accounts for 0.5% of all rhabdomyosarcomas (Spunt et al. 2000). The majority of these patients are young (median age 3.4 years) and have large tumors. Gross surgical resection at diagnosis was feasible in only 24% of patients. The outcome of these patients when treated with combined modality therapy and avoidance of extensive surgical resection is excellent; 13 or 14 patients with gross residual disease who survive the early postoperative period remain disease free (Spunt et al. 2000). These results emphasize that the role of surgery in these patients should be limited to establishing the diagnosis and assessing the extent of disease. Since multimodal therapy will achieve cure in the majority of these children, the IRSG committee has reclassified these tumors as low risk.

6.10.2 Perineal and Perianal Rhabdomyosarcoma (Blakely et al. 2003)

This anatomic site accounts for approximately 2% of cases of rhabdomyosarcoma. The median age at diagnosis is 6 years and nearly two-thirds of children present with advanced stage disease (clinical Group III and IV disease) and alveolar or undifferentiated tumors (Raney et al. 1990a). Half of the patients have nodal involvement. The estimated 5-year failure-free survival and survival for all patients enrolled in IRSG-I–IV was 45% and 49% respectively. The outcome for these patients has not significantly changed over time. Patients with clinical Group I and II, lower stage, negative nodes, and age under 10 years have a significant survival advantage. This group might benefit from routine evaluation of ilioinguinal nodes and intensified therapies. Very aggressive surgery is not indicated given the critical adjacent structures located in the anatomic location.

6.10.3 Pelvic and Retroperitoneal Rhabdomyosarcoma (Blakely et al. 1999; Raney et al. 2004)

Rhabdomyosarcoma of the non-genitourinary pelvis and retroperitoneum is relatively rare, accounting for approximately 5–6% of all rhabdomyosarcomas. The majority of patients present with advanced stage disease and up to a third may have metastases at the time of diagnosis. Results of IRSG-I and II revealed that the median age at presentation is approximately 6 years. And two-thirds of tumors had embryonal histology. For patients with Group III and IV disease the overall 5-year survival is 60%. Resection of more than 50% of the tumor at the time of initial diagnosis or debulking surgery appears to improve outcome in these patients.

6.11 Acute and Long Term Effects of Therapy

The use of intensified chemotherapy and local therapeutic approaches has improved the outcome of patients with rhabdomyosarcoma; however, these therapeutic interventions have produced significant acute and long-term side effects.

The administration of dose intensified chemotherapy has been associated with a toxic death rate as high as 12 (regimen 37a of IRSG III) (Crist et al. 1995), and intensification of alkylating agents without the use of growth factor support in an IRS-IV pilot was associated with a toxic death rate of 9% (Ruymann et al. 1995). Other toxicities reported in IRSG trials have included adult respiratory distress syndrome, cardiac toxicity, radiotherapy associated toxicity, metabolic complications and bleeding secondary to thrombocytopenia. Over 90% of patients treated with VAC chemotherapy experience significant myelosuppression and 55% have developed infectious complications. Renal toxicity secondary to administration of ifosfamide has been reported in approximately 2% of patients (Crist et al. 2001).

The administration of high doses of cyclophosphamide in combination with vincristine and actinomycin has been linked to the development of hepatopathy and thrombocytopenia in approximately 6% of patients. The majority of these events were seen in patients younger than 3 years of age (14% vs. 4%) and occurred during the first 12 weeks of therapy. Death was recorded in 4 of the 18 cases, 3 of whom were younger than 3 years of age (Arndt et al. 2004b). Age-appropriate dose modifications have been instituted in current protocols in an attempt to decrease the incidence of this complication.

The estimated cumulative incidence at 20 years for the development of second malignant neoplasms after therapy for rhabdomyosarcoma in IRS-I–IV is 3.5% (Spunt et al. 2001b). The median age at the time of the diagnosis of rhabdomyosarcoma was 5 years and the median time for the development of a second malignancy was 5.5 years. Twenty-seven of the 67 malignancies (40%) were leukemias and lymphomas, 27 (40%) were soft tissue and bone sarcomas (most commonly osteosarcoma) and 13 were due to other various cancers. The estimated 5-year survival after the development of a second malignancy was only 20%. The median time for the development of secondary leukemias was shorter than that of solid tumors (3.4 years vs. 9 years) and the administration of a melphalan-containing regimen was associated with a very high incidence of secondary leukemias. Protocol modifications including the avoidance of etoposide and melphalan and the administration of doses of radiotherapy based on initial tumor response are expected to decrease the incidence of this devastating complication.

A retrospective study examined the incidence of late events in children who survived 5 years event free and who were enrolled in IRSG-III, IV pilot and IV. In this study, the estimated 10-year rate for developing a late event (defined as second cancer, relapse, or death from other cause) was 9%. Nearly half (46%) of the late events were due to relapse and one-third (35%) were due to second malignancies. Patients with Group III/IV tumors and those with large primary tumors had a higher risk (19%) of a late event than those with limited disease (clinical Group I and II disease) and small tumors (3%) (Sung et al. 2004b).

Although eye preservation is possible in over 85% of patients with orbital rhabdomyosarcoma, 82% of patients developed cataracts, 70% had reduced vision of the affected eye, 59% had orbital hypoplasia and about one-fourth of patients have problems with keratitis, dry eyes, or conjunctivitis. Statural growth was affected in 24% of patients who were irradiated (Raney et al. 2000). Two complications, orbital hypoplasia and cataracts, were more frequently reported in IRSG trials when compared to European trials in which 50% of patients did not receive radiotherapy (Oberlin et al. 2001).

Among 213 long term survivors of head and neck rhabdomyosarcoma who were treated in the IRS-II and III trials, 77% developed one or more complications after completion of therapy (Raney et al. 1999). Nearly half of the patients under the age of 15 years failed to maintain their height velocity and 19% were receiving growth hormone replacements. Other complications included hypoplasia and asymmetry of the irradiated tissues (35%), poor dentition (29%), impaired vision secondary to cataracts (17%), corneal changes and optic atrophy, decreased hearing acuity (17%) and learning disabilities (16%).

Following initial staging laparotomy, approximately 12% of patients with paratesticular rhabdomyosarcoma developed bowel obstruction. A small proportion of patients also developed a hydrocele, lymphedema, or antegrade ejaculatory problems (Heyn et al. 1992). Following radiotherapy, a small proportion of patients developed chronic diarrhea, bone or soft tissue hypoplasia, and urethral strictures. Among patients who were treated with cyclophosphamide, one-third developed hemorrhagic cystitis and over half had elevated follicle stimulating hormone levels or azoospermia (Heyn et al. 1992).

Satisfactory bladder function was found to be present in 73% of patients who retained their bladders as a consequence of bladder and prostate rhabdomyosarcoma and who were treated in IRSG-I and II (Raney et al. 1993). Nearly one-third of patients who had follow-up renal imaging studies had a structural abnormality, most commonly hydronephrosis.

Abnormalities of irradiated bone and bowel were infrequently observed and approximately 10% of patients had significant growth deceleration. In IRSG-IV, bladder function was preserved in 55% of patients who survived event free (Arndt et al. 2004a).

6.12 Future Directions

The lack of improvements in survival among patients with metastatic disease and in selected patients with localized disease has stimulated the search for more effective therapies for these patients. The Intergroup Rhabdomyosarcoma Study Group has conducted several pilot trials using promising drug pairs for the treatment of high-risk rhabdomyosarcoma. These agents have been selected by their mechanism of action and anti-tumor activity profile in tumor cell lines. In addition, in an attempt to circumvent the problem of drug resistance seen in multiply relapsed patients, promising drugs identified through the xenograft model (see Chap. 5) have been administered "up-front" to previously untreated patients. Some of the drug pairs that have been tested in a series of IRSG pilots have included the combination of vincristine and melphalan, ifosfamide and etoposide, and ifosfamide and doxorubicin (Breitfeld et al. 2001; Sandler et al. 2001). Response rates exceeding 70% at week 12 were reported for all regimens but an overall survival advantage has only been documented for the ifosfamide and etoposide pair (Breitfeld et al. 2001). The value of adding one or more of these drug pairs to standard VAC therapy in patients with high-risk metastatic disease will be prospectively tested in the upcoming IRSG trial. In recent years, given the excellent activity in preclinical models when administered in a low-dose protracted schedule, the IRSG has conducted a series of window trials with the topoisomerase I inhibitors topotecan and irinotecan (Houghton et al. 1996). Topotecan alone or when combined with cyclophosphamide produced responses in approximately 50% of untreated patients with metastatic rhabdomyosarcoma (Pappo et al. 2001; Walterhouse et al. 2004). This combination is being compared in a randomized study to standard VAC therapy (protocol D9803) in patients with intermediate risk disease. Irinotecan either alone or in combination with vincristine has also been recently evaluated by the committee with promising results (Pappo 2002). The development of a preclinical testing program as proposed by the National Cancer Institute and the Children's Oncology Group will likely facilitate identification and prioritization of agents for this disease (Houghton et al. 2002).

Other approaches aimed at improving the outcome of patients with rhabdomyosarcoma have included cyclophosphamide dose-intensification and the use of high dose therapy with stem cell support. In a trial for patients with intermediate risk disease, cyclophosphamide doses were escalated to 4.5 g/m^2 during induction therapy without an improvement in outcome (Spunt et al. 2002). The experience with the use of high-dose therapy and end-intensification with stem cell transplantation was recently reviewed by Weigel B, Breitfeld P et al. 2001. In this review of 389 patients with rhabdomyosarcoma, this approach failed to improve survival in patients with metastatic or relapsed disease.

Other therapies under active investigation include tumor specific peptide vaccination (Dagher et al. 2002) and mTOR inhibitors (Bjornsti and Houghton 2004).

6.13 Outcome and Therapy of Relapse

The 5-year survival for patients who sustain a relapse is only 20%. Among 605 patients enrolled in IRSG-III and IV pilot who sustained a first relapse, those with botryoid tumors, stage 1 Group I embryonal tumors and Group I alveolar tumors had a relatively favorable outcome following relapse (survival of 50%) (Pappo et al. 1999). In contrast, the survival for the remaining 80% of patients who relapse is only 10%. These findings prompted the development of a multi-institutional risk-based relapse protocol which will stratify patients into favorable and unfavorable groups; those with favorable features will receive intensive multiagent chemotherapy with radiotherapy and surgery whereas those with unfavorable prognosis will receive a phase II window of vincristine and irinotecan followed by dose intensified therapy and maintenance therapy with agents such as etoposide, doxorubicin and ifosfamide.

Acknowledgements. I would like to thank Drs. Bev Raney and Jim Anderson for their helpful suggestions and critical review of the manuscript.

References

Arndt CA, Donaldson SS et al. (2001) What constitutes optimal therapy for patients with rhabdomyosarcoma of the female genital tract? Cancer 91(12):2454–2468

Arndt C, Rodeberg D et al. (2004a) Does bladder preservation (as a surgical principle) lead to retaining bladder function in bladder/prostate rhabdomyosarcoma? Results from Intergroup Rhabdomyosarcoma Study IV. J Urol 171(6):2396–2403

Arndt C, Hawkins D et al. (2004b) Age is a risk factor for chemotherapy-induced hepatopathy with vincristine, dactinomycin, and cyclophosphamide. J Clin Oncol 22(10):1894–1901

Baker KS, Anderson JR et al. (2000) Benefit of intensified therapy for patients with local or regional embryonal rhabdomyosarcoma: results from the Intergroup Rhabdomyosarcoma Study IV. J Clin Oncol 18(12):2427–2434

Barr FG, Galili N et al. (1993) Rearrangement of the PAX3 paired box gene in the paediatric solid tumour alveolar rhabdomyosarcoma. Nat Genet 3(2):113–117

Barr FG, Xiong QB et al. (1995) A consensus polymerase chain reaction-oligonucleotide hybridization approach for the detection of chromosomal translocations in pediatric bone and soft tissue sarcomas. Am J Clin Pathol 104(6):627–633

Barr FG, Nauta LE et al. (1996) In vivo amplification of the PAX3-FKHR and PAX7-FKHR fusion genes in alveolar rhabdomyosarcoma. Hum Mol Genet 5(1):15–21

Bennicelli JL, Edwards RH et al. (1996) Mechanism for transcriptional gain of function resulting from chromosomal translocation in alveolar rhabdomyosarcoma. Proc Natl Acad Sci USA 93(11):5455–5459

Bennicelli JL, Advani S et al. (1999) PAX3 and PAX7 exhibit conserved cis-acting transcription repression domains and utilize a common gain of function mechanism in alveolar rhabdomyosarcoma. Oncogene 18(30):4348–4356

Bernasconi M., Remppis A et al. (1996) Induction of apoptosis in rhabdomyosarcoma cells through down-regulation of PAX proteins. Proc Natl Acad Sci USA 93(23):13164–13169

Biegel JA, Meek RS et al. (1991) Chromosomal translocation t(1;13) (p36;q14) in a case of rhabdomyosarcoma. Genes Chromosomes Cancer 3(6):483–484

Bjornsti MA, Houghton PJ (2004) The TOR pathway: a target for cancer therapy. Nat Rev Cancer 4(5):335–348

Blakely ML, Lobe TE et al. (1999) Does debulking improve survival rate in advanced-stage retroperitoneal embryonal rhabdomyosarcoma? J Pediatr Surg 34(5):736–741

Blakely ML, Andrassy RJ et al. (2003) Prognostic factors and surgical treatment guidelines for children with rhabdomyosarcoma of the perineum or anus: a report of Intergroup Rhabdomyosarcoma Studies I through IV, 1972 through 1997. J Pediatr Surg 38(3):347–353

Breitfeld PP, Lyden E et al. (2001) Ifosfamide and etoposide are superior to vincristine and melphalan for pediatric metastatic rhabdomyosarcoma when administered with irradiation and combination chemotherapy: a report from the Intergroup Rhabdomyosarcoma Study Group. J Pediatr Hematol Oncol 23(4):225–233

Breneman JC, Lyden E et al. (2003) Prognostic factors and clinical outcomes in children and adolescents with metastatic rhabdomyosarcoma – a report from the Intergroup Rhabdomyosarcoma Study IV. J Clin Oncol 21(1):78–84

Bridge JA, Liu J et al. (2000) Novel genomic imbalances in embryonal rhabdomyosarcoma revealed by comparative genomic hybridization and fluorescence in situ hybridization: an intergroup rhabdomyosarcoma study. Genes Chromosomes Cancer 27(4):337–344

Bridge JA, Liu J et al. (2002) Genomic gains and losses are similar in genetic and histologic subsets of rhabdomyosarcoma, whereas amplification predominates in embryonal with anaplasia and alveolar subtypes. Genes Chromosomes Cancer 33(3):310–321

Crist WM, Garnsey L et al. (1990) Prognosis in children with rhabdomyosarcoma: a report of the intergroup rhabdomyosarcoma studies I and II. Intergroup Rhabdomyosarcoma Committee. J Clin Oncol 8(3):443–452

Crist W, Gehan EA et al. (1995) The Third Intergroup Rhabdomyosarcoma Study. J Clin Oncol 13(3):610–630

Crist WM, Anderson JR et al. (2001) Intergroup rhabdomyosarcoma study-IV: results for patients with nonmetastatic disease. J Clin Oncol 19(12):3091–3102

Dagher R, Long LM et al. (2002) Pilot trial of tumor-specific peptide vaccination and continuous infusion interleukin-2 in patients with recurrent Ewing sarcoma and alveolar rhabdomyosarcoma: An inter-institute NIH study. Med Pediatr Oncol 38(3):158–164

Davis RJ, Barr FG (1997) Fusion genes resulting from alternative chromosomal translocations are overexpressed by gene-specific mechanisms in alveolar rhabdomyosarcoma. Proc Natl Acad Sci USA 94(15):8047–8051

Davis RJ, D'Cruz CM et al. (1994) Fusion of PAX7 to FKHR by the variant t(1;13) (p36;q14) translocation in alveolar rhabdomyosarcoma. Cancer Res 54(11):2869–2872

DeBaun MR (2002) Screening for cancer in children with Costello syndrome. Am J Med Genet 108(1):88–90

Diller L, Sexsmith E et al. (1995) Germline p53 mutations are frequently detected in young children with rhabdomyosarcoma. J Clin Invest 95(4):1606–1611

Donaldson SS, Meza J et al. (2001) Results from the IRS-IV randomized trial of hyperfractionated radiotherapy in children with rhabdomyosarcoma – a report from the IRSG. Int J Radiat Oncol Biol Phys 51(3):718–728

Driman D, Thorner PS et al. (1994) MYCN gene amplification in rhabdomyosarcoma. Cancer 73(8):2231–2237

Epstein JA, Lam P et al. (1995) Pax3 inhibits myogenic differentiation of cultured myoblast cells. J Biol Chem 270(20): 11719–11722

Ferrari A, Casanova M et al. (2003) Rhabdomyosarcoma in infants younger than one year old: a report from the Italian Cooperative Group. Cancer 97(10):2597–2604

Flamant F, Luboinski B, Couanet D, McDowell H (1991) Rhabdomyosarcoma in children: Clinical symptoms, diagnosis, and staging. CRC Press, Boca Raton, FL

Galili N, Davis RJ et al. (1993) Fusion of a fork head domain gene to PAX3 in the solid tumour alveolar rhabdomyosarcoma. Nat Genet 5(3):230–235

Goodman KA, Wolden SL et al. (2003) Intraoperative high-dose-rate brachytherapy for pediatric solid tumors: a 10-year experience. Brachytherapy 2(3):139–146

Goodrich LV, Milenkovic L et al. (1997) Altered neural cell fates and medulloblastoma in mouse patched mutants. Science 277(5329):1109–1113

Gordon AT, Brinkschmidt C et al. (2000) A novel and consistent amplicon at 13q31 associated with alveolar rhabdomyosarcoma. Genes Chromosomes Cancer 28(2):220–226

Gripp KW, Scott CI Jr et al. (2002) Five additional Costello syndrome patients with rhabdomyosarcoma: proposal for a tumor screening protocol. Am J Med Genet 108(1):80–87

Grosfeld JL, Clatworthy HW Jr, Newton WA Jr (1969) Combined therapy in childhood rhabdomyosarcoma: an analysis of 42 cases. J Pediatr Surg 4:637–645

Grufferman S, Schwartz AG et al. (1993) Parents' use of cocaine and marijuana and increased risk of rhabdomyosarcoma in their children. Cancer Causes Control 4(3):217–224

Hahn H, Wojnowski L et al. (1998) Rhabdomyosarcomas and radiation hypersensitivity in a mouse model of Gorlin syndrome. Nat Med 4(5):619–622

Hartley AL, Birch JM et al. (1993) Patterns of cancer in the families of children with soft tissue sarcoma. Cancer 72(3): 923–930

Hays DM, Raney RB Jr et al. (1982) Primary chemotherapy in the treatment of children with bladder-prostate tumors in the Intergroup Rhabdomyosarcoma Study (IRS-II) J Pediatr Surg 17(6):812–820

Hennekam RC (2003) Costello syndrome: an overview. Am J Med Genet 117C(1):42–48

Heyn RM, Holland R, Newton WA Jr, Tefft M, Breslow N, Hartmann JR (1974) The role of combined chemotherapy in the treatment of rhabdomyosarcoma in children. Cancer 34:2128–2142

Heyn R, Beltangady M et al. (1989) Results of intensive therapy in children with localized alveolar extremity rhabdomyosarcoma: a report from the Intergroup Rhabdomyosarcoma Study. J Clin Oncol 7(2):200–207

Heyn R, Raney RB Jr et al. (1992) Late effects of therapy in patients with paratesticular rhabdomyosarcoma. Intergroup Rhabdomyosarcoma Study Committee. J Clin Oncol 10(4): 614–623

Heyn R, Haeberlen V et al. (1993) Second malignant neoplasms in children treated for rhabdomyosarcoma. Intergroup Rhabdomyosarcoma Study Committee. J Clin Oncol 11(2): 262–270

Heyn R, Newton WA et al. (1997) Preservation of the bladder in patients with rhabdomyosarcoma. J.Clin Oncol 15(1):69–75

Hill DA, Dehner LP et al. (2002) Perianal rhabdomyosarcoma presenting as a perirectal abscess: A report of 11 cases. J Pediatr Surg 37(4):576–581

Houghton PJ, Stewart CF et al. (1996) Schedule-dependent efficacy of camptothecins in models of human cancer. Ann N Y Acad Sci 803:188–201

Houghton PJ, Adamson PC et al. (2002) Testing of new agents in childhood cancer preclinical models: meeting summary. Clin Cancer Res 8(12):3646–3657

Hug EB, Sweeney RA et al. (2002) Proton radiotherapy in management of pediatric base of skull tumors. Int J Radiat Oncol Biol Phys 52(4):1017–1024

Iolascon A, Faienza MF et al. (1996) Analysis of cyclin-dependent kinase inhibitor genes (CDKN2A, CDKN2B, and CDKN2C) in childhood rhabdomyosarcoma. Genes Chromosomes Cancer 15(4):217–222

Jacks T, Remington L et al. (1994) Tumor spectrum analysis in p53-mutant mice. Curr Biol 4(1):1–7

Joshi D, Anderson JR et al. (2004) Age is an independent prognostic factor in rhabdomyosarcoma: a report from the Soft Tissue Sarcoma Committee of the Children's Oncology Group. Pediatr Blood Cancer 42(1):64–73

Khan J, Bittner ML et al. (1999) cDNA microarrays detect activation of a myogenic transcription program by the PAX3-FKHR fusion oncogene. Proc Natl Acad Sci USA 96(23): 13264–13269

Khatib ZA, Matsushime H et al. (1993) Coamplification of the CDK4 gene with MDM2 and GLI in human sarcomas. Cancer Res 53(22):5535–5541

Kodet R, Newton WA Jr et al. (1993) Childhood rhabdomyosarcoma with anaplastic (pleomorphic) features. A report of the Intergroup Rhabdomyosarcoma Study. Am J Surg Pathol 17(5):443–453

Koi M, Johnson LA et al. (1993) Tumor cell growth arrest caused by subchromosomal transferable DNA fragments from chromosome 11. Science 260(5106):361–364

Koufos A, Hansen MF et al. (1985) Loss of heterozygosity in three embryonal tumours suggests a common pathogenetic mechanism. Nature 316(6026):330–334

Kuttesch JF Jr, Wexler LH et al. (1996) Second malignancies after Ewing's sarcoma: radiation dose-dependency of secondary sarcomas. J Clin Oncol 14(10):2818–2825

Lam PY, Sublett JE et al. (1999) The oncogenic potential of the Pax3-FKHR fusion protein requires the Pax3 homeodomain recognition helix but not the Pax3 paired-box DNA binding domain. Mol Cell Biol 19(1):594–601

Lavigueur A, Maltby V et al. (1989) High incidence of lung, bone, and lymphoid tumors in transgenic mice overexpressing mutant alleles of the p53 oncogene. Mol Cell Biol 9(9):3982–3991

Lawrence W Jr, Jegge G, Foote FW Jr (1964) Embryonal rhabdomyosarcoma. A clinicopathologic study. Cancer 17:361–376

Lawrence W Jr, Gehan EA et al. (1987) Prognostic significance of staging factors of the UICC staging system in childhood rhabdomyosarcoma: a report from the Intergroup Rhabdomyosarcoma Study (IRS-II). J Clin Oncol 5(1):46–54

Lawrence W Jr, Anderson JR et al. (1997) Pretreatment TNM staging of childhood rhabdomyosarcoma: a report of the Intergroup Rhabdomyosarcoma Study Group. Children's Cancer Study Group. Pediatric Oncology Group. Cancer 80(6):1165–1170

Loh WE Jr, Scrable HJ et al. (1992) Human chromosome 11 contains two different growth suppressor genes for embryonal rhabdomyosarcoma. Proc Natl Acad Sci USA 89(5): 1755–1759

Malkin D, Li FP et al. (1990) Germ line p53 mutations in a familial syndrome of breast cancer, sarcomas, and other neoplasms. Science 250(4985):1233–1238

Maurer HM, Beltangady M et al. (1988) The Intergroup Rhabdomyosarcoma Study-I. A final report. Cancer 61(2): 209–220

Maurer HM, Gehan EA et al. (1993) The Intergroup Rhabdomyosarcoma Study-II. Cancer 71(5):1904–1922

Michalski JM, Sur RK et al. (1995) Three dimensional conformal radiation therapy in pediatric parameningeal rhabdomyosarcomas. Int J Radiat Oncol Biol Phys 33(5):985–991

Michalski JM, Meza J et al. (2004) Influence of radiation therapy parameters on outcome in children treated with radiation therapy for localized parameningeal rhabdomyosarcoma in Intergroup Rhabdomyosarcoma Study Group trials II through IV. Int J Radiat Oncol Biol Phys 59(4):1027–1038

Moutou C, Le Bihan C et al. (1996) Genetic transmission of susceptibility to cancer in families of children with soft tissue sarcomas. Cancer 78(7):1483–1491

Nanni P, Nicoletti G et al. (2003) Development of rhabdomyosarcoma in HER-2/neu transgenic p53 mutant mice. Cancer Res 63(11):2728–2732

Neville HL, Andrassy RJ et al. (2000) Preoperative staging, prognostic factors, and outcome for extremity rhabdomyosarcoma: a preliminary report from the Intergroup Rhabdomyosarcoma Study IV (1991–1997). J Pediatr Surg 35(2):317–321

Newton WA Jr, Gehan EA et al. (1995) Classification of rhabdomyosarcomas and related sarcomas. Pathologic aspects and proposal for a new classification – an Intergroup Rhabdomyosarcoma Study. Cancer 76(6):1073–1085

Oberlin O, Rey A et al. (2001) Treatment of orbital rhabdomyosarcoma: survival and late effects of treatment – results of an international workshop. J Clin Oncol 19(1): 197–204

Olivier M, Goldgar DE et al. (2003) Li-Fraumeni and related syndromes: correlation between tumor type, family structure, and TP53 genotype. Cancer Res 63(20):6643–6650

Pappo AS, Crist WM et al. (1993) Tumor-cell DNA content predicts outcome in children and adolescents with clinical group III embryonal rhabdomyosarcoma. The Intergroup Rhabdomyosarcoma Study Committee of the Children's Cancer Group and the Pediatric Oncology Group. J Clin Oncol 11(10):1901–1905

Pappo AS, Shapiro DN et al. (1995) Biology and therapy of pediatric rhabdomyosarcoma. J Clin Oncol 13(8):2123–2139

Pappo AS, Anderson JR et al. (1999) Survival after relapse in children and adolescents with rhabdomyosarcoma: A report from the Intergroup Rhabdomyosarcoma Study Group. J Clin Oncol 17(11):3487–3493

Pappo AS, Lyden E et al. (2001) Up-front window trial of topotecan in previously untreated children and adolescents with metastatic rhabdomyosarcoma: an intergroup rhabdomyosarcoma study. J Clin Oncol 19(1):213–219

Pappo AS, Lyden E, Breitfeld PP, Houghton P, Parham D, Donaldson SS, Meyer W, Crist W (2002) Irinotecan (CPT-11) is active against pediatric rhabdomyosarcoma (RMS): a phase II window trial from the Soft Tissue Sarcoma Committee (STS) of the Children's Oncology Group (COG). American Society of Clinical Oncology, Orlando, FL

Pappo AS, Meza JL et al. (2003) Treatment of localized nonorbital, nonparameningeal head and neck rhabdomyosarcoma: lessons learned from intergroup rhabdomyosarcoma studies III and IV. J Clin Oncol 21(4):638–645

Peydro-Olaya A, Llombart-Bosch A et al. (2003) Electron microscopy and other ancillary techniques in the diagnosis of small round cell tumors. Semin Diagn Pathol 20(1):25–45

Pinkel D, Pickren J (1961) Rhabdomyosarcoma in children. JAMA 175:293–298

Porterfield JF, Zimmerman LE (1962) Rhabdomyosarcoma of the orbit. A clinicopathologic study of 55 cases. Virchows Arch Path Anat 335:329–344

Pratt CB (1969) Response of childhood rhabdomyosarcoma to combination chemotherapy. J Pediatr 74:791–794

Pratt CB, Hustu HO, Fleming ID, Pinkel D (1972) Coordinated treatment of childhood rhabdomyosarcoma with surgery, radiotherapy, and combination chemotherapy. Cancer Res 32:606–610

Qualman SJ, Coffin CM et al. (1998) Intergroup Rhabdomyosarcoma Study: update for pathologists. Pediatr Dev Pathol 1(6):550–561

Raney RB Jr, Tefft M et al. (1987) Paratesticular sarcoma in childhood and adolescence. A report from the Intergroup Rhabdomyosarcoma Studies I and II, 1973–1983. Cancer 60(9):2337–2343

Raney RB Jr, Crist W et al. (1990a) Soft tissue sarcoma of the perineal region in childhood. A report from the Intergroup Rhabdomyosarcoma Studies I and II, 1972 through 1984. Cancer 65(12):2787–2792

Raney RB Jr, Gehan EA et al. (1990b) Primary chemotherapy with or without radiation therapy and/or surgery for children with localized sarcoma of the bladder, prostate, vagina, uterus, and cervix. A comparison of the results in Intergroup Rhabdomyosarcoma Studies I and II. Cancer 66(10): 2072–2081

Raney B, Tefft M et al. (1992) Ascending myelitis after intensive chemotherapy and radiation therapy in children with cranial parameningeal sarcoma. Cancer 69(6):1498–1506

Raney B Jr, Heyn R et al. (1993) Sequelae of treatment in 109 patients followed for 5 to 15 years after diagnosis of sarcoma of the bladder and prostate. A report from the Intergroup Rhabdomyosarcoma Study Committee. Cancer 71(7):2387–2394

Raney RB, Asmar L et al. (1999) Late complications of therapy in 213 children with localized, nonorbital soft-tissue sarcoma of the head and neck: A descriptive report from the Intergroup Rhabdomyosarcoma Studies (IRS)–II and –III. IRS Group of the Children's Cancer Group and the Pediatric Oncology Group. Med Pediatr Oncol 33(4):362–371

Raney RB, Anderson JR et al. (2000) Late effects of therapy in 94 patients with localized rhabdomyosarcoma of the orbit: Report from the Intergroup Rhabdomyosarcoma Study (IRS)–III, 1984–1991. Med Pediatr Oncol 34(6):413–420

Raney RB, Anderson JR et al. (2001) Rhabdomyosarcoma and undifferentiated sarcoma in the first two decades of life: a selective review of intergroup rhabdomyosarcoma study group experience and rationale for Intergroup Rhabdomyosarcoma Study V. J Pediatr Hematol Oncol 23(4): 215–220

Raney RB, Meza J et al. (2002) Treatment of children and adolescents with localized parameningeal sarcoma: experience of the Intergroup Rhabdomyosarcoma Study Group protocols IRS-II through -IV, 1978–1997. Med Pediatr Oncol 38(1):22–32

Raney RB, Stoner JA et al. (2004) Results of treatment of fifty-six patients with localized retroperitoneal and pelvic rhabdomyosarcoma: a report from The Intergroup Rhabdomyosarcoma Study-IV, 1991–1997. Pediatr Blood Cancer 42(7):618–625

Ries LA, Smith MA et al. (1999) Cancer incidence and survival among children and adolescents: United States SEER Program 1975–1995. SEER program Pub No 99–4649. National Cancer Institute, Bethesda, MD

Ruymann FB, Maddux HR et al. (1988) Congenital anomalies associated with rhabdomyosarcoma: an autopsy study of 115 cases. A report from the Intergroup Rhabdomyosarcoma Study Committee (representing the Children's Cancer Study Group, the Pediatric Oncology Group, the United Kingdom Children's Cancer Study Group, and the Pediatric Intergroup Statistical Center). Med Pediatr Oncol 16(1): 33–39

Ruymann FB, Vietti T et al. (1995) Cyclophosphamide dose escalation in combination with vincristine and actinomycin-D (VAC) in gross residual sarcoma. A pilot study without hematopoietic growth factor support evaluating toxicity and response. J Pediatr Hematol Oncol 17(4):331–337

Ruymann FGS (1991) Introduction and epidemiology of soft tissue sarcomas. CRC Press, Boca Raton, FL

Sandler E, Lyden E et al. (2001) Efficacy of ifosfamide and doxorubicin given as a phase II "window" in children with newly diagnosed metastatic rhabdomyosarcoma: a report from the Intergroup Rhabdomyosarcoma Study Group. Med Pediatr Oncol 37(5):442–448

Scheidler S, Fredericks WJ et al. (1996) The hybrid PAX3-FKHR fusion protein of alveolar rhabdomyosarcoma transforms fibroblasts in culture. Proc Natl Acad Sci USA 93(18): 9805–9809

Schuck A, Mattke AC et al. (2004) Group II rhabdomyosarcoma and rhabdomyosarcomalike tumors: is radiotherapy necessary? J Clin Oncol 22(1):143–149

Scrable HJ, Witte DP et al. (1987) Chromosomal localization of the human rhabdomyosarcoma locus by mitotic recombination mapping. Nature 329(6140):645–647

Scrable H, Cavenee W et al. (1989) A model for embryonal rhabdomyosarcoma tumorigenesis that involves genome imprinting. Proc Natl Acad Sci USA 86(19):7480–7484

Sebire NJ, Malone M (2003) Myogenin and MyoD1 expression in paediatric rhabdomyosarcomas. J Clin Pathol 56(6):412–416

Sharp R, Recio JA et al. (2002) Synergism between INK4a/ARF inactivation and aberrant HGF/SF signaling in rhabdomyosarcomagenesis. Nat Med 8(11):1276–1280

Smith AC, Squire JA et al. (2001a) Association of alveolar rhabdomyosarcoma with the Beckwith-Wiedemann syndrome. Pediatr Dev Pathol 4(6):550–558

Smith LM, Anderson JR et al. (2001b) Which patients with microscopic disease and rhabdomyosarcoma experience relapse after therapy? A report from the soft tissue sarcoma committee of the children's oncology group. J Clin Oncol 19(20):4058–4064

Sorensen PH, Lynch JC et al. (2002) PAX3-FKHR and PAX7-FKHR gene fusions are prognostic indicators in alveolar rhabdomyosarcoma: a report from the children's oncology group. J Clin Oncol 20(11):2672–2679

Soule EH, Mahour GH, Mills SD, Lynn HB (1968) Soft tissue sarcomas of infants and children: A clinicopathologic study of 135 cases. Mayo Clinic Proc 43:313–326

Spunt SL, Lobe TE, et al. (2000) Aggressive surgery is unwarranted for biliary tract rhabdomyosarcoma. J Pediatr Surg 35(2):309–316

Spunt SL, Anderson JR et al. (2001a) Routine brain imaging is unwarranted in asymptomatic patients with rhabdomyosarcoma arising outside of the head and neck region that is metastatic at diagnosis: a report from the Intergroup Rhabdomyosarcoma Study Group. Cancer 92(1):121–125

Spunt SL, Meza JL, Anderson JR, Donaldson SS, Qualman SJ, Robison LL, Ruymann FB, Crist WM, Pappo AS (2001b) Second malignant neoplasms (SMN) in children treated for rhabdomyosarcoma: A report from the Intergroup Rhabdomyosarcoma Studies (IRS) I–IV. Proceedings of the American Society of Clinical Oncology, San Francsico, CA

Spunt SL, Smith LM, Ruymann FB, Qualman SJ, Donaldson SS, Rodeberg DA, Anderson JR, Crist WM, Link MP (2002) Cyclophosphamide dose intensification during induction therapy is feasible but does not appear to improve the outcome of children and adolescents with intermediate risk rhabdomyosarcoma (RMS): a report from the Children's Oncology Group Soft Tissue Sarcoma Committee D9502 Study. American Society of Clinical Oncology, Orlando, FL

Stratton MR, Fisher C et al. (1989) Detection of point mutations in N-ras and K-ras genes of human embryonal rhabdomyosarcomas using oligonucleotide probes and the polymerase chain reaction. Cancer Res 49(22):6324–6327

Sung L, Anderson JR, Arndt C, Raney B, Meyer WH, Pappo AS (2004a) Neurofibromatosis in children with rhabdomyosarcoma: A report from the intergroup rhabdomyosarcoma study IV. J Pediatr 144(5):666–668

Sung L, Anderson JR et al. (2004b) Late events occurring five years or more after successful therapy for childhood rhabdomyosarcoma: a report from the Soft Tissue Sarcoma Committee of the Children's Oncology Group. Eur J Cancer 40(12):1878–1885

Sutow WW, Berry DH, Haddy TB, Sullivan MP, Watkins WL, Windmiller J (1966) Vincristine sulfate therapy in children with metastatic soft tissue sarcoma. Pediatrics 38:465–472

Takayama H, LaRochelle WJ et al. (1997) Diverse tumorigenesis associated with aberrant development in mice overexpressing hepatocyte growth factor/scatter factor. Proc Natl Acad Sci USA 94(2):701–706

Taylor AC, Shu L et al. (2000) P53 mutation and MDM2 amplification frequency in pediatric rhabdomyosarcoma tumors and cell lines. Med Pediatr Oncol 35(2):96–103

Tefft M, Fernandez C et al. (1978) Incidence of meningeal involvement by rhabdomyosarcoma of the head and neck in children: a report of the Intergroup Rhabdomyosarcoma Study (IRS) Cancer 42(1):253–258

Turc-Carel C, Lizard-Nacol S et al. (1986) Consistent chromosomal translocation in alveolar rhabdomyosarcoma. Cancer Genet Cytogenet 19(3–4):361–362

Walterhouse DO, Pappo AS et al. (2001) Rhabdomyosarcoma of the parotid region occurring in childhood and adolescence. A report from the Intergroup Rhabdomyosarcoma Study Group. Cancer 92(12):3135–3146

Walterhouse DO, Lyden ER et al. (2004) Efficacy of topotecan and cyclophosphamide given in a phase II window trial in children with newly diagnosed metastatic rhabdomyosarcoma: a Children's Oncology Group Study. J Clin Oncol 22(8):1398–1403

Weber-Hall S, Anderson J et al. (1996) Gains, losses, and amplification of genomic material in rhabdomyosarcoma analyzed by comparative genomic hybridization. Cancer Res 56(14):3220–3224

Weksberg R, Smith AC et al. (2003) Beckwith-Wiedemann syndrome demonstrates a role for epigenetic control of normal development. Hum Mol Genet 12 Spec No 1:R61–8

Weigel B, Breitfeld P et al. (2001) Role of high dose chemotherapy with hematoporetic stem cell rescue in the treatment of metastate or recurrent rhabtomyosarcoma. J Pediatr Hematol Oncol 23(5):272–276

Wiener ES, Anderson JR et al. (2001) Controversies in the management of paratesticular rhabdomyosarcoma: is staging retroperitoneal lymph node dissection necessary for adolescents with resected paratesticular rhabdomyosarcoma? Semin Pediatr Surg 10(3):146–152

Wilbur JR (1974) Combination chemotherapy for embryonal rhabdomyosarcoma. Cancer Chemother Rep 58:281–284

Wolden SL, Anderson JR et al. (1999) Indications for radiotherapy and chemotherapy after complete resection in rhabdomyosarcoma: A report from the Intergroup Rhabdomyosarcoma Studies I to III. J Clin Oncol 17(11):3468–3475

Wolden SL, La TH et al. (2003) Long-term results of three-dimensional conformal radiation therapy for patients with rhabdomyosarcoma. Cancer 97(1):179–185

Non-Rhabdomyosarcoma Soft Tissue Sarcomas

Sheri L. Spunt, Suzanne L. Wolden, Deborah E. Schofield, Stephen X. Skapek

Contents

7.1 Epidemiology/Pathogenesis

The non-rhabdomyosarcoma soft tissue sarcomas (NRSTS) are a heterogeneous group of neoplasms of mesenchymal cell origin that occur throughout childhood and adolescence. Most are named for the mature tissue which the neoplasm most closely resembles, though these tumors often arise at sites where the mature tissue does not exist. For example, synovial sarcoma is named based on its resemblance to synovium, though it frequently arises distant from joints. Because each of the NRSTS is individually quite rare in pediatrics, little is known about their biology and natural history. There have been few prospective clinical trials in pediatric NRSTS, so most treatment and outcome data are derived from single institution retrospective studies. Published information in adults with soft tissue sarcomas contributes to our understanding of these diseases in childhood. However, the clinical behavior of certain pediatric tumors differs from the same tumor in adults. Therapeutic considerations also differ in childhood, where therapy may have an deleterious impact on normal growth and development.

This chapter focuses on the pediatric soft tissue sarcomas other than rhabdomyosarcoma, which is the most common soft tissue malignancy of childhood. Also not included in this chapter is extraosseous Ewing's sarcoma, which is described in Chap. 9.

7.1.1 Incidence

In the United States, the age-adjusted incidence of soft tissue sarcomas is approximately 11 cases per million children less than 20 years of age (Ries et al. 1999). Of these, about 40% are rhabdomyosarcoma (RMS) and 60% are NRSTS. The 500–550 children diagnosed with NRSTS each year in the United States represent about 4% of pediatric cancer cases.

In childhood, the incidence of soft tissue sarcomas is marginally higher in males than in females; blacks are affected slightly more often than whites. The incidence of soft tissue sarcoma subtypes differs significantly by age. RMS accounts for 60% of soft tissue sarcomas in children less than 5 years of age, but its relative frequency decreases in each successive 5-year age group. The NRSTS contribute to the high incidence of soft tissue sarcomas in infancy. However, their incidence declines after the first year of life and then increases progressively throughout childhood and adolescence. Among the NRSTS, the most common histologic subtypes (dermatofibrosarcoma, malignant fibrous histiocytoma, synovial sarcoma, fibrosarcoma, and malignant peripheral nerve sheath tumor) occur with increasing frequency with advancing age. Infantile fibrosarcoma and infantile hemangiopericytoma occur exclusively in children younger than 5 years of age.

7.1.2 Risk Factors

Most cases of NRSTS have no obvious cause, though certain genetic syndromes and environmental exposures are associated with the development of NRSTS. Germline mutation of the *p53* gene (Li-Fraumeni syndrome) predisposes individuals to the development of various malignancies including NRSTS and rhabdomyosarcoma, as well as osteosarcoma, breast cancer, brain tumors, leukemia, and adrenocortical carcinoma (Li et al. 1988; Malkin et al. 1990). A chief tumor suppressor function of the p53 protein is to act as the "guardian" of the genome. In response to a number of DNA damaging insults, p53 causes cell proliferation arrest or programmed cell death to prevent the propagation of a cell with damaged genetic material that may give rise to malignant behavior. Germline mutation of one *p53* allele, as in the Li-Fraumeni syndrome, allows tumor progression when the second allele is mutated as a somatic event.

Individuals with germline mutation of the retinoblastoma susceptibility gene, *RB*, are also at increased risk for a variety of cancers, including NRSTS. Radiotherapy administered for the treatment of retinoblastoma further increases the risk of developing a second malignant neoplasm; the relative risk increases with radiotherapy dose (Wong et al. 1997). The *RB* gene product apparently functions as a tumor suppressor by preserving irreversible cell cycle arrest, thereby functioning as a "brake" to cell proliferation. As with the *p53* gene, germline loss of one *RB* allele facilitates tumor cell proliferation when the second allele is mutated in a somatic cell.

Germline mutation of the *NF-1* gene, which causes the neurofibromatosis type I syndrome, predisposes to the development of a variety of malignancies, including malignant peripheral nerve sheath tumors (MPNST). The most common malignancies in individuals with neurofibromatosis occur in the central nervous system; about 2% of patients with neurofibromatosis develop MPNST (Sorensen et al. 1986). Like *RB* loss, mutation of one *NF-1* allele confers a proliferative advantage to a cell because its protein product, Neurofibromin, normally functions to downregulate the functional activity of the RasRAS proto-oncogene product.

Exposure to ionizing radiation predisposes to the development of NRSTS, though fewer than 5% of NRSTS are radiation related. Ionizing radiation facilitates sarcoma formation by causing damage to key genes regulating aspects of the malignant tumor "phenotype" (discussed further below). Although NRSTS have been reported following radiotherapy for treatment for childhood cancer, no studies have systematically evaluated the magnitude of this risk. However, the risk of radiation-induced sarcomas appears to be dose related (Kuttesch et al. 1996). In a review of over 3,000 adults with bone or soft tissue sarcomas, 2.6% were believed to be radiation related and developed at a median latency of 10.3 years from the antecedent malignancy (Brady et al. 1992). Osteosarcoma, malignant fibrous histiocytoma, and angiosarcoma/lymphangiosarcoma were the most common histologic subtypes, and most of the tumors (87%) were high grade. Overall survival was poor, but patients with small tumors and those with tumors that were completely resected had a more favorable prognosis.

Despite the fact that fundamentally important insights into the molecular causes of cancer came from studies of the avian Rous sarcoma virus, there is limited evidence that viruses play a role in the genesis of sarcomas in humans. A major exception is Kaposi's sarcoma, once a very rare tumor that is now common in patients infected with the human immunodeficiency virus 1 (HIV). Infection by the human herpesvirus-8 (HHV-8) is closely linked to the development of Kaposi's sarcoma in HIV-infected patients. Individuals infected with HIV also have an excess risk of leiomyosarcoma, which may develop during childhood. Epstein-Barr virus appears to play a role in the pathogenesis of these HIV-related tumors (McClain et al. 1995).

A number of other risk factors for soft tissue sarcomas have been identified, though few of these factors play a role in pediatric NRSTS. Chronic lymphedema, whether following breast cancer treatment or following filarial infection, predisposes to the development of lymphangiosarcoma (Stewart et al. 1981). Vinyl chloride, inorganic arsenic, Thorotrast, and androgenic-anabolic steroid exposure are causally related to hepatic angiosarcoma (Falk et al. 1981). The phenoxy acid herbicides and their contaminant 2, 3, 7, 8-tetrachlorodibenzo-*p*-dioxin (dioxin) have been implicated in the development of soft tissue sarcomas, though conflicting findings in various studies make this relationship somewhat controversial (Dich et al. 1997).

7.2 Pathology/Molecular Pathology

A broad array of histologic subtypes of NRSTS can occur in children. The most common subtypes, reported in a prospective study from the Pediatric Oncology Group and retrospective series from St. Jude Children's Research Hospital, include synovial sarcoma, malignant fibrous histiocytoma, malignant peripheral nerve sheath tumor, and fibrosarcoma (Pratt et al. 1999; Spunt et al. 1999). In some instances, histologic subtype is closely related to clinical behavior; hence, the Pediatric Oncology Group (POG) grading system incorporates histologic subtype (Table 7.1) (Parham et al. 1995). In other cases, morphologic criteria like necrosis comprising >15% of the tumor area or a mitotic count greater than 5 per 10 high-power fields are considered high-grade features, independent of histologic subtype. Most NRSTS in children have a clinical behavior that is similar to that in adults. Notable exceptions are infantile fibrosarcoma and infantile hemangiopericytoma, defined as occurring in a child <4 years of age. In the POG grading system, these are considered low-grade tumors de-

Table 7.1. Pediatric Oncology Group (POG) non-rhabdomyosarcoma soft tissue sarcoma grading system [Reprinted by permission from *Modern Pathology* (Parham DM et al. 1995: Nonrhabdomyosarcomatous soft tissue sarcomas of childhood: Formulation of a simplified system for grading. Mod Pathol 8:705–710), copyright 1995, Macmillan Publishers Ltd.]

Grade I
Myxoid and well-differentiated liposarcoma
Deep-seated dermatofibrosarcoma protuberans
Well-differentiated or infantile (≤4 years old) fibrosarcoma
Well-differentiated or infantile (≤4 years old) hemangiopericytoma
Well-differentiated malignant peripheral nerve sheath tumor
Extraskeletal myxoid chondrosarcoma
Angiomatoid malignant fibrous histiocytoma
Grade II
Sarcomas not specifically included in Grade I and III, and in which <15% of the surface area shows necrosis. Mitotic count is ≤5/10 high-power fields (hpf) using a ×40 objective. As secondary criteria, nuclear atypia is not marked and the tumor is not markedly cellular
Grade III
Pleomorphic or round cell liposarcoma
Mesenchymal chondrosarcoma
Extraskeletal osteosarcoma
Malignant triton tumor
Alveolar soft part sarcoma
Sarcomas not included in Grade I and with >15% of surface area with necrosis, or with ≥5 mitoses/10 hpf using a ×40 objective
Marked atypia or cellularity are less predictive but may assist in placing tumors in this category

spite their histologic appearance due to their benign behavior in young children (Parham et al. 1995). Recent molecular genetic studies provide some insight into the unusual biology of infantile fibrosarcoma (see below).

NRSTS, like other sarcomas, represent tumors derived from mesenchymal cells. In some cases, like malignant peripheral nerve sheath tumor arising from a preexisting benign neurofibroma, the cellular origin of the sarcoma is easy to explain. In most types of NRSTS, the exact cell(s) of origin is not known. NRSTS cells express proteins normally found in connective tissue, smooth and skeletal muscle, cartilage, vasculature, adipose, or nervous system. Conceptually, different histologic subtypes of NRSTS could originate from different types of mesenchymal cells "transformed" at some stage to recapitulate a stage in development. For example, analogous to the expression of the MyoD family of transcription factors in rhabdomyosarcoma, liposarcomas express PPARγ, a transcription factor involved in adipocyte differentiation. This scenario predicts that histologically different NRSTS likely originate from distinct types of cell. An alternative possibility is that a more-or-less common mesenchymal progenitor cell could give rise to different types of NRSTS. In this case, the histology of individual tumors may then depend on the genes expressed within the tumor cell. In support of this, the expression of distinct, abnormal transcription factors generated by a balanced chromosomal translocation essentially defines many NRSTS histologic subtypes. For example, the different fusion proteins EWS-CHOP, EWS-ATF1, and EWS-WT1 are exclusively expressed in myxoid liposarcoma, malignant melanoma of soft parts (or clear cell sarcoma), and desmoplastic small round cell tumor, respectively (reviewed in Skapek et al. 2000). That a single transcription factor could alter complex cell biology is certainly reasonable – witness the capacity of MyoD expression to define skeletal muscle lineage and induce complete skeletal muscle differentiation in cell culture models. Elucidating the cellular origin for NRSTS may provide new insight into novel therapeutic targets and increase our understanding of their fundamental biology.

The complex phenotype of malignant cancer cells, including NRSTS cells, depends on what has been described to be six essential "hallmarks" of cancer (Hanahan et al. 2000). These include: (1) self-sufficiency in cell proliferation signals, (2) resistance to antiproliferative signals, (3) resistance to proapoptotic death signals, (4) angiogenic capacity, (5) potential for locally invasive and metastatic growth, and (6) limitless replication potential. Clearly, no single genetic or epigenetic "event" confers all these properties on a mesenchymal cell to cause a sarcoma and there are probably many means to these ends during sarcomagenesis. Two key tumor suppressor pathways involve the *p53* and retinoblastoma susceptibility (*RB*) genes. Their loss impacts directly on the first three "hallmarks" involving cell proliferation, cell cycle arrest, and cell death machinery. It is likely that all cancers, including sarcomas, have defects in these two pathways. Functional loss of p53 may occur by loss or mutation of the *p53* gene or of the growing list of key effectors; overexpression of the p53 inhibitor Hdm2; loss of p14ARF, which inhibits Hdm2; or loss or dysfunction of p53 activators like the ATM kinase. Loss of RB function could be accomplished by *RB* gene mutation (as can occur in osteosarcoma), excess activity of its negative regulators like cyclins and cyclin-dependent kinases (cdks), or loss of function of the p21Waf/Cip1 and/or p16Ink4 families of cyclin/cdk inhibitors. As for other solid tumors, the capacity of NRSTS for large, invasive, and metastatic tumor growth likely depends on the relative expression of tumor-derived pro- and anti-angiogenic factors, such as vascular endothelial factor (VEGFs), fibroblast growth factor (FGFs), angiopoietins 1 and 2, thrombospondins (TSP1); and the relative expression of various matrix metalloproteinases (MMPs) and matrix metalloproteinase inhibitors. The capacity for cancer cells to replicate indefinitely is typically conferred by mechanisms to prevent loss of DNA from the ends (telomeres) of chromosomes with each cell division. This is usually due to induction of the telomerase enzyme but in some cases it is accomplished by an alternative mechanism to maintain telomeric ends through homologous recombination. Osteosarcoma is one notable example in which the alternative mechanism seems to predominate (Scheel et al. 2001). The relative importance of each mechanism for NRSTS has not been well established.

7.2.1 Molecular Pathogenesis

As noted above (Sect. 7.1.2, "Risk Factors"), the cause of an individual's sarcoma is usually unknown but certain environmental (e.g., ionizing radiation) and host genetic factors (e.g., germline mutations of *RB, p53, NF-1*) are important in some cases. The genetic host susceptibility factors discussed above hinge on the presence or absence of specific DNA aberrations in the germline as heritable traits. By far, most childhood NRSTS are not part of heritable syndromes. Instead, the genetic or epigenetic "events" driving sarcoma development are more likely to be somatic cell events that occur during or after development. Much insight into the nature of these factors has been uncovered by studying the sarcoma tissue or cells themselves.

Many biology studies of NRSTS initially focused on evaluating the cells for gross chromosomal abnormalities detectable by analysis of the karyotype of cultured sarcoma cells. The aggregate of NRSTS cytogenetics studies indicate that the tumors can by divided into those with complex genomic abnormalities – manifested by large increases in chromosome number, numerous chromosomal breaks and translocations, end-to-end chromosome fusions – and those with very specific chromosomal abnormalities but relatively few global genomic abnormalities (Helman and Meltzer 2003). Unifying mechanisms leading to global genomic abnormalities are not established for NRSTS. Dysfunction of a component of the p53 pathway leads to genomic instability in cultured cells and likely also plays a role in sarcomagenesis. If not as a germline trait discussed above, this could be in a somatic cell during sarcoma development. It has long been established that mice lacking p53 or p19Arf (which activates p53) frequently develop sarcomas. In principle and in certain experimental models, dysfunction of DNA repair or telomere maintenance enzymes could also lead to complex karyotypic abnormalities in NRSTS cells. For example, mice predisposed to develop tumors because of loss of the *Ink4a/Arf* gene locus (disrupting both RB and p53 pathways) develop a wide range of soft tissue sarcomas when they are also deficient in DNA ligase IV, an enzyme involved in DNA end joining (Sharp-

Table 7.2. Recurring chromosomal translocations in non-rhabdomyosarcoma soft tissue sarcomas

Tumor	Translocation	Fusion protein
Alveolar soft part sarcoma	der(17)t(X;17)(p11;q25)	TFE3-ASPL
Clear cell sarcoma of tendons and aponeuroses	t(12;22)(q13;q12)	EWS-ATF1
Dermatofibrosarcoma protuberans	t(17;22)(q22;q13)	COL1A1-PDGFB
Desmoplastic small round cell tumor	t(11;22)(p13;q12)	EWS-WT1
Endometrial stromal sarcoma	t(7;17)(p15;q21)	JAZF1-JJAZ1
Extraskeletal myxoid chondrosarcoma	t(9;22)(q22;q12) t(9;17)(q22;q11) t(9;15)(q22;q21)	EWS-CHN RBP56-CHN TCF12-CHN
Infantile fibrosarcoma	t(12;15)(p13;q25)	ETV6-NTRK3
Inflammatory myofibroblastic tumor	t(1;2)(q22;p23) t(2;19)(p23;p13)	TPM3-ALK TPM4-ALK
Low-grade fibromyxoid sarcoma	t(7;16)(q33;p11)	FUS-CREB3L2
Myxoid liposarcoma	t(12;16)(q13;p11) t(12;22)(q13;q12) t(12;22;20)(q13;q12;q11)	TLS-CHOP EWS-CHOP EWS-CHOP
Synovial sarcoma	t(X;18)(p11;q11)	SYT-SSX1 or SYT-SSX2 or SYT-SSX4

less et al. 2001). Strikingly, spectral karyotyping and comparative genomic hybridization show clonal chromosomal translocations, amplifications and deletions, analogous to what occurs in human NRSTS. Mice lacking one *p53* allele engineered to also have dysfunctional, short telomeres due to telomerase deficiency develop tumors with complex chromosomal abnormalities; however, there is a preponderance of epithelial tumors in these mice (Artandi et al. 2000). Conceptually, early loss of pro-apoptotic cell-death machinery (like p53) and loss of DNA repair enzymes that prevent random chromosomal losses and gains would provide the perfect cellular environment for tumor cells to acquire the features required for malignant biology.

NRSTS without global genomic derangements are likely to be fundamentally different with respect to the machinery to maintain chromosomal integrity. Many of these have specific chromosomal defects initially detectable by routine karyotype analysis (Table 7.2). In many cases, these specific chromosomal abnormalities are now detectable using more sensitive molecular techniques (see chapter 2) even when the karyotype appears grossly normal. The striking correlation between histologic subtype and specific chromosomal rearrangement implies that the rearrangements likely drive the biology of a particular sarcoma. Nonetheless, much evidence from mouse models supports the concept that a single genetic event is not sufficient to cause a malignancy. Therefore, even in these cases of NRSTS with specific chromosomal translocations, occult abnormalities in other genes are likely present and will hopefully become detectable using newer approaches to identify secondary and tertiary cooperative genetic events.

Other studies have provided important insights into the biology of specific sarcomas. These were often based on initial observations from karyotype studies of sarcoma-derived cells. In other cases, like the association of *NF-1* mutations with MPNST, clinical associations provided important clues. Finally, some advances were extensions of studies initially developed in other tumor types. Relevant examples are outlined below.

7.2.2 Synovial Sarcoma and the SYT/SSX Translocation

Some synovial sarcoma-derived cells were identified to have non-random translocations between chromosomes X and 18 [t(X;18)(p11.2; q11.2)]. Cloning of the translocation breakpoint and subsequent molecular studies revealed that the translocation generates a novel fusion protein containing all but the last eight amino acids of SYT fused to the carboxyl terminus of either of the closely related SSX1 or SSX2 proteins. Cloning the breakpoint facilitated molecular testing for *SYT/SSX1* and *SYT/SSX2* gene translocations in synovial sarcoma tissue samples by reverse transcriptase polymerase chain reaction (RT-PCR) and FISH in situations where karyotype analysis was not possible. The presence of an *SYT/SSX* fusion transcript is a remarkably sensitive and specific test for synovial sarcoma as it is present in over 90% of synovial sarcomas and very few (if any) other soft tissue sarcomas.

How the presence of either the *SYT/SSX1* or the *SYT/SSX2* fusion transcript influences synovial sarcoma biology is a subject of great interest. Functional motifs in the fusion protein and results from experimental models indicate that SYT/SSX fusion protein likely functions as a transcriptional regulator by interacting with other nuclear proteins (reviewed in Skapek et al. 2000). Importantly, SYT/SSX1 protein may be functionally distinct from SYT/SSX2 because either fusion transcript can occur in the monophasic subtype of synovial sarcoma, whereas biphasic tumors nearly always express the *SYT/SSX1* transcript. The correlation implies a potential cause-effect relationship: for example, the presence of the SYT/SSX1 fusion protein may be required (but is apparently not sufficient) to promote epithelial differentiation within a biphasic tumor. Moreover, some studies suggest that the presence of a particular fusion protein may have clinical significance as well (Ladanyi et al. 2002).

7.2.3 Infantile Fibrosarcoma and ETV6-NTRK3

Molecular genetic studies have provided new insight into the biology of infantile fibrosarcoma, which has a distinctly good prognosis despite aggressive histologic features. Cells from these tumors were previously described to have trisomies of several chromosomes 8, 11, 17, and 20. Careful cytogenetics studies revealed that they also have a consistent translocation involving chromosomes 12 and 15 [t(12;15)(p13;q25)] (reviewed in Skapek et al. 2000). Molecular analysis demonstrated that the translocation creates a novel fusion protein containing the protein-protein interaction domain of ETV6 (also known as TEL) and the tyrosine kinase domain of NTRK3, resulting in a constitutively active enzyme capable of transforming cultured fibroblasts. Strikingly, the same molecular translocation has also been described in congenital mesoblastic nephroma and secretory breast carcinoma, both of which often carry a good prognosis in children. However, this translocation does not occur in adult-type fibrosarcoma or in other fibroblastic lesions. The presence of the same fusion protein in histologically different tumors suggests that it may play a primary role in the malignant transformation process that is not necessarily cell-lineage specific. Whether and by what mechanism it may also contribute to the favorable biology of these tumors is not established.

7.2.4 Rhabdoid Tumor and INI1

Rhabdoid tumors are high-grade neoplasms that occur in the kidney, brain, and soft tissues. Irrespective of their anatomic location, these are highly aggressive tumors. Despite similar clinical behavior, their wide range of histologic features, somewhat dependent on anatomic location, made classification of this group of tumors difficult. Molecular genetic findings, based on earlier karyotypic findings of frequent loss of chromosome 22q11.2, largely clarified this problem. All rhabdoid tumors are thought to contain disruptions of the *SNF5/INI1* gene (Versteege et al. 1998). *SNF5/INI1* mutations range from complete gene deletions to small mutations disrupting the gene reading frame. They occur as somatic mutations and as germline mutations in a smaller fraction of patients. Mice engineered to lack one *Snf5* allele are viable and frequently develop tumors histologically similar to rhabdoid tumors (Roberts et al. 2000).

The *SNF5/INI1* gene encodes a protein that is a component of the SWI/SNF complex. The SWI/SNF complex functions as a chromatin-remodeling machine, which ultimately alters the expression of other genes. Presumably, loss of *SNF5/INI1* significantly alters the function of this protein complex, but the exact mechanisms for how this leads to rhabdoid tumors in both mice and humans are not known.

7.2.5 Inflammatory Myofibroblastic Tumor and ALK

A similar theme encompasses recent molecular insight into inflammatory myofibroblastic tumor (IMT). This tumor presented nosological confusion because it was not clear whether it represented a reactive or truly neoplastic process. Clonal cytogenetics abnormalities confirmed its neoplastic nature and led to the identification of consistent translocations involving the anaplastic lymphoma kinase, *ALK*, at chromosome 2p23 (reviewed in Duyster et al. 2001). Translocations in IMT generate fusion proteins in which the tyrosine kinase domain of ALK is connected to tropomyosin 3 (TPM3), tropomyosin 4 (TPM4), or clathrin heavy chain (CLTC). These fusion partners likely allow protein-protein interactions to constitutively activate the ALK kinase. Analogous to the evolving story for ETV6-NTRK3, ALK fusion proteins have been described in other types of tumors like anaplastic large cell lymphoma, where ALK is usually fused with nucleophosmin (NPM). Hence, the transforming activity of activated ALK is, like ETV6-NTRK3, not cell-lineage specific.

7.2.6 Gastrointestinal Stromal Tumors and the KIT Transferase

Although uncommon in children, gastrointestinal stromal tumors (GISTs) provide an elegant example of the clinical relevance of molecular understanding of sarcoma biology. Over 90% of a large series of GISTs were noted to express the KIT receptor tyrosine kinase encoded by the *KIT* proto-oncogene (Hirota et al. 1998). Analysis of the *KIT* mRNA sequence demonstrated point mutations that rendered the KIT enzyme constitutively active, implying a functional role in the biology of this tumor.

In parallel to these studies, imatinib mesylate (STI571), developed as a selective tyrosine kinase inhibitor, was found to inhibit the activity of KIT. Recent clinical trials demonstrate prolonged disease control in patients with high-risk GIST treated with imatinib mesylate (Eisenberg et al. 2004).

7.2.7 Dermatofibrosarcoma Protuberans and PDGF

Dermatofibrosarcoma protuberans (DFSP) is a low-grade sarcoma that is relatively common in children. It is associated with chromosomal abnormalities, resulting in juxtaposition of the collagen 1A1 (*COL1A1*) and *PDGF* B genes. The resulting constitutive expression of PDGF protein causes autocrine or paracrine stimulation of its cognate receptor in the tumor cells. The capacity of imatinib to interfere with the PDGF receptor raises the possibility that it may also be effective treatment for DFSP, a possibility supported by a recent case report (Rubin et al. 2002). Examples of this type of targeted therapy have effectively launched an era in which better understanding of NRSTS biology may lead directly to better therapy.

7.3 Histologic Classification

There are two clinically important aspects to the pathology of the NRSTS. The first and most obvious aspect is to render a diagnosis, usually by establishing the underlying histogenesis of the sarcoma. The second important aspect is histologic grading of the tumor, which is more controversial and will be discussed separately.

The approach to the microscopic diagnosis of sarcomas is systematic and begins with a solid knowledge of the basic histologic diversity between and within each entity, along with the clinical context and anatomic site in which the tumor is arising. Although the NRSTS are heterogeneous, they share the unifying microscopic features of at least moderate cellularity and at least a subpopulation of cells with spindled morphology. The number of mitotic figures varies widely from tumor to tumor and they may be inconspicuous. Based upon the phenotypic appearance, a differential diagnosis is generated for a given tumor. Ancillary tools are then used to establish or confirm the specific diagnosis as needed. These ancillary tools traditionally include immunohistochemistry, electron microscopy and, in some cases, molecular genetic analyses. In the future, it is likely that information gathered from microarray studies currently underway will further refine our current classification systems.

7.3.1 Synovial Sarcoma

Most synovial sarcomas arise within the deep soft tissue of extremities, particularly in the region of the knee. The cell of origin from which they evolve, however, is unclear as fewer than 5% arise within a joint or bursa. Synovial sarcoma is characterized by a wide spectrum of histologic appearances ranging from purely mesenchymal, spindle cell morphology (monophasic synovial sarcoma) to tumors that are predominantly epithelial and mimic adenocarcinoma to tumors with features of both epithelial and mesenchymal differentiation (biphasic synovial sarcoma). Dystrophic calcification/ossification is not uncommon. In addition, there is a poorly differentiated variant of synovial sarcoma comprising cells with less spindled morphology that resembles the group of pediatric small round blue cell tumors. In children and adolescents, the monophasic mesenchymal synovial sarcoma is relatively common and is characterized by densely cellular sheets or poorly formed fascicles of spindle-shaped cells. The number of mitotic figures ranges from sparse to abundant.

Immunohistochemistry is helpful in establishing the diagnosis of synovial sarcoma as cytokeratin (CK) and epithelial membrane antigen (EMA) expression are documented in the vast majority of tumors. In the monophasic mesenchymal synovial sarcoma, this may be sparse and limited to isolated cells or small cords/nests of cells. Although the expression of many subtypes of CK can be seen in other sarcomas, expression of cytokeratins 7 and 19 seems to be unique to synovial sarcoma and may be particularly useful (Miettinen 1991). Expression of CD99, S100 protein and, occasionally, muscle specific or smooth muscle actin are also seen in a significant number of tumors.

Ultrastructural examination of biphasic or epithelial synovial sarcoma, not surprisingly, reveals classic epithelial features such as external lamina, tonofilaments, terminal bar complexes and microvilli, in areas with an epithelial appearance by light microscopy. In contrast, the mesenchymal or poorly differentiated areas display no distinctive features other than a rare wisp of cell-associated external lamina.

Due to the almost universal presence of an *SSX/SYT* fusion in cases of synovial sarcoma, molecular studies (usually RT-PCR) are frequently very useful in confirming the diagnosis (Coindre et al. 2003; Hill et al. 2003). It has been shown that greater than 90% of synovial sarcomas are cytogenetically characterized by t(X;18)(p11;q11), fusing one of the *SSX* genes on chromosome X (all situated at band p11) with the *SYT/SS18* gene on chromosome 18. The most common *SSX* genes that have been reported as translocation partners with the *SYT* gene are *SSX1* and *SSX2,* accounting for approximately 60% and 35% of cases respectively. *SSX4* (rarely including only exon 6) has also been observed as a fusion partner with *SYT*. In addition, fusion of the *SS18L1* gene on chromosome 20 with the *SSX1* gene has been reported, illustrating the rare occurrence of variant translocations that may characterize the minority of these tumors (Storlazzi et al. 2003; Tornkvist et al. 2002).

Within the group of synovial sarcomas, it has been reported that the prognosis may be better for completely resectable tumors that measure less than 5 cm in diameter, have fewer than 10 mitoses per 10 high-power fields, have prominent ossification and have no necrosis. The prognosis may be worse for the poorly differentiated synovial sarcomas, particularly those with >50% necrosis and/or rhabdoid cells. In addition to these clinical/histologic features, the *SSX/SYT* fusion type has been associated with prognosis (Kawai et al. 1998; Ladanyi et al. 2002; Panagopoulos et al. 2001). Retrospective studies have shown that localized tumors with an *SSX2/SYT* fusion are associated with a better prognosis than those with the *SSX1/SYT*.

7.3.2 Malignant Peripheral Nerve Sheath Tumor

Malignant peripheral nerve sheath tumors (MPNSTs) often arise in association with a large peripheral nerve, or in patients with NF1, within a preexisting neurofibroma. Microscopically, they are most commonly characterized by a densely cellular proliferation of cells, frequently arranged in fascicles. In some cases, these cellular areas are intermixed with hypocellular myxoid areas, while in other cases the cells form whorled structures suggestive of tactoid differentiation. The neoplastic cells are usually spindled in shape with irregular, wavy nuclei, although round cell areas can be seen. Formation of heterotopic elements, most commonly cartilage and bone – less commonly skeletal muscle or epithelial structures such as mucin-secreting glands – are seen in a minority of cases.

At an immunohistochemical level, the majority of MPNSTs express S100 protein, although it is usually focal and limited to isolated cells or small clusters of cells. Leu-7 and myelin basic protein are also expressed in a significant percentage of tumors, although less commonly than S100. Expression of epithelial antigens, such as keratin, is infrequent and may be useful if the differential diagnosis includes a monophasic synovial sarcoma. In addition, expression of p53, Mib-1 and TopoIIα seem to be limited to high-grade MPNST (vs. low-grade MPNST or neurofibroma) (Skotheim et al. 2003; Zhou et al. 2003).

Ultrastructurally, the cells of MPNSTs have cell processes and contain microtubules and neurofilaments. Cell-associated basal lamina formation ranges from well developed to incomplete.

MPNSTs are characterized by certain features at a molecular genetic level, including chromosome 7p, 9p, 17q and 22q abnormalities. Although not globally useful from a diagnostic standpoint, some of these abnormalities may be diagnostically useful in select cases – for example hemizygous or homozygous p16 (chromosome 9p) deletions are seen in the majority of MPNSTs, but not in benign nerve sheath tumors, and *NF-1* deletions (chromosome 17q) are seen in the majority of MPNSTs, but not synovial sarcoma (Perry et al. 2002).

Tumor-specific features that appear to have prognostic import include tumor size, age greater than 7 years, tumor necrosis >25% and the underlying presence of neurofibromatosis (usually NF1). In addition, there is preliminary array data to suggest that upregulation of topoisomerase II alpha may be associated with an adverse outcome.

7.3.3 Infantile Fibrosarcoma

Infantile fibrosarcomas (IFS) occur almost exclusively in infants and young children and a significant proportion are congenital. Although they can arise at almost any site, they most commonly present in the extremities or the trunk and head/neck region. Histologically, they are densely cellular tumors characterized by interlacing fascicles or sheets of relatively homogeneous, ovoid to spindle-shaped cells associated with minimal collagen production. Mitoses are readily identified and necrosis is frequently seen.

Immunohistochemical staining of IFS is nonspecific. All tumors express vimentin and a significant minority express neuron specific enolase and actin. Desmin, S100 protein, CD34, CD57, CD68, and CAM5.2 keratin can also be expressed, although stains for other cytokeratins and EMA are negative.

Ultrastructurally, the neoplastic cells of IFS show features of fibroblasts or myofibroblasts with abundant rough endoplasmic reticulum, variable numbers of lysosomes and cytoplasmic filaments. Focal cell-associated basal lamina can also be seen.

IFSs are uniformly characterized by the presence of a t(12;15)(p13;q25) translocation that results in fusion of the *TEL/ETV6* gene on chromosome 12 to the *TRKC/NTRK3* gene on chromosome 15. Other than a subset of mesoblastic nephromas, this translocation appears to be unique to this tumor. It is not seen in other fibroblastic or myofibroblastic lesions, including adult-type fibrosarcoma and, therefore, molecular analysis, usually by RT-PCR, for t(12;15) is diagnostically useful (Sandberg and Bridge 2002).

Although occasional cases of IFS have been reported to spontaneously regress or not recur following subtotal resection, occasional cases metastasize, leading to the overall acceptance that these tumors are low-grade malignancies. To date, there are no histologic or molecular features that have been identified that correlate with the variable clinical behavior.

7.3.4 Adult Type Fibrosarcoma

Adult fibrosarcoma (AFS) is uncommonly encountered in children and adolescents, but it is in the differential diagnosis of other tumors, particularly IFS, IMT and even cellular fibromatosis. When diagnosed in the pediatric age group, AFS usually has a relatively homogeneous histologic appearance. It is a densely cellular tumor comprising long, interlacing fascicles of spindle-shaped cells, giving it a herringbone appearance.

Immunohistochemical staining of AFS reveals the presence of vimentin and, in occasional cases, focal staining for smooth muscle actin. Expression of other muscle antigens, S100 protein and epithelial antigens is not seen.

The cells of AFS are ultrastructurally fibroblasts with rough endoplasmic reticulum and a lack of other differentiating features such as cell junctions, myofilaments, or cell-associated basal lamina.

Neither diagnostically nor prognostically useful molecular genetic features of AFS have been identified. Older studies, prior to segregation of AFS, IFS and IMT, suggested that tumor size, resectability and grade (based on cellularity/mitosis/necrosis – see separate discussion below) may correlate with prognosis.

7.3.5 Rhabdoid Tumor

Rhabdoid tumors are well-defined entities in both the kidney and brain. Due to their histologic overlap with other soft tissue tumors, it has taken longer to define this entity in soft tissue. However, as our repertoire of ancillary diagnostic tools has expanded, so has our ability to identify and define these biologically aggressive tumors that occur primarily in infants and young children. These densely cellular neoplasms comprise sheets or solid trabeculae of neoplastic cells with large, vesicular nuclei, prominent centrally located eosinophilic nucleoli and abundant eosinophilic cytoplasm. The cytoplasm coalesces to form large, distinctive, eosinophilic hyaline inclusions in variable numbers of these cells, giving them the appearance of rhabdomyoblasts – hence the designation of "rhabdoid" tumor. While these diagnostic "rhabdoid cells" are usually numerous, they may be isolated and inconspicuous in occasional tumors, presenting a diagnostic challenge and potential diagnostic pitfall in small biopsy samples.

As a variety of tumors may express the rhabdoid phenotype, immunohistochemistry may provide invaluable information when considering a diagnosis of rhabdoid tumor. The majority of rhabdoid tumors coexpress vimentin and an epithelial antigen such as keratin, epithelial membrane antigen and/or CAM 5.2. In addition, a significant percentage of tumors express neuroectodermal antigens such as CD33, synaptophysin, and/or neuron specific enolase. Expression of muscle specific actin and focal S-100 positivity is also not uncommon. Despite this polyphenotypic appearance, however, rhabdoid tumors do not express desmin, myoglobin or CD34.

Ultrastructurally, the cytoplasmic inclusions of rhabdoid cells are whorls of intermediate filaments that measure 8–10 µm in diameter. It has been shown that the filamentous whorls may comprise cytokeratin, while vimentin forms a filamentous network throughout the cytoplasm. In addition, neoplastic cells contain scattered organelles and occasional lipid droplets. Variably developed intercellular junctions may be present, but true desmosomes are not seen.

It has been shown that the majority of rhabdoid tumors are characterized by cytogenetic abnormalities involving the q11.2 band of chromosome 22. At a molecular level, this observation translates into homozygous deletions or mutations of the *SMARCB1* (also known as *hSNF5* or *INI1*) gene. Similar abnormalities are seen in rhabdoid tumors of the kidney and central nervous system, along with a few other central nervous system tumors. However, they have not been reported in other soft tissue sarcomas, other than a rare rhabdomyosarcoma, making this a potentially useful diagnostic feature of these tumors (Biegel et al. 2002; Judkins et al. 2004).

Rhabdoid tumors are highly malignant neoplasms, regardless of the site of their occurrence. Neither histologic nor molecular genetic features that correlate with prognosis or therapeutic responsiveness have been identified.

7.3.6 Inflammatory Myofibroblastic Tumor

Inflammatory myofibroblastic tumor (IMT) usually is diagnosed in the first 2 decades of life and can arise in a variety of locations including lung and mesentery/omentum. Microscopically, IMT is characterized by variable combinations of proliferating fibroblasts or myofibroblasts and inflammatory cells, the latter primarily consisting of lymphocytes, plasma cells and/or eosinophils. Collagen deposition may be prominent and neovascularization may give some cases the deceptive appearance of granulation tissue.

IMTs are one of the tumors in which immunohistochemistry may be helpful in establishing a diagnosis. In addition to the strong expression of vimentin, approximately half of these tumors express ALK1 protein (Cessna et al. 2002). Although ALK1 expression is not specific to IMT and is seen in a significant percentage of MPNST and rhabdomyosarcoma, it is usually not expressed in other myofibroblastic tumors. In addition to vimentin and ALK1, desmin and focal expression of keratin, along with actin, are not uncommonly seen in IMT. Expression of S100 protein, CD117 (KIT), myoglobin, myogenin, CD21, CD23 and CD34 are not seen in IMT.

The ultrastructural features of IMT are not specific and are the same as other fibroblastic/ myofibroblastic tumors. Abundant rough endoplasmic reticulum, variable numbers of cytoplasmic filaments and extracellular collagen production are characteristically seen.

The expression of ALK1 protein in IMT frequently correlates with the presence of rearrangement of the *ALK* receptor tyrosine kinase gene, located on chromosome 2, band p23. Unlike many of the other genomic alterations present in pediatric soft tissue sarcomas, however, *ALK* gene rearrangements are heterogeneous in that translocations fuse this gene with a number of different partners, including *TMP3*, *TMP4*, *CLTC*, *CARS*, *ATIC*, and *RANBP2*, whose protein products that share putative N-terminal oligomerization motifs. For this reason, routine cytogenetic analysis or FISH using a probe for the *ALK* gene are more helpful diagnostic adjuncts than standard RT-PCR assays (Coffin et al. 2001; Li et al. 2004).

The heterogeneity that characterizes IMT at the microscopic and genetic level is also seen in terms of clinical behavior. Generally considered a low-grade malignancy, occasional tumors may regress or metastasize. To date, there are no tumor specific features that predict into which end of the clinical spectrum a given tumor will fall.

7.3.7 Gastrointestinal Stromal Tumor

Gastrointestinal stromal tumors (GIST) arise both in association with the wall of the gastrointestinal tract and in intra-abdominal soft tissue, primarily the omentum and mesentery. The vast majority of GISTs are characterized by overexpression of KIT (CD117) and most by expression of CD34. This is in contrast to other smooth muscle and myofibroblastic tumors, including inflammatory myofibroblastic tumor, that might be in the differential diagnosis. A significant percentage of GIST also express smooth muscle actin. Although rare tumors may express desmin or S100 protein, these antigens are typically not expressed, making them useful in ruling out smooth muscle and neural tumors respectively. Immunoperoxidase stains, combined with the light microscopic and clinical appearances, should provide a definitive diagnosis in the vast majority of cases.

Many GISTs are characterized by mutations in the c-kit tyrosine kinase oncogene, not surprising in light of its consistent overexpression in these tumors. In addition, a significant minority of tumors are characterized by mutation in the platelet-derived growth factor receptor-alpha (*PDGF*α) gene (Heinrich et al. 2003). Abnormalities in these genes have provided a therapeutic target for these tumors in the form of imatinib mesylate, thus influencing prognosis. In addition, some have reported that tumors with a high Ki-67 labeling index and mitotic count may have a worse prognosis (Yamamoto et al. 2004; Yan et al. 2003).

7.3.8 Infantile Hemangiopericytoma

Hemangiopericytomas are neoplasms that in the past have been diagnosed by their typical routine light microscopic appearance (Rodriguez-Galindo C, Ramsey K et al. 2000). As similar patterns of growth are seen in a variety of other tumors, the definition of this lesion as a distinct clinicopathologic entity has evolved over time. The majority of these tumors occur in older patients and it is currently believed that most represent solitary fibrous tumors. However, a significant minority (approximately 5–10%) of hemangiopericytomas occur in the first 2 decades of life, primarily at birth and within the first year. These lesions are associated with a better prognosis and have been termed infantile hemangiopericytoma. It is currently believed that most of these lesions probably fall within the spectrum of infantile myofibromatosis and, as such, carry similar clinical features. Although they most commonly present as solitary lesions, usually arising within the superficial or deep soft tissue (and frequently the oral cavity), a significant minority are multifocal or generalized. Visceral lesions may be seen, particularly in multifocal or generalized cases (Rodriguez-Galindo C, Ramsey K et al. 2000).

Regardless of clinical presentation, hemangiopericytomas are microscopically characterized by thin-walled, frequently stag-horn to stellate-shaped, vascular channels within a densely cellular proliferation of stromal cells. These cells are relatively uniform, spindle- to polygonal-shaped cells with oval to round nuclei and inconspicuous cytoplasm. Mitoses are generally few, although they may rarely number up to 10 per 10 high power fields. The lesion may have a nodular appearance, diffusely infiltrate adjacent soft tissue and form perivascular satellite nodules. Subendothelial vascular infiltration is not uncommon and should not be mistaken as a feature of malignancy. Few smooth muscle bundles or less cellular, fibroblastic-appearing foci may be present.

Immunohistochemical staining is variably helpful. The neoplastic cells express vimentin and variable amounts of muscle specific actin. A significant percentage may express CD34.

Ultrastructural examination of infantile hemangiopericytoma is generally not helpful from a diagnostic standpoint. The neoplastic cells have few cytoplasmic organelles, occasional arrays of microfilaments and poorly developed cell junctions.

Although infantile hemangiopericytoma is generally considered a benign lesion, few cases of spontaneous regression and occasional cases of recurrence and even metastasis occur. Histologic features that will identify these tumors with atypical clinical behavior have not been established in infantile hemangiopericytoma.

7.3.9 Desmoplastic Small Round Cell Tumor

Desmoplastic small round cell tumors (DSRCT) are uncommon, but clinically aggressive tumors that were first described within the abdomen; however, they have since been found to occur in a variety of other locations, including the central nervous system. This tumor was first identified by a combination of its routine light microscopic appearance and immunohistochemical pattern of antigen expression. By routine H&E staining, the classic DSRCT comprises islands of small round cells within a prominent desmoplastic stroma. These islands of neoplastic cells show features of polyphenotypic differentiation in that they coexpress epithelial (keratin, epithelial membrane antigen), mesenchymal (vimentin, desmin) and neural markers (neuron specific enolase). In addition, virtually all of these tumors express WT1, an antigen that is only rarely seen in other small round blue cell tumors such as rhabdomyosarcoma, Ewing's sarcoma/primitive neuroectodermal tumor, neuroblastoma and rhabdoid tumor.

Ultrastructurally, DSRCTs are characterized by paranuclear aggregates of intermediate filaments, occasional desmosomes and basal lamina.

The diagnostic hallmark of DSRCT is the cytogenetic/molecular genetic presence of a t(11;22)(p13;q12). This translocation results in fusion of the *EWS* gene on chromosome 22 with the *WT1* gene on chromosome 11 – hence the universal expression of WT1 in these tumors. This same translocation has not been described in any other tumors, making it a particularly useful tool in those rare cases in which the divergent phenotype is not documented (Gerald et al. 1998).

Currently, there are no histologic or genetic features that have been shown to correlate with prognosis in these highly malignant tumors.

7.3.10 Grading Systems

Approaches to the grading of soft tissue sarcomas over the years have varied, particularly in the pediatric age group (Oliveira et al. 2001; Parham et al. 1995). Although it makes intuitive sense that features such as mitotic index, necrosis, cellularity, nuclear atypia and vascular invasion would/should correlate with prognosis, it is well known that these features may not carry the same significance in all tumor types, particularly those arising within the first 2 years of life. In addition, most studies assessing these attributes have varied with respect to the percentage of various tumors covered, patient selection, clinicopathologic information provided, therapeutic approaches and a variety of other features. With these caveats in mind, and incorporating the unique clinical features of some pediatric tumors, a grading system for pediatric sarcomas has been proposed (Parham et al. 1995). This classification begins with the acceptance that certain lesions, such as infantile fibrosarcoma and infantile hemangiopericytoma, are generally clinically benign, while other lesions, such as alveolar soft part sarcoma and extraskeletal osteosarcoma, are uniformly clinically aggressive. The remaining lesions are classified into grades II or III based upon the standard criteria of necrosis, mitoses, cellularity and atypia. Although grade has correlated with prognosis in pediatric NRSTS using this system, no prospective clinical trials have yet used this system to stratify patients for therapy assignment.

7.4 Clinical Presentation and Diagnosis

7.4.1 Presenting Features

NRSTS can occur in any anatomic site except, by definition, in bone. As in adults, about half of pediatric NRSTS arise in the extremities (Pappo et al. 1999; Pratt et al. 1999; Spunt et al. 1999, 2002). The remaining cases are relatively evenly divided among trunk wall, head and neck, and visceral/retroperitoneal sites. A painless mass is the most common presenting symptom. Depending on the anatomic location, however, the tumor may impinge on normal structures, thereby resulting in other symptoms. Systemic complaints such as fever and weight loss are rare, except in patients with widely disseminated disease.

Approximately 15% of patients have metastatic disease at the time of initial presentation (Pappo et al. 1999). The lung is the most common site of distant metastasis. Regional lymph node involvement is quite uncommon, except in certain histologic subtypes such as epithelioid sarcoma and clear cell sarcoma (Fong et al. 1993). Bone, liver, subcutaneous and brain metastases occur in a small percentage of patients (Pappo et al. 1999). Bone marrow involvement is exceedingly rare.

7.4.2 Differential Diagnosis

Identifying a child with soft tissue sarcoma may be challenging for the primary care provider because painless masses are easily ignored and because the rarity of these tumors results in a low index of suspicion. In a retrospective study of 315 children with solid tumors, the median interval between the onset of symptoms and the diagnostic biopsy for children with soft tissue sarcomas was 9.5 weeks (Haimi et al. 2004). Only children with epithelial and bone tumors had a longer lag time between symptom onset and diagnosis (11 and 13.5 weeks, respectively). In a second study of 100 children and adults with soft tissue sarcomas, the interval between the first physician visit and the diagnostic procedure was more than 1 month in 27% of the patients (Brouns et al. 2003). In these cases, the delay lasted a median of 6 months and an erroneous clinical impression from the outset was the most frequent cause of the delay.

In pediatrics, the differential diagnosis of a soft tissue mass includes a variety of malignant and benign entities. Besides NRSTS, primary or metastatic rhabdomyosarcoma, Ewing's sarcoma, and neuroblastoma are the predominant malignant entities to be considered; osteosarcoma only rarely arises in soft tissues (Wodowski et al. 2003). One or more soft tissue chloromas may be the presenting feature of a hematologic malignancy. Other lesions that typically present as a soft tissue mass include aggressive fibromatosis and other fibrohistiocytic entities, Langerhans cell histiocytosis, benign tumors such as lipoma and neurofibroma, and non-proliferative entities such as cysts and abscesses.

Once a tumor is categorized as a NRSTS, there may be considerable disagreement among pathologists regarding the precise histologic diagnosis. In an Eastern Cooperative Oncology Group study of pathologic specimens from 424 adults enrolled on soft tissue sarcoma trials, a panel of expert pathologists found that the institutional pathologist's diagnosis was correct in only 74% of cases; 10% of the tumors were not sarcoma and the specific diagnosis in the remaining 16% differed from that reported by the institutional pathologist (Shiraki et al. 1989). A similar study of 216 adults by the Southeastern Cancer Study Group established that 6% did not have sarcoma and 27% had a specific diagnosis that differed from that rendered by the institutional pathologist (Presant et al. 1986). Discordant diagnoses were more common when the tumor was of higher grade.

7.4.3 The Diagnostic Biopsy

Procurement of an adequate biopsy specimen is critical to accurately identifying the histologic subtype and grade of NRSTS present. Diagnosis may also be aided by obtaining adequate tissue for molecular pathologic studies to identify chromosomal translocations specific for certain histologic subtypes of NRSTS.

Incisional tumor biopsy is the gold standard approach. However, multiple core needle biopsies may be a justifiable option, particularly in centers with pathologic expertise in interpreting these specimens. In a single-institution study that evaluated 60 core needle biopsies of extremity soft tissue sarcomas, the correlation with the final diagnosis at the time of definitive resection was 95% for malignancy, 88% for grade, and 75% for histologic subtype (Heslin et al. 1997). Fine needle aspiration (FNA) cytology is inadequate for establishing an accurate diagnosis at initial presentation. However, FNA cytology may be useful to confirm or exclude the presence of tumor at the time of suspected local recurrence (Miralles et al. 1986).

7.4.4 Evaluation of Disease Extent

Among the primary goals of the disease assessment at the time of initial presentation is to determine the anatomic boundaries of the primary tumor for surgical planning and for the evaluation of treatment response in the event that neoadjuvant therapy is contemplated. The primary site should generally be evaluated with magnetic resonance imaging (MRI), which provides optimal soft tissue definition. For tumors arising within the chest and abdominal cavities, however, computed tomography (CT) may be more useful. CT also may be helpful in defining the extent of skull base erosion and intracranial tumor extension in cranial parameningeal tumors. The role of positron emission tomography (PET) imaging remains unclear. A meta-analysis of studies evaluating PET scans in soft tissue sarcomas showed that this modality was capable of reliably discriminating between high-grade lesions and low-grade or benign lesions (Ioannidis and Lau 2003). However, PET imaging was unable to adequately discriminate between low-grade and benign lesions.

The metastatic workup depends to some extent on the histologic subtype of the tumor and its location. Imaging of regional lymph nodes is indicated for tumors associated with a significant likelihood of lymphatic metastasis, such as epithelioid sarcoma and clear cell sarcoma (Fong et al. 1993). Sentinel lymph node mapping may be a more sensitive technique than diagnostic imaging for identifying occult nodal disease (Paganelli et al. 2000). Since the lungs are the most common site of distant tumor spread, a chest X-ray or CT scan is a routine component of the evaluation. However, several studies in adults have questioned whether routine chest CT scans in newly diagnosed patients with soft tissue sarcomas are necessary or cost-effective. Chest X-rays appear to be as effective as CT scans in identifying the rare patient with a small (≤5 cm) soft tissue sarcoma and pulmonary metastases (Fleming et al. 2001). In patients with large (>5 cm) soft tissue sarcomas, chest CT imaging identifies more patients with pulmonary metastases than does chest X-ray, but at considerably higher cost (Porter et al. 2002). Bone scintigraphy may be restricted to patients with bone pain or other sites of metastatic disease involvement (Jager et al. 2000). Imaging to detect liver metastases is necessary only in patients with intra-abdominal and retroperitoneal primary tumors. Brain metastases are very rare; brain imaging is warranted only in symptomatic patients and perhaps in those with widespread metastatic disease (Espat et al. 2002). Bone marrow aspirates and biopsies are not indicated in the evaluation of patients with NRSTS.

7.5 Prognostic Factors and Clinical Staging

7.5.1 Prognostic Factors

Few prospective studies have been undertaken in pediatric NRSTS, so much of what is known about the factors that influence prognosis in childhood is derived from retrospective analyses and studies in adults with soft tissue sarcomas. The factors with the most consistent relationship to event-free and overall survival include disease extent and the histologic grade and size of the primary tumor.

In a retrospective evaluation of prognostic factors in pediatric NRSTS, patients with tumors that were surgically resected at the time of initial presentation fared better than those with unresected tumors, who in turn fared better than those with metastatic disease (5-year overall survival 89% vs. 56% vs. 15%) (Spunt et al. 2002). The extent of resection (resected vs. unresected) was an independently significant predictor of both event-free and overall survival. Among patients whose tumor was resected at the time of initial presentation, positive microscopic margins was an independent predictor of poorer event-free and overall survival (Spunt et al. 1999). Prospective pediatric studies confirm the observation that patients with metastatic disease fare extremely poorly, though there is no prospective evidence that there is a relationship between extent of tumor resection and outcome (Pappo et al. 2001; Pratt et al. 1998). However, many studies in adult soft tissue sarcomas indicate that the extent of resection has an influence on survival (Lewis et al. 1998; Pisters et al. 1996a).

High histologic grade and large (>5 cm) tumor size are consistently associated with inferior survival in pediatric (Marcus et al. 1997; Pratt et al. 1999; Spunt et al. 1999) and adult soft tissue sarcomas (Lewis et al. 1998; Pisters et al. 1996a). Other factors that have been correlated with survival in childhood NRSTS include primary site and age. Patients with surgically resected intra-abdominal primary tumors had an inferior event-free and overall survival compared to those with primary tumors at other sites in a retrospective analysis (Spunt et al. 1999). Age ≥10 years was associated with a lower likelihood of survival in patients whose tumors were not surgically resected at the time of initial presentation (Spunt et al. 2002). Other factors related to survival in studies of adults with extremity soft tissue sarcomas include site (upper vs. lower extremity), depth (superficial vs. deep), and histologic subtype (Pisters et al. 1996a).

The risk of distant tumor recurrence in both pediatric and adult populations depends predominantly on tumor grade and size; patients with large, high-grade tumors are at high risk (Lewis et al. 1998; Pisters et al. 1996a; Spunt et al. 1999). Tumor invasiveness also predicted the development of distant metastases in pediatric NRSTS (Spunt et al. 1999). The extent of resection, tumor histology, primary site, and the use of chemotherapy did not have an impact on the likelihood of distant tumor recurrence.

Unlike distant recurrence, local tumor recurrence in pediatric NRSTS appears to depend primarily on the extent of resection rather than on tumor grade and size. Local control following gross total tumor resection is superior to that of unresected tumors (Marcus et al. 1997; Spunt et al. 1999, 2002). Among patients whose tumor is surgically resected at the time of initial presentation, a negative microscopic surgical margin confers a lower risk of local recurrence (Pisters et al. 1996a; Spunt et al. 1999). Patients treated with radiotherapy following gross total tumor resection also are at significantly lower risk for local disease recurrence (Marcus et al. 1997; Spunt et al. 1999).

Little is known about the predictors of survival in pediatric NRSTS patients who experience disease recurrence or progression following treatment. In a retrospective single-institution analysis of children and adolescents with resected NRSTS, the outcome of patients with local tumor recurrence was superior to that of patients with distant (or both local and distant) recurrence (5-year postrelapse survival 77% vs. 36%) (Spunt et al. 1999). Although the small number of patients precluded definitive conclusions about other prognostic factors, high histologic grade also appeared to have a negative impact on survival. Although patients with a local recurrence of resected NRSTS fared better than those with a distant recurrence, the opposite was true in patients with unresected NRSTS. In these patients, 5-year postrelapse survival after local recurrence was only 9%, compared to 29% after distant recurrence (Spunt et al. 2002). The dismal outcome noted after local recurrence of initially unresected NRSTS likely reflects the fact that recurrent tumor is rarely resectable and that prior radiation therapy generally precludes adequate radiotherapy at the time of recurrence.

7.5.2 Clinical Staging

There is no standard staging system in common use for pediatric NRSTS. Historically, the surgicopathologic staging system developed by the Intergroup Rhabdomyosarcoma Study Group (IRSG) for childhood rhabdomyosarcoma has been used for NRSTS (Maurer et al. 1988). However, this system accounts only for the presence or absence of metastatic disease and the extent of surgery at the time of initial presentation. Other prognostic factors with a significant impact on survival, such as tumor size and histologic grade, are not included in this staging system. These deficiencies limit the usefulness of the IRS staging system for pediatric NRSTS. For example, the overall survival of IRS clinical group I or II NRSTS approaches 90% (Pratt et al. 1999; Spunt et al. 1999). However, the survival of patients in this category whose tumor is either larger than 5 cm in diameter or of high histologic grade is in the 75% range, whereas the survival of those with small or low-grade tumors exceeds 95% (Spunt et al. 1999). Because the IRS clinical group designation does not adequately categorize patients by survival likelihood, it is of limited utility in staging pediatric NRSTS.

Staging systems commonly used in adults with soft tissue sarcomas include those of the International Union Against Cancer/American Joint Committee on Cancer (UICC/AJCC) (American Joint Committee on Cancer 2002), the Memorial Sloan-Kettering Cancer Center (MSKCC) (Hajdu et al. 1988), and the Musculoskeletal Tumor Society (MTS) (Enneking et al. 1980). All of these staging systems incorporate histologic grade and the presence or absence of metastatic disease. The UICC/AJCC and MSKCC systems also account for tumor size (≤5 cm or >5 cm) and depth [superficial (exclusively above the superficial fascia) or deep (invading the superficial fascia or located below the superficial fascia)]. Particular combinations of tumor grade, size, depth, and metastatic involvement create the six stages in the UICC/AJCC system. The MSKCC system assigns one of five stages based on the number of unfavorable prognostic signs (high grade, large size, deep site, and metastatic spread) present. The five stages of the MTS system are based on histologic grade, the presence or absence of metastatic disease, and the "surgical site," which is divided into intracompartmental and extracompartmental locations.

None of the soft tissue sarcoma staging systems developed for adults has been validated in pediatric NRSTS. However, a comparison of staging systems in adults with localized extremity soft tissue sarcomas showed that the MSKCC system was superior to the AJCC and MTS systems in predicting systemic disease recurrence (Wunder et al. 2000). Which system will prove most useful for pediatric NRSTS remains to be seen.

Among the difficulties inherent in staging pediatric NRSTS is determining which grading system to use in assigning stage, since grade has a significant impact on outcome. Although a variety of systems exist for grading soft tissue sarcomas in adults, none of these accounts for the unique histologic subtypes that occur in childhood. For example, fibrosarcoma and hemangiopericytoma, when they occur in very young children, have a very favorable clinical outcome despite an aggressive histologic appearance. Thus, assigning a histologic grade to these tumors using a system designed for adults would erroneously categorize these as high-grade neoplasms. In an effort to address this problem, the Pediatric Oncology Group (POG) developed and prospectively validated a pediatric NRSTS grading system (Parham et al. 1995) based largely on the National Cancer Institute (NCI) system developed by Costa et al. The POG grading system incorporates mitotic index, necrosis, cellularity, and nuclear pleomorphism in the assessment of grade for most tumors, while assigning certain histologic subtypes categorically to a grade based on their clinical behavior. Although the POG system is most commonly used to grade pediatric NRSTS, a study suggesting that the French Federation of Cancer Centers Sarcoma Group (FNCLCC) grading system may be superior to the NCI system (on which the POG grading system is based) suggests that a modification of the FNCLCC for pediatric use may be warranted.

7.6 Treatment

7.6.1 Surgery

Surgical resection is an integral component of effective therapy for pediatric NRSTS. A retrospective analysis of children and adolescents with NRSTS showed that patients whose tumor can be grossly resected at the time of initial diagnosis fare better than those with tumors that are initially unresected (Spunt et al. 2002). Wide en bloc resection of all sites of disease is the optimal local therapeutic approach for NRSTS. Unfortunately, the proximity of neurovascular, bony, and other vital structures often precludes adequate resection. Even when feasible, wide surgical resection may result in unacceptable functional deficits or cosmesis. Thus, the extent of surgery must be considered carefully in the context of other adjuvant therapies.

7.6.1.1 Surgical Management of the Primary Tumor

The goal of surgical intervention is to excise the primary tumor with widely negative margins. If this is not feasible, then gross tumor resection leaving microscopic residual tumor behind is the next best option. For extremity NRSTS, amputation is a surgical option. This procedure should only rarely be utilized, however, since limb-sparing operations are possible in the vast majority of cases. Amputation should be reserved for patients whose tumor cannot be grossly resected by any other means or who are likely to have a poor functional outcome following limb-sparing surgery. Children and adolescents who undergo amputation appear to adapt well psychosocially following this procedure (Hudson et al. 1998).

Amputation was compared to conservative resection with adjuvant radiotherapy in a prospective, randomized trial of adults with soft tissue sarcomas (Rosenberg et al. 1982). In this study, there was a trend toward improved local control for amputation ($p=0.06$). However, overall survival in patients undergoing limb-sparing surgery was no different than that of patients who had an amputation. A matched-pair analysis of adults undergoing limb-sparing operation or amputation for recurrent extremity soft tissue sarcoma also showed a higher local recurrence rate following limb-sparing surgery, but overall survival was similar in the two groups (Stojadinovic et al. 2001).

The deleterious long-term effects of adjuvant radiotherapy in children and adolescents include soft tissue and bone growth impairment, functional mobility restrictions, and secondary malignancies developing within the radiation field. Thus, minimizing radiotherapy exposure in pediatric patients is an important goal. Several retrospective studies in adults with soft tissue sarcomas suggest that certain patient subsets may be safely treated without adjuvant radiotherapy. At a median follow-up of 126 months, the 10-year actuarial local control rate was 93±4% in 74 adults treated with surgery alone for non-metastatic trunk or extremity soft tissue sarcoma (Baldini et al. 1999). In this study, tumor grade, size, site (extremity vs. trunk), and depth did not significantly influence the local recurrence rate. A similar study of 56 adults with soft tissue sarcoma (84% high grade) treated with wide resection alone reported a 7% incidence of local recurrence (Rydholm et al. 1991). These findings suggest that omitting adjuvant radiotherapy in pediatric patients who undergo wide resection of NRSTS may be a viable option. However, the safety of this approach will need to be confirmed in prospective pediatric trials.

Patients with microscopic residual low-grade NRSTS following maximal surgery are another group for whom adjuvant radiotherapy may reasonably be omitted. The local recurrence rate for patients in this category ranges from 25% to 50% (Brennan 1997; Spunt et al. 1999). Although this rate is relatively high, virtually all patients can be salvaged after local recurrence with further surgery, with or without radiotherapy (Spunt et al. 1999). With this approach, about three-quarters of children with microscopic residual low-grade NRSTS may be spared radiotherapy and its long-term consequences.

Since the local control approach (amputation or limb sparing surgery with radiotherapy) does not influence survival, the decision regarding which approach to use in a particular patient with resectable NRSTS may be individualized. Issues to be considered include functional outcome, psychosocial adjustment, and the risk of radiotherapy-induced secondary cancers.

7.6.1.2 Surgical Management of Metastases

Complete excision of all distant metastases is critical to cure in the small proportion of patients with metastatic disease who can be cured. The indications for surgical resection of pulmonary metastases are evolving and depend in part on individual tumor and patient characteristics. The goal of pulmonary metastasectomy should be cure, so this procedure should be avoided in patients with widespread parenchymal metastases and those with extensive mediastinal or chest wall involvement. In addition, there should be no evidence of residual tumor at the primary site, no extrapulmonary metastatic disease, no significant comorbidity, and adequate pulmonary function. The ability to completely resect all visible metastases is prognostically more important than the number of tumors removed (Girard et al. 1997); thus, metastasectomy should be considered in patients with multiple nodules if they can be safely approached surgically.

For patients whose tumor recurs in the lungs following pulmonary metastasectomy, repeat resection may be warranted. Those with one or fewer adverse risk factors (high-grade tumor, more than three nodules, any lesion larger than 2 cm) have a disease-specific survival of 65 months, compared to 10 months for those with three adverse risk factors (Weiser et al. 2000).

7.6.2 Radiation Therapy

Radiation therapy plays an important adjuvant role in the multimodality management for many patients with NRSTS. Unlike rhabdomyosarcoma and Ewing's sarcoma where radiotherapy can be used instead of surgery, local control with radiotherapy alone for unresectable soft-tissue sarcomas is reported to be no higher than 25–30%. Most of the useful data regarding treatment for NRSTS is derived from studies in adults since large clinical trials for children with these tumors have been lacking. In addition to defining the role for radiotherapy in the pediatric population, future investigations will need to answer basic questions relating to the necessary radiation dose and margin in pediatric NRSTS.

The current standard for high-grade soft tissue sarcomas is limb-preserving resection, when possible, in conjunction with radiotherapy. In a well known prospective randomized trial from the National Cancer Institute (NCI), this approach was shown to produce disease-free and overall survival rates similar to those achieved with amputation (Rosenberg et al. 1982). All patients in that study received chemotherapy. Subsequently, the NCI has reported another prospective randomized trial comparing limb-preserving surgery with or without postoperative radiation. Radiotherapy was shown to significantly decrease the risk of local relapse for both high-grade and low-grade sarcomas (Yang et al. 1998). Only those patients with high-grade tumors received chemotherapy. Radiation therapy did not affect overall survival in this trial. There are single institution series of highly selected patients indicating that some patients with high-grade tumor less than 5 cm may have excellent local control with wide resection alone (Alektiar et al. 2002; Baldini et al. 1999).

The role of adjuvant radiotherapy for low-grade sarcomas is controversial. Most series support the assertion that local control following wide surgical resection alone is excellent and therefore radiotherapy is not indicated (Baldini et al. 1999). However, postoperative radiation may be considered for low-grade sarcomas in the case of involved surgical margins, tumor that has recurred following initial wide resection, large tumor size (>5 cm), or in a case where surgery for recurrence would be unacceptably morbid (i.e., amputation).

At this time, no histology-specific guidelines exist for the use of radiotherapy. It is generally believed though not proven that synovial sarcoma may be more sensitive to radiotherapy than other histologies, based on its improved responsiveness to chemotherapy. Nonetheless, maximal surgical resection is still recommended. Some tumors that are relatively unresponsive to chemotherapy, for instance alveolar soft part sarcoma, are known to be sensitive to radiotherapy. The least responsive tumors are thought to be the low-grade tumors. The development of multi-institutional clinical trials will hopefully allow investigators to gain more understanding about the relationship between tumor histology and radiation therapy.

Whole lung radiation therapy is not recommended for patients with lung metastases from NRSTS. This is very different than the paradigm for rhabdomyosarcoma and Ewing's sarcoma where whole lung radiotherapy is used routinely and is thought to contribute to the low but still significant cure rates in patients with metastatic disease. Unfortunately, almost all patients with metastatic NRSTS are incurable with current therapies. Because of reduced sensitivity of these histologies to radiation, the therapeutic ratio of efficacy versus toxicity is too unfavorable to consider whole lung radiotherapy to be of benefit.

7.6.2.1 Radiation Planning

For patients who will likely require radiotherapy, it is ideal for the radiation oncologist to evaluate the patient as soon as the diagnosis is made. Radiation fields are based on the initial extent of disease, prior to chemotherapy or surgery. The radiation oncologist may suggest interventions that may only be possible before definitive surgery is performed. Such options include preoperative radiotherapy, intraoperative radiation therapy, or brachytherapy. There may be other considerations at the time of surgery such as the need to move ovaries or sling bowel out of the planned radiation field.

Before beginning a course of radiotherapy, a simulation must be preformed. During this session, the patient is positioned properly for radiation treatment, an immobilization cast may be made, and small permanent dots are made on the skin. This allows the patient to be positioned in precisely the same way each day for treatment. Simple treatments may be designed with blocks drawn on X-rays taken at the time of simulation. More complex or conformal radiotherapy requires a treatment planning CT scan. In this case, treatment fields are designed in three dimensions on a computer. New technology enables the radiation oncologist to fuse diagnostic MRI scans and functional imaging studies such as positron emission tomography (PET) scans with the treatment planning CT scan. This allows an ideal view of the anatomy in three dimensions.

The radiation target volume consists of the tumor volume at diagnosis plus a margin. While a standard sarcoma margin in adults is 5 cm, an effort is made in pediatric patients to reduce the margin to 2 cm so that more normal tissue is spared. Traditionally, the entire operative bed and all scars have been included in the initial treatment volume. This concept has recently been challenged because of the excellent results achieved with brachytherapy where all of these areas are not necessarily included. In the 1980s, the Pediatric Oncology Group randomized patients with Ewing's sarcoma to involved field (tumor plus 2 cm margin) versus whole bone or whole muscle bundle radiotherapy. With recently reported mature results, there was no difference in event free survival between the groups (Donaldson et al. 1998). It is preferred not to irradiate across a joint space when possible. It is also imperative that a strip of normal tissue be spared when treating an extremity since circumferential radiation can result in severe lymphedema.

In adults, radiation doses of 63–70 Gy are typically used for adjuvant treatment of NRSTS. While these doses may be reasonable for older teenagers, there is concern that such high doses will cause severe morbidity in younger patients. There is no reliable data to confirm what dose is adequate for various histologies and clinical situations. Some rhabdomyosarcoma and Ewing's sarcoma trials that include NRSTS have used doses as low as 40–50 Gy. The planned Children's Oncology Group NRSTS has proposed a neoadjuvant dose of 45 Gy (with a boost to a total dose of 55.8 Gy for positive microscopic margins at the time of surgery) and an adjuvant dose of 55.8 Gy. Outside of an investigational trial, factors such as the patient's age, tumor histology and site, as well as surgical margin status should be considered when choosing a dose.

7.6.2.2 Timing of Radiotherapy

The timing of radiation treatment depends upon a number of factors including diagnosis, location, extent of disease and the details of surgery and/or chemotherapy. Postoperative radiotherapy is most commonly used and should begin as soon as adequate would healing is achieved. This is usually 3–6 weeks after surgery. Any further delay may increase the risk of a local recurrence. Radiation therapy should not be given concurrently with doxorubicin chemotherapy because of the severe radiosensitizing effect on normal tissues such as skin.

Preoperative radiotherapy may be given with or without chemotherapy in cases where shrinking the tumor may significantly improve the possibility or quality of resection. Aside from potentially increasing resectability, preoperative radiation may decrease the risk of tumor contamination at the time of surgery. Preoperative radiation often allows for smaller radiotherapy treatment fields, particularly if extensive surgery is planned. Pelvic tumors are very well suited for preoperative treatment because the dose limiting normal structures (bladder, bowel, etc.) are often pushed out of the field by the tumor and receive less radiation than they would postoperatively when they fall back into the treatment field. A lower dose of radiation may theoretically be given preoperatively since the biological effectiveness is expected to be higher in the well-oxygenated intact tumor than in a hypoxic tumor bed. Potential disadvantages of preoperative radiation are the delay in surgery, increased risk of wound healing complications, and less information on tumor extent and pathology. Nonetheless, long-term function appears to be better in patients receiving preoperative therapy (DeLaney et al. 2003; O'Sullivan et al. 2002).

7.6.2.3 Brachytherapy

Brachytherapy refers to the insertion of radiation sources into tissues. These implants can be temporary or permanent. In experienced hands, brachytherapy may be an excellent postoperative treatment for soft tissue sarcomas. This technique was pioneered at Memorial Sloan-Kettering Cancer Center (MSKCC). In a prospective randomized trial, adjuvant brachytherapy was associated with a dramatic improvement in local control for high-grade lesions (89% with brachytherapy compared to 66% with no radiation) (Pisters et al. 1996b). A second study from the same center showed that external beam radiotherapy should be added to brachytherapy for tumors that are resected with involved surgical margins. Local control was 90% with external beam plus brachytherapy versus 59% with brachytherapy alone (Alekhteyar et al. 1996).

Brachytherapy is performed by the radiation oncologist at the time of tumor resection. Catheters are aligned at 1-cm intervals across the entire open operative bed following tumor removal. The catheters are sutured in place prior to the surgeon closing the wound. The following day, radiation localization films are taken in order to plan the brachytherapy dosing. For low-dose-rate treatment, cesium or iodine radioactive sources are placed inside the catheters on postoperative day 5. Earlier placement of sources was found to delay wound healing. The sources remain in place for 2–5 days depending on the prescribed dose. The recommended doses are 45 Gy for patients with negative margins and 15–20 Gy plus 45–50 Gy external beam for those with positive margins. The sources are then removed from the patient and the catheters are pulled. Alternatively, fractionated high-dose-rate therapy with iridium may be used. Early experience at MSKCC with a definitive regimen of ten fractions of 3.4 Gy/day over 5 days has been promising. This option is especially attractive for pediatric patients because it does not require radiation safety restrictions on visitors to the child's hospital room.

Brachytherapy is most useful for extremity tumors. The advantages of this technique over external beam radiation include a much more rapid and convenient treatment and increased sparing of normal tissues. Another form of brachytherapy called intraoperative radiotherapy (IORT) has been shown to produce encouraging rates of local control of 74% for primary retroperitoneal sarcomas when combined with external beam radiotherapy (Alektiar et al. 2000).

7.6.2.4 New Technologies

Intensity modulated radiation therapy and proton beam therapy may be used in pediatric sarcomas in an effort to decrease late side-effects of radiation. Selective avoidance of critical normal tissues near the tumor may be achieved with these modalities. For instance, in a child with a tumor surrounding a growing bone, the bone dose can often be reduced so that the bone can continue to grow normally. Patients with tumors in almost all anatomical sites can potentially benefit from this advanced technology.

7.6.2.5 Acute Side Effects of Radiotherapy

External beam radiotherapy is typically given once daily, 5 days/week. A course of radiation for sarcoma may take 6–7 weeks depending upon the total dose required. Acute side effects of treatment generally begin after the first 2 weeks and increase as treatment continues. Most patients report fatigue during radiation therapy and the majority develop a grade 1–3 skin reaction, especially with extremity treatment. Provided that adequate wound healing is achieved prior to beginning radiation, it is uncommon for wound dehiscence to occur. Epilation in the treatment portals is expected. Radiation only suppresses blood counts if large volumes of bone marrow are included in the field, as in the case of large pelvic tumors. Other acute side effects are less common and depend upon the anatomical site.

7.6.2.6 Long-Term Side Effects of Radiotherapy

The long-term complications of radiation therapy in children can be severe and debilitating depending on the site treated and upon the dose and technique used. Thus, radiation should only be prescribed when absolutely indicated. It is the responsibility of the radiation oncologist to do everything possible to minimize the risk of long-term side effects. Months to years after receiving radiation therapy, patients may experience muscle fibrosis. This may be asymptomatic or in more severe cases may inhibit function. Stretching exercises are recommended to combat this problem. If the growth plates of a bone receive more than 20–25 Gy, arrest of growth will occur. In a prepubescent child, this can lead to significant cosmetic and functional problems, with the severity depending upon the age of the child, the radiation dose and the anatomic site. Care must be taken to irradiate bones such as vertebral bodies symmetrically to prevent iatrogenic scoliosis. Higher doses of radiation can weaken bones or cause joint dysfunction. Only in rare cases does this lead to a serious complication such as fracture or the need for joint replacement. Edema distal to the irradiated site in an extremity may occur as a result of radiation. This risk depends upon the extent of surgery as well as the amount of soft tissue that is spared during radiotherapy. For this reason, the full circumference of a limb should never be treated to a high dose.

The risk of a second malignancy, typically more than 20 years after radiation, should be mentioned in the consent for radiotherapy in children. A recent paper (Hawkins et al. 1996) showed that the rate of secondary bone cancer after treatment for all childhood cancers was less than 1%. For those treated for Ewing's sarcoma, the risk was 5.4%. Children requiring radiotherapy should always be treated at a cancer center with an experienced pediatric radiation oncologist in order to minimize the risk and severity of long-term complications.

7.6.3 Chemotherapy

Although surgery and radiotherapy are known to be effective for the local treatment of soft tissue sarcomas, the role of chemotherapy in the management of pediatric patients with NRSTS remains controversial. In children and adolescents who have undergone gross tumor resection at the time of initial presentation, only 12% experience metastatic tumor recurrence (Spunt et al. 1999). However, patients with large (>5 cm), invasive, or high-grade tumors have a significantly higher (25–35%) risk of distant disease recurrence. Furthermore, survival following the development of metastatic disease is poor. For patients at high risk of developing distant metastases following local tumor control, and for those with tumors that are unresectable or metastatic at the time of initial presentation, chemotherapy must be considered.

The two agents that have exhibited the greatest activity in adult soft tissue sarcomas are doxorubicin and ifosfamide (Demetri and Elias 1995). Controversy surrounds the optimal dose and schedule of these drugs, which often have been studied in combination with other agents, such as dacarbazine. Translating the data from adult soft tissue sarcoma studies into recommendations for the treatment of pediatric patients is troublesome for several reasons. First, few studies in adults have utilized dose-intensive regimens that would be well tolerated in pediatric patients. Thus, response rates and outcomes might be superior in pediatric populations treated with higher-dose regimens compared to those reported in adults. Second, the predominant histologic subtypes in adults (liposarcoma, malignant fibrous histiocytoma, leiomyosarcoma) differ from those that are most prevalent in childhood (synovial sarcoma, malignant peripheral nerve sheath tumor, fibrosarcoma). The extent to which differences in the distribution of histologic subtype influence the response to chemotherapy is unclear. However, synovial sarcoma, the most common NRSTS in childhood, is among the most chemosensitive subtypes. Thus, the indications for chemotherapy in children may differ from those in adults. Finally, the long-term consequences of chemotherapy exposure must be considered carefully in children and young adults, for whom life expectancy may be decades longer than in many adult patients.

7.6.3.1 Adjuvant Chemotherapy

The only published pediatric adjuvant chemotherapy study, conducted by the Pediatric Oncology Group in the late 1980s, was a randomized comparison of VACA (vincristine, actinomycin D, cyclophosphamide, and doxorubicin) to observation alone (Pratt et al. 1999). Unfortunately, only 30 of the 81 eligible patients accepted randomization; the remaining 51 were treated according to their preference. Among the patients who accepted randomization, event-free and overall survival were inferior in the group that received chemotherapy. The findings were similar in the group as a whole; patients who received chemotherapy had event-free and overall survival estimates that were inferior to those of patients who were observed. However, in both the randomized and non-randomized subsets there was an imbalance in patients with high-grade tumors between the two treatment arms, with a greater proportion of patients with high-grade tumors assigned to the chemotherapy arm. The differences in outcomes between patients randomized to chemotherapy and to observation disappeared when the analyses of event-free and overall survival were stratified by tumor grade. Event-free survival was found to be significantly worse in patients with high-grade tumors, regardless of their randomization status. Further analysis of patients with high-grade tumors showed that outcome did not differ depending on whether or not chemotherapy was administered.

This clinical trial did not adequately determine whether or not adjuvant chemotherapy is beneficial in pediatric patients with grossly resected soft tissue sarcomas. However, it did confirm an important finding from studies in adults, namely that high histologic grade is a major determinant of the risk of distant metastatic spread. The difficulties inherent in randomized comparisons of chemotherapy to observation alone make future pediatric studies to firmly establish the role of adjuvant chemotherapy unlikely. Thus, conclusions must be drawn by extrapolating findings from studies in adults with soft tissue sarcomas.

Many clinical trials of adjuvant chemotherapy for soft tissue sarcomas in adults have been conducted. As anthracyclines are among the most active agents in sarcomas, they are a component of virtually all of these adjuvant chemotherapy regimens. Fewer studies have included ifosfamide, which has recently shown significant activity in soft tissue sarcomas. These adjuvant chemotherapy trials in adults have important limitations. First, most of these studies are small and are inadequately powered to identify small improvements in outcome. Many of the trials enrolled relatively heterogeneous patient populations (for example, patients with both low-grade and high-grade tumors), making their interpretation more difficult. Finally, the anthracycline dose-intensity in many of these studies was suboptimal, raising the question of whether outcomes might improve with the use of more intensive chemotherapy regimens. A recent randomized clinical trial by an Italian cooperative group contributed important data to the debate about the role of adjuvant chemotherapy (Frustaci et al. 2001). In this study, 104 adults with high-grade extremity soft tissue sarcomas were randomized, after locoregional treatment, to high-dose epirubicin/ifosfamide chemotherapy or observation. At a median follow-up of 59 months, the median disease-free survival was 48 vs. 16 months (p=.04) and overall survival 75 vs. 46 months (p=.03) for the chemotherapy and observation groups, respectively. Although this was a well-designed study, its small size precludes drawing definitive conclusions from its findings.

Due to the limitations of the published randomized clinical trials, several meta-analyses have been performed. The most rigorous of these was an analysis of 1,568 patients treated on 14 randomized adjuvant trials (doxorubicin-based chemotherapy vs. observation) (Sarcoma Meta-analysis Collaboration 1997). The overall hazard ratio for recurrence-free survival was 0.75 (95% CI 0.64–0.87) (p=0.0001) in favor of adjuvant chemotherapy, translating to an absolute improvement of 10% (from 45% to 55%) at 10 years. Although there was a trend toward improved overall survival in chemotherapy-treated patients, the hazard ratio of 0.89 (95% CI 0.76–1.03) was not significant (p=0.12). This meta-analysis has many shortcomings, namely the inclusion of patients with tumors at all anatomic locations and tumors of both high and low grade, as well as the fact that only one of the studies analyzed included ifosfamide in the chemotherapy regimen. Despite these limitations it appears that chemotherapy carries some benefit, at least for certain patients with non-metastatic NRSTS.

7.6.3.2 Neoadjuvant Chemotherapy

Two pediatric clinical trials have evaluated neoadjuvant chemotherapy for the treatment of unresectable or metastatic NRSTS. The first, which opened in 1986, was a randomized comparison of VACA (vincristine, actinomycin D, cyclophosphamide, doxorubicin) to VACAD (VACA plus dacarbazine) (Pratt et al. 1998). The study was closed prematurely (after nearly 8 years) due to slow accrual and a high rate of refusal of randomization among patients enrolled. Ultimately a total of 61 patients were treated, of whom 50 were randomized (25 to each treatment arm). The remaining 11 patients were non-randomly assigned to VACA due to a shortage of dacarbazine. Of the entire group of 61 patients, only 28 (46%) experienced a complete or partial response to neoadjuvant chemotherapy. Among randomized patients, the addition of dacarbazine to VACA did not lead to an improved response rate (p=0.4) or event-free survival (p=0.7).

The second neoadjuvant chemotherapy trial for pediatric patients with unresected or metastatic NRSTS tested the combination of vincristine, ifosfamide (9 g/m^2/cycle), and doxorubicin (60 mg/m^2/cycle) (Pappo 2005 all updated reference). This regimen was well tolerated, and the overall rate of complete or partial response following two courses of chemotherapy was 40%. Patients with synovial sarcoma and undifferentiated sarcoma experienced a slightly higher rate of response. One shortcoming of this clinical trial was the use of relatively modest doses of doxorubicin (60 mg/m^2/cycle).

The published experience in adults with soft tissue sarcomas treated with neoadjuvant chemotherapy mirrors that of childhood NRSTS. Preoperative chemotherapy is generally tolerable and appears to have no significant impact on postoperative morbidity (Meric et al. 2000). Rates of response range from about 30% to 50%, depending on the study population and the chemotherapy regimen used (Elias et al. 1989; Gortzak et al. 2001). Dose-intensive regimens may induce objective responses in up to two-thirds of patients (Patel et al. 1998). Although tumor responses are documented in a significant fraction of patients, it is unclear what proportion of those with initially unresectable primary tumors are able to undergo gross tumor resection following induction chemotherapy. Furthermore, up to 20% of patients experience tumor progression following neoadjuvant chemotherapy. Thus, outside of a clinical trial setting, neoadjuvant chemotherapy should be considered only for children with unresectable or metastatic NRSTS.

7.6.3.3 Other Approaches to the Use of Standard Chemotherapy

Studies in adults have explored a variety of other methods of delivering standard chemotherapy. Intra-arterial chemotherapy has the potential advantage of providing higher chemotherapy exposure for extremity tumors than intravenous therapy. However, complications associated with intra-arterial chemotherapy include arterial thromboembolism, infection, gangrene, and poor wound healing. This technique, which has a limited role in adult soft tissue sarcomas, has not been well studied in childhood NRSTS.

Isolated limb perfusion, with or without hyperthermia, has also been studied in adult soft tissue sarcomas. In this technique, the arterial and venous supplies of the limb are connected to an extracorporeal circulation system to isolate the limb from the systemic circulation. Chemotherapy, with or without biologic agents (such as tumor necrosis factor), is then infused into the circuit. Blood in the circuit may be warmed to 39° to 40 °C to enhance the efficacy of chemotherapy. Complications of this technique include thrombosis, infection, damage to soft tissue structures, lymphedema, and systemic complications related to leakage of tumor necrosis factor into the systemic circulation. Published experience with this technique in pediatric NRSTS is limited to case reports.

Whole body hyperthermia via extracorporeal heating of blood has been used in a small number of adult studies in an effort to enhance the effects of chemotherapy. Although this technique has shown some promise, it has not been used for childhood NRSTS.

7.6.3.4 High-Dose Chemotherapy

The poor outcome of patients with high-risk NRSTS has led to the evaluation of chemotherapy dose escalation as a strategy to improve outcome. A number of phase I and II clinical trials in adults have shown that dose escalation of known active agents can modestly improve response rates in soft tissue sarcomas, providing the rationale for studying more intensive chemotherapy with hematopoietic stem cell rescue. Very few studies have been conducted to date (Reichardt 2002). These studies are hampered by their small size, heterogeneous patient population, and the fact that they were not randomized. Thus, dose-intensive chemotherapy with stem cell rescue must be considered investigational at this time. There have been no studies evaluating high-dose chemotherapy with stem cell support for pediatric NRSTS.

7.6.3.5 Novel Agents

Several novel chemotherapeutic and biologic agents have become available in the last few years that show promise in adults with soft tissue sarcomas. Ecteinascidin-743 (ET-743) has aroused considerable interest based on the findings of two multicenter phase II studies showing a 14% objective response rate in untreated patients and a median duration of response of 11 months (Demetri 2002). Side effects were mild, manageable, and transient. Both gemcitabine and docetaxel have shown some efficacy in single-agent phase II studies; a recent retrospective evaluation of the combination demonstrated responses in adults with leiomyosarcoma, malignant peripheral nerve sheath tumor, malignant fibrous histiocytoma, and angiosarcoma (Leu et al. 2004).

The identification of imatinib mesylate for patients with gastrointestinal stromal tumor (GIST) illustrates the potential advantage of therapy targeted to tumor biology. Prior to the development of imatinib mesylate, outcome for adults with unresectable or metastatic GIST was dismal since standard chemotherapy was only rarely effective. The observation that many GISTs overexpress the tyrosine kinase c-kit led to clinical trials of imatinib mesylate, a potent inhibitor of this protein. Imatinib, which is very well tolerated, has shown considerable activity in GIST and has transformed the treatment of this soft tissue sarcoma (Eisenberg et al. 2004). Similarly, clinical response to imatinib mesylate has been seen in metastatic dermatofibrosarcoma protuberans, presumably due to imatinib-induced inhibition of the related PDGFB kinase (Rubin et al. 2002).

Other categories of drugs still in early phase clinical trials that hold potential promise for soft tissue sarcomas include the anti-angiogenic agents, epidermal growth factor receptor inhibitors, mTOR (mammalian target of rapamycin) inhibitors, and matrix metalloproteinase inhibitors. Targeted therapy may prove more effective and less toxic than treatments currently available for childhood NRSTS.

7.6.3.6 Late Effects of Chemotherapy

The long-term side effects of standard chemotherapy may be severe and even life-threatening. Doxorubicin can cause cardiomyopathy, which may be worsened by concomitant radiotherapy to the heart. Efforts to replace doxorubicin with other chemotherapeutic agents or to prevent its cardiotoxic effects (for example, with dexrazoxane) may diminish the risk of long-term cardiac compromise. Ifosfamide is associated with a variety of long-term complications including renal impairment (glomerular and/or tubular toxicity), osteopenia/osteoporosis, gonadal hormonal failure/infertility, and chronic hemorrhagic cystitis with resulting bladder fibrosis. Both doxorubicin and ifosfamide have been etiologically related to the development of second malignant neoplasms, the risk of which is further increased by radiotherapy.

7.7 Current Problems and Future Challenges

Because each of the childhood NRSTS is rare and these tumors have not been studied as systematically as have other more common childhood cancers, our understanding of these tumors remains quite limited. Careful laboratory investigations may identify novel biologic prognostic factors as well as targets for therapeutic intervention. Prospective pediatric clinical trials are needed to confirm reported clinical prognostic features, since these will form the basis of risk-based therapy. Identifying a histologic grading system for pediatric NRSTS that will allow comparison with results of studies in adults is critical. Similarly, identifying a standard staging system for pediatric NRSTS will be important.

Among the most critical therapeutic questions is which patients fare well without adjuvant therapy. For the remaining patients who do require treatment beyond surgery alone, the optimal application of modalities currently in use must be evaluated. The minimum dose and field of radiotherapy necessary for adequate local control in pediatric NRSTS must be identified, and the least toxic and most effective chemotherapy regimen(s) must be ascertained. How to best use chemotherapy and radiotherapy to achieve gross tumor resection in patients with unresectable disease is another important research priority. Finally, novel therapies devoid of the toxicity of chemotherapy and radiotherapy must be found. In the coming years, laboratory investigations will surely identify relevant therapeutic targets; the challenge will be to develop effective targeted therapies and to learn how best to utilize these agents.

References

Alekhteyar KM, Leung DH, Brennan MF, Harrison LB (1996) The effect of combined external beam radiotherapy and brachytherapy on local control and wound complications in patients with high-grade soft tissue sarcomas of the extremity with positive microscopic margin. Int J Radiat Oncol Biol Phys 36(2):321–324

Alektiar KM, Hu K, Anderson L, Brennan MF, Harrison LB (2000) High-dose-rate intraoperative radiation therapy (HDR-IORT) for retroperitoneal sarcomas. Int J Radiat Oncol Biol Phys 47(1):157–163

Alektiar KM, Leung D, Zelefsky MJ, Brennan MF (2002) Adjuvant radiation for stage II-B soft tissue sarcoma of the extremity. J Clin Oncol 20(6):1643–1650

American Joint Committee on Cancer (2002) Chapter 22. In: Greene FL, Page DL, Fleming ID, Fritz AG, Balch CM, Haller DG, Morrow M (eds) AJCC Cancer Staging Handbook. Springer, New York

Artandi SE, Chang S, Lee SL et al. (2000) Telomere dysfunction promotes non-reciprocal translocations and epithelial cancers in mice. Nature 406(6796):641–645

Baldini EH, Goldberg J, Jenner C et al. (1999) Long-term outcomes after function-sparing surgery without radiotherapy for soft tissue sarcoma of the extremities and trunk. J Clin Oncol 17(10):3252–3259

Biegel JA, Tan L, Zhang F, Wainwright L, Russo P, Rorke LB (2002) Alterations of the hSNF5/INI1 gene in central nervous system atypical teratoid/rhabdoid tumors and renal and extrarenal rhabdoid tumors. Clin Cancer Res 8(11): 3461–3467

Brady MS, Gaynor JJ, Brennan MF (1992) Radiation-associated sarcoma of bone and soft tissue. Arch Surg 127(12):1379–1385

Brennan MF (1997) The enigma of local recurrence. The Society of Surgical Oncology. Ann Surg Oncol 4(1):1–12

Brouns F, Stas M, De Wever I (2003) Delay in diagnosis of soft tissue sarcomas. Eur J Surg Oncol 29(5):440–445

Cessna MH, Zhou H, Sanger WG et al. (2002) Expression of ALK1 and p80 in inflammatory myofibroblastic tumor and its mesenchymal mimics: a study of 135 cases. Mod Pathol 15(9):931–938

Coffin CM, Patel A, Perkins S, Elenitoba-Johnson KS, Perlman E, Griffin CA (2001) ALK1 and p80 expression and chromosomal rearrangements involving 2p23 in inflammatory myofibroblastic tumor. Mod Pathol 14(6):569–576

Coindre JM, Pelmus M, Hostein I, Lussan C, Bui BN, Guillou L (2003) Should molecular testing be required for diagnosing synovial sarcoma? A prospective study of 204 cases. Cancer 98(12):2700–2707

DeLaney TF, Spiro IJ, Suit HD et al. (2003) Neoadjuvant chemotherapy and radiotherapy for large extremity soft-tissue sarcomas. Int J Radiat Oncol Biol Phys 56(4): 1117–1127

Demetri GD (2002) ET-743: the US experience in sarcomas of soft tissues. Anticancer Drugs 13 Suppl 1:S7–9

Demetri GD, Elias AD (1995) Results of single-agent and combination chemotherapy for advanced soft tissue sarcomas. Implications for decision making in the clinic. Hematol Oncol Clin North Am 9(4):765–785

Dich J, Zahm SH, Hanberg A, Adami HO (1997) Pesticides and cancer. Cancer Causes Control 8(3):420–443

Donaldson SS, Torrey M, Link MP et al. (1998) A multidisciplinary study investigating radiotherapy in Ewing's sarcoma: end results of POG #8346. Pediatric Oncology Group. Int J Radiat Oncol Biol Phys 42(1):125–135

Duyster J, Bai RY, Morris SW (2001) Translocations involving anaplastic lymphoma kinase (ALK). Oncogene 20(40): 5623–5637

Eisenberg BL, Judson I (2004) Surgery and imatinib in the management of GIST: emerging approaches to adjuvant and neoadjuvant therapy. Ann Surg Oncol 11(5):465–475

Elias A, Ryan L, Sulkes A, Collins J, Aisner J, Antman KH (1989) Response to mesna, doxorubicin, ifosfamide, and dacarbazine in 108 patients with metastatic or unresectable sarcoma and no prior chemotherapy. J Clin Oncol 7(9): 1208–1216

Enneking WF, Spanier SS, Goodman MA (1980) A system for the surgical staging of musculoskeletal sarcoma. Clin Orthop 153:106–120

Espat NJ, Bilsky M, Lewis JJ, Leung D, Brennan MF (2002) Soft tissue sarcoma brain metastases. Prevalence in a cohort of 3829 patients. Cancer 94(10):2706–2711

Falk H, Herbert J, Crowley S et al. (1981) Epidemiology of hepatic angiosarcoma in the United States: 1964–1974. Environ Health Perspect 41:107–113

Fleming JB, Cantor SB, Varma DG et al. (2001) Utility of chest computed tomography for staging in patients with T1 extremity soft tissue sarcomas. Cancer 92(4):863–868

Fong Y, Coit DG, Woodruff JM, Brennan MF (1993) Lymph node metastasis from soft tissue sarcoma in adults. Analysis of data from a prospective database of 1772 sarcoma patients. Ann Surg 217(1):72–77

Frustaci S, Gherlinzoni F, De Paoli A et al. (2001) Adjuvant chemotherapy for adult soft tissue sarcomas of the extremities and girdles: results of the Italian randomized cooperative trial. J Clin Oncol 19(5):1238–1247

Gerald WL, Ladanyi M, de Alava E et al. (1998) Clinical, pathologic, and molecular spectrum of tumors associated with t(11;22)(p13;q12): desmoplastic small round-cell tumor and its variants. J Clin Oncol 16(9):3028–3036

Girard P, Spaggiari L, Baldeyrou P et al. (1997) Should the number of pulmonary metastases influence the surgical decision? Eur J Cardiothorac Surg 12(3):385–391; discussion 392

Gortzak E, Azzarelli A, Buesa J et al. (2001) A randomised phase II study on neo-adjuvant chemotherapy for 'high-risk' adult soft-tissue sarcoma. Eur J Cancer 37(9):1096–1103

Haimi M, Peretz Nahum M, Ben Arush MW (2004) Delay in diagnosis of children with cancer: a retrospective study of 315 children. Pediatr Hematol Oncol 21(1):37–48

Hajdu SI, Shiu MH, Brennan MF (1988) The role of the pathologist in the management of soft tissue sarcomas. World J Surg 12(3):326–331

Hanahan D, Weinberg RA (2000) The hallmarks of cancer. Cell 100(1):57–70

Hawkins MM, Wilson LM et al. (1996) Radiotherapy, alkylating agents, and risk of bone cancer after childhood cancer. J Nat Cancer Inst 88(5):270–278

Heinrich MC, Corless CL, Duensing A et al. (2003) PDGFRA activating mutations in gastrointestinal stromal tumors. Science 299(5607):708–710

Helman LJ, Meltzer P (2003) Mechanisms of sarcoma development. Nat Rev Cancer 3(9):685–694

Heslin MJ, Lewis JJ, Woodruff JM, Brennan MF (1997) Core needle biopsy for diagnosis of extremity soft tissue sarcoma. Ann Surg Oncol 4(5):425–431

Hill DA, Riedley SE, Patel AR et al. (2003) Real-time polymerase chain reaction as an aid for the detection of SYT-SSX1 and SYT-SSX2 transcripts in fresh and archival pediatric synovial sarcoma specimens: report of 25 cases from St. Jude Children's Research Hospital. Pediatr Dev Pathol 6(1):24–34

Hirota S, Isozaki K, Moriyama Y et al. (1998) Gain-of-function mutations of c-kit in human gastrointestinal stromal tumors. Science 279(5350):577–580

Hudson MM, Tyc VL, Cremer LK et al. (1998) Patient satisfaction after limb-sparing surgery and amputation for pediatric malignant bone tumors. J Pediatr Oncol Nurs 15(2):60–69; discussion 70–61

Ioannidis JP, Lau J (2003) 18F-FDG PET for the diagnosis and grading of soft-tissue sarcoma: a meta-analysis. J Nucl Med 44(5):717–724

Jager PL, Hoekstra HJ, Leeuw J, van Der Graaf WT, de Vries EG, Piers D (2000) Routine bone scintigraphy in primary staging of soft tissue sarcoma. Is it worthwhile? Cancer 89(8): 1726–1731

Judkins AR, Mauger J, Ht A, Rorke LB, Biegel JA (2004) Immunohistochemical analysis of hSNF5/INI1 in pediatric CNS neoplasms. Am J Surg Pathol 28(5):644–650

Kawai A, Woodruff J, Healey JH, Brennan MF, Antonescu CR, Ladanyi M (1998) SYT-SSX gene fusion as a determinant of morphology and prognosis in synovial sarcoma. N Engl J Med 338(3):153–160

Kuttesch JF Jr, Wexler LH, Marcus RB et al. (1996) Second malignancies after Ewing's sarcoma: radiation dose-dependency of secondary sarcomas. J Clin Oncol (10):2818–2825

Ladanyi M, Antonescu CR, Leung DH et al. (2002) Impact of SYT-SSX fusion type on the clinical behavior of synovial sarcoma: a multi-institutional retrospective study of 243 patients. Cancer Res 62(1):135–140

Leu KM, Ostruszka LJ, Shewach D et al. (2004) Laboratory and clinical evidence of synergistic cytotoxicity of sequential treatment with gemcitabine followed by docetaxel in the treatment of sarcoma. J Clin Oncol 22(9):1706–1712

Lewis JJ, Leung D, Woodruff JM, Brennan MF (1998) Retroperitoneal soft-tissue sarcoma: analysis of 500 patients treated and followed at a single institution. Ann Surg 228(3):355–365

Li FP, Fraumeni JF Jr, Mulvihill JJ et al. (1988) A cancer family syndrome in twenty-four kindreds. Cancer Res 48(18): 5358–5362

Li XQ, Hisaoka M, Shi DR, Zhu XZ, Hashimoto H (2004) Expression of anaplastic lymphoma kinase in soft tissue tumors: an immunohistochemical and molecular study of 249 cases. Hum Pathol 35(6):711–721

Malkin D, Li FP, Strong LC et al. (1990) Germ line p53 mutations in a familial syndrome of breast cancer, sarcomas, and other neoplasms. Science 250(4985):1233–1238

Marcus KC, Grier HE, Shamberger RC et al. (1997) Childhood soft tissue sarcoma: a 20-year experience. J Pediatr 131(4): 603–607

Maurer HM, Beltangady M, Gehan EA et al. (1988) The Intergroup Rhabdomyosarcoma Study-I. A final report. Cancer 61(2):209–220

McClain KL, Leach CT, Jenson HB et al. (1995) Association of Epstein-Barr virus with leiomyosarcomas in children with AIDS. N Engl J Med 332(1):12–18

Meric F, Milas M, Hunt KK et al. (2000) Impact of neoadjuvant chemotherapy on postoperative morbidity in soft tissue sarcomas. J Clin Oncol 18(19):3378–3383

Miettinen M (1991) Keratin subsets in spindle cell sarcomas. Keratins are widespread but synovial sarcoma contains a distinctive keratin polypeptide pattern and desmoplakins. Am J Pathol 138(2):505–513

Miralles TG, Gosalbez F, Menendez P, Astudillo A, Torre C, Buesa J (1986) Fine needle aspiration cytology of soft-tissue lesions. Acta Cytol 30(6):671–678

Oliveira AM, Nascimento AG (2001) Grading in soft tissue tumors: principles and problems. Skeletal Radiol 30(10):543–559

O'Sullivan B, Davis AM, Turcotte R et al. (2002) Preoperative versus postoperative radiotherapy in soft-tissue sarcoma of the limbs: a randomised trial. Lancet 359(9325):2235–2241

Paganelli G, De Cicco C, Chinol M (2000) Sentinel node localization by lymphoscintigraphy: a reliable technique with widespread applications. Recent Results Cancer Res 157: 121–129

Panagopoulos I, Mertens F, Isaksson M et al. (2001) Clinical impact of molecular and cytogenetic findings in synovial sarcoma. Genes Chromosomes Cancer 31(4):362–372

Pappo AS, Rao BN, Jenkins JJ et al. (1999) Metastatic nonrhabdomyosarcomatous soft-tissue sarcomas in children and adolescents: the St. Jude Children's Research Hospital experience. Med Pediatr Oncol 33(2):76–82

Pappo AS, Devidas M, Jenkins J et al. (2005) Phase II trial of neoadjuvant vincristine, ifosfamide, and doxorubicin with granulocyte colony-stimulating factor support in children and adolescents with advanced-stage nonrhabdomyosarcomatous soft tissue sarcomas: a pediatric oncology group study. J Clin Oncol 23(18):4031–4038

Parham DM, Webber BL, Jenkins JJ 3rd, Cantor AB, Maurer HM (1995) Nonrhabdomyosarcomatous soft tissue sarcomas of childhood: formulation of a simplified system for grading. Mod Pathol 8(7):705–710

Patel SR, Vadhan-Raj S, Burgess MA et al. (1998) Results of two consecutive trials of dose-intensive chemotherapy with doxorubicin and ifosfamide in patients with sarcomas. Am J Clin Oncol 21(3):317–321

Perry A, Kunz SN, Fuller CE et al. (2002) Differential NF1, p16, and EGFR patterns by interphase cytogenetics (FISH) in malignant peripheral nerve sheath tumor (MPNST) and morphologically similar spindle cell neoplasms. J Neuropathol Exp Neurol 61(8):702–709

Pisters PW, Leung DH, Woodruff J, Shi W, Brennan MF (1996a) Analysis of prognostic factors in 1,041 patients with localized soft tissue sarcomas of the extremities. J Clin Oncol 14(5):1679–1689

Pisters PW, Harrison LB, Leung DH, Woodruff JM, Casper ES, Brennan MF (1996b) Long-term results of a prospective randomized trial of adjuvant brachytherapy in soft tissue sarcoma. J Clin Oncol 14(3):859–868

Porter GA, Cantor SB, Ahmad SA et al. (2002) Cost-effectiveness of staging computed tomography of the chest in patients with T2 soft tissue sarcomas. Cancer 94(1):197–204

Pratt CB, Maurer HM, Gieser P et al. (1998) Treatment of unresectable or metastatic pediatric soft tissue sarcomas with surgery, irradiation, and chemotherapy: a Pediatric Oncology Group study. Med Pediatr Oncol 30(4):201–209

Pratt CB, Pappo AS, Gieser P et al. (1999) Role of adjuvant chemotherapy in the treatment of surgically resected pediatric nonrhabdomyosarcomatous soft tissue sarcomas: A Pediatric Oncology Group Study. J Clin Oncol 17(4):1219

Presant CA, Russell WO, Alexander RW, Fu YS (1986) Soft-tissue and bone sarcoma histopathology peer review: the frequency of disagreement in diagnosis and the need for second pathology opinions. The Southeastern Cancer Study Group experience. J Clin Oncol 4(11):1658–1661

Reichardt P (2002) High-dose chemotherapy in adult soft tissue sarcoma. Crit Rev Oncol Hematol 41(2):157–167

Ries LA, Smith MA, Gurney JG et al. (1999) Cancer incidence and survival among children and adolescents: United States SEER Program 1975–1995. NCI, SEER Program. NIH Pub. No. 99-4649. Bethesda, MD, pp 99–4649

Roberts CW, Galusha SA, McMenamin ME, Fletcher CD, Orkin SH (2000) Haploinsufficiency of Snf5 (integrase interactor 1) predisposes to malignant rhabdoid tumors in mice. Proc Natl Acad Sci USA 97(25):13796–13800

Rodriguez-Galindo C, Ramsey K et al. (2000) Hemangiopericytoma in children and infants. Cancer 88(1):198–204.

Rosenberg SA, Tepper J, Glatstein E et al. (1982) The treatment of soft-tissue sarcomas of the extremities: prospective randomized evaluations of (1) limb-sparing surgery plus radiation therapy compared with amputation and (2) the role of adjuvant chemotherapy. Ann Surg 196(3):305–315

Rubin BP, Schuetze SM, Eary JF et al. (2002) Molecular targeting of platelet-derived growth factor B by imatinib mesylate in a patient with metastatic dermatofibrosarcoma protuberans. J Clin Oncol 20(17):3586–3591

Rydholm A, Gustafson P, Rooser B et al. (1991) Limb-sparing surgery without radiotherapy based on anatomic location of soft tissue sarcoma. J Clin Oncol 9(10):1757–1765

Sandberg AA, Bridge JA (2002) Updates on the cytogenetics and molecular genetics of bone and soft tissue tumors: congenital (infantile) fibrosarcoma and mesoblastic nephroma. Cancer Genet Cytogenet 132(1):1–13

Sarcoma Meta-analysis Collaboration (1997) Adjuvant chemotherapy for localised resectable soft-tissue sarcoma of adults: meta-analysis of individual data. Lancet 350(9092): 1647–1654

Scheel C, Schaefer KL, Jauch A et al. (2001) Alternative lengthening of telomeres is associated with chromosomal instability in osteosarcomas. Oncogene 20(29):3835–3844

Sharpless NE, Ferguson DO, O'Hagan RC et al. (2001) Impaired nonhomologous end-joining provokes soft tissue sarcomas harboring chromosomal translocations, amplifications, and deletions. Mol Cell 8(6):1187–1196

Shiraki M, Enterline HT, Brooks JJ et al. (1989) Pathologic analysis of advanced adult soft tissue sarcomas, bone sarcomas, and mesotheliomas. The Eastern Cooperative Oncology Group (ECOG) experience. Cancer 64(2):484–490

Skapek SX, Chui CH (2000) Cytogenetics and the biologic basis of sarcomas. Curr Opin Oncol 12(4):315–322

Skotheim RI, Kallioniemi A, Bjerkhagen B et al. (2003) Topoisomerase-II alpha is upregulated in malignant peripheral nerve sheath tumors and associated with clinical outcome. J Clin Oncol 21(24):4586–4591

Sorensen SA, Mulvihill JJ, Nielsen A (1986) Long-term follow-up of von Recklinghausen neurofibromatosis. Survival and malignant neoplasms. N Engl J Med 314(16):1010–1015

Spunt SL, Poquette CA, Hurt YS et al. (1999) Prognostic factors for children and adolescents with surgically resected nonrhabdomyosarcoma soft tissue sarcoma: an analysis of 121 patients treated at St Jude Children's Research Hospital. J Clin Oncol 17(12):3697–3705

Spunt SL, Hill DA, Motosue AM et al. (2002) Clinical features and outcome of initially unresected nonmetastatic pediatric nonrhabdomyosarcoma soft tissue sarcoma. J Clin Oncol 20(15):3225–3235

Stewart FW, Treves N (1981) Classics in oncology: lymphangiosarcoma in postmastectomy lymphedema: a report of six cases in elephantiasis chirurgica. CA Cancer J Clin 31(5):284–299

Stojadinovic A, Jaques DP, Leung DH, Healey JH, Brennan MF (2001) Amputation for recurrent soft tissue sarcoma of the extremity: indications and outcome. Ann Surg Oncol 8(6): 509–518

Storlazzi CT, Mertens F, Mandahl N et al. (2003) A novel fusion gene, SS18L1/SSX1, in synovial sarcoma. Genes Chromosomes Cancer 37(2):195–200

Tornkvist M, Brodin B, Bartolazzi A, Larsson O (2002) A novel type of SYT/SSX fusion: methodological and biological implications. Mod Pathol 15(6):679–685

Versteege I, Sevenet N, Lange J et al. (1998) Truncating mutations of hSNF5/INI1 in aggressive paediatric cancer. Nature 394(6689):203–206

Weiser MR, Downey RJ, Leung DH, Brennan MF (2000) Repeat resection of pulmonary metastases in patients with soft-tissue sarcoma. J Am Coll Surg 191(2):184–190; discussion 190–181

Wodowski K, Hill DA, Pappo AS, Shochat SJ, Kun LE, Spunt SL (2003) A chemosensitive pediatric extraosseous osteosarcoma: case report and review of the literature. J Pediatr Hematol Oncol 25(1):73–77

Wong FL, Boice JD Jr, Abramson DH et al. (1997) Cancer incidence after retinoblastoma. Radiation dose and sarcoma risk. JAMA 278(15):1262–1267

Wunder JS, Healey JH, Davis AM, Brennan MF (2000) A comparison of staging systems for localized extremity soft tissue sarcoma. Cancer 88(12):2721–2730

Yamamoto H, Oda Y, Kawaguchi K et al. (2004) c-kit and PDGFRA mutations in extragastrointestinal stromal tumor (gastrointestinal stromal tumor of the soft tissue). Am J Surg Pathol 28(4):479–488

Yan H, Marchettini P, Acherman YI, Gething SA, Brun E, Sugarbaker PH (2003) Prognostic assessment of gastrointestinal stromal tumor. Am J Clin Oncol 26(3):221–228

Yang JC, Chang AE, Baker AR et al. (1998) Randomized prospective study of the benefit of adjuvant radiation therapy in the treatment of soft tissue sarcomas of the extremity. J Clin Oncol 16(1):197–203

Zhou H, Coffin CM, Perkins SL, Tripp SR, Liew M, Viskochil DH (2003) Malignant peripheral nerve sheath tumor: a comparison of grade, immunophenotype, and cell cycle/growth activation marker expression in sporadic and neurofibromatosis 1-related lesions. Am J Surg Pathol 27(10):1337–1345

Fibrous and Fibrohistiocytic Tumors

Diane Nam, Benjamin A. Alman

Contents

8.1 Fibrous and Fibrohistiocytic Tumors

Fibrous and fibrohistiocytic tumors are a diverse group of lesions with a wide range of clinical behavior. Despite their disparate behaviors, lesions within each of these tumor types are composed of cells that share nearly identical cytological appearance. For instance, soft tissue fibrous tumors range from lesions that are unable to invade into outside of the anatomic structure of origin, such as in the case of palmar fibromatosis or Dupuytren's contracture, to locally invasive lesions that can cause mortality by impinging on vital organs, such as aggressive fibromatosis. However, both of these lesions are composed of cells that are difficult to tell apart based on cytology alone. To further confound things there is no uniformly accepted nomenclature, and several terms are used for the same tumor type. In the case of a locally invasive soft tissue fibrous lesion, often called aggressive fibromatosis, terms such as desmoid tumor, deep fibromatosis, and myofibromatosis are also used to describe an identical lesion. In this chapter, the fibrous tumors and fibrohistiocytic tumors will be considered separately, while within each type lesions with similar clinical behavior will be grouped together in a way that simplifies clinical decision making.

8.2 Soft Tissue Fibrous Tumors

Soft tissue fibrous lesions can be grouped based on clinical behavior into two broad groups according to their anatomic location: superficial and deep (Montgomery et al. 2001; Anthony et al. 1996). Such a classification is useful clinically, as it helps to guide the clinician to an appropriate therapeutic course for a given tumor. Unfortunately there is sometimes an overlap between these groups, especially in some cases of aponeurotic fibromatosis. As a general rule, one should consider using therapeutic management principles for a deep lesion if it is difficult to accurately classify a particular lesion into one of these two categories.

Superficial lesions are tumors that are characterized by being limited to the fascial structures overlaying the muscles (the superficial fascia), and these lesions seem to push the surrounding structures out of the way of the expanding fascia, which now contains the lesion (Anthony et al. 1996). In most cases the tumor extends primarily outwards towards the skin; however, in some cases, it will extend into the deep fascia. In distinction to deep fibromatosis, the cells in these lesions do not infiltrate into the normal muscle cells deep to the fascial layer. Superficial lesions located in the palm and the sole of the foot are often referred to by their eponyms, Dupuytren's and Ledderhose disease. Dupuytren's disease is palmar fibromatosis involving the hand, while Ledderhose disease is plantar fibromatosis involving the foot. These lesions are more common in adults than in children, especially in the case of palmar fibromatosis. Treatment for superficial fibromatosis is directed at symptoms. In the case of plantar fibromatosis of the foot, this may be as simple as modifying shoe wear to take pressure off the region. Occasionally a lesion that clinically presents as a plantar fibromatosis in a child will progress to a more invasive tumor. In some of these cases, the lesions initially may be associated with a larger proportion that is deep to the fascia and infiltration into the musculature of the sole of the foot. As such, they may actually have presented as a deep fibromatosis.

Deep fibromatoses are located deep to the superficial fascial layer overlying the muscles. They invade local structures, infiltrate between surrounding normal cells, and have a high recurrence rate after surgery, giving rise to the name aggressive fibromatosis. Such lesions can be associated with significant morbidity due to invasion of surrounding structures such as nerves, tendons, and muscles. When located in the retroperitoneal area, abdominal cavity, or chest, they can cause mortality which is associated with invasion into vital structures. These lesions are rather problematic to manage, with frequent recurrences being common. The difficulty in management despite their relatively occurrence results in patients with deep fibromatosis frequently being more memorable for physicians who manage patients with musculoskeletal tumors.

8.2.1 Epidemiology/Pathogenesis

The deep fibromatosis occurs with an incidence of less than one per million in the general population. There are, however, two syndromes in which this tumor type is substantially more prevalent. In familial adenomatous polyposis, which is a premalignant condition associated with the development of hundreds of colonic polyps, there is at least a 15% chance of developing a deep fibromatosis. Since most patients with this condition are managed with early colectomy, a leading cause of mortality is related to deep fibromatosis tumors (Clark and Phillips 1996; Clark et al. 1999; Gurbuz et al. 1994; Heiskanen et al. 1996; Parc et al. 2004; Jarvinen 1987). Familial infiltrating fibromatosis is an autosomal dominant condition, in which the development of deep fibromatosis is a cardinal feature. Both of these conditions are caused by germline mutations in the adenomatous polyposis coli (APC) gene (Eccles et al. 1996; Groden et al. 1991; Kinzler et al. 1991; Rodriguez-Bigas et al. 1994). Most APC mutations in these conditions result in an early stop codon and a truncated protein product. The location of the mutation differs from those

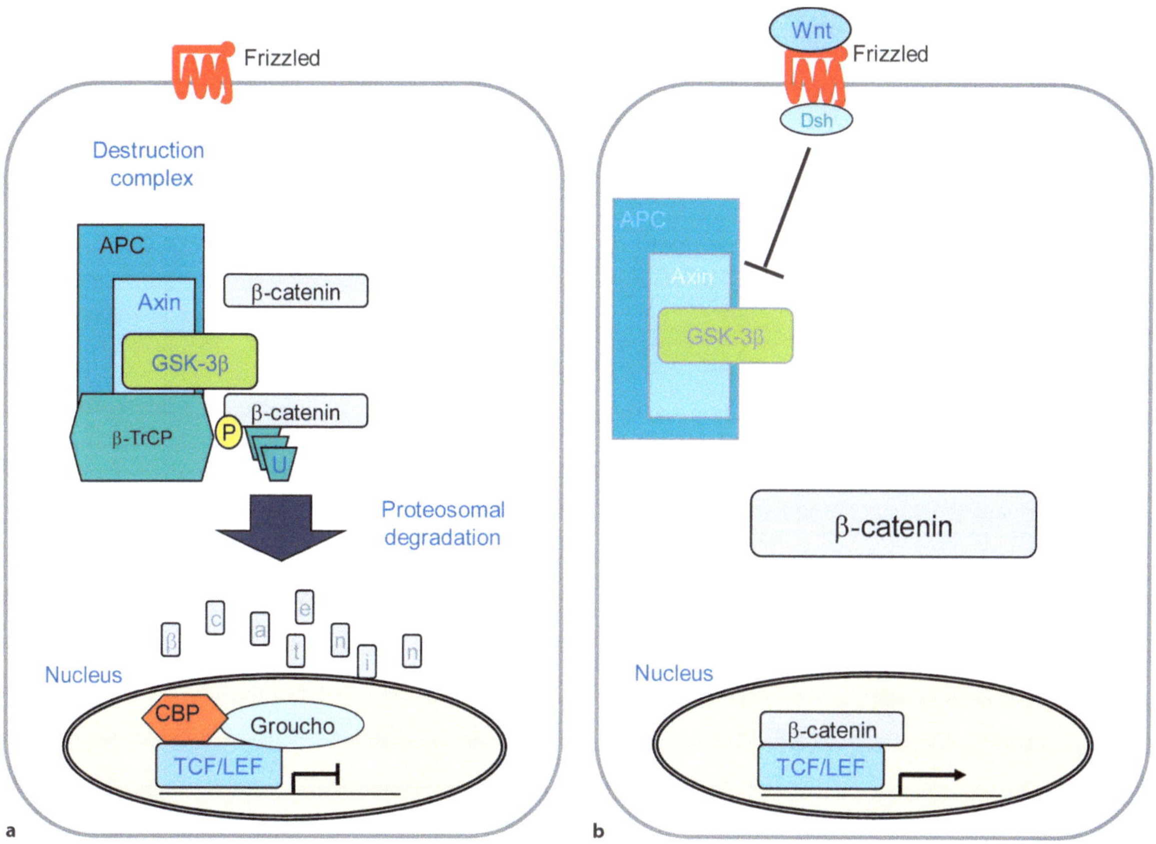

Figure 8.1 a,b

β-Catenin regulation and function. **a** When Wnt signaling is quiescent, a multiprotein complex phosphorylates amino-terminal serine and threonine residues, resulting in β-catenin degradation. **b** Wnt activation, mutations or activation of members in the multiprotein complex, or mutations in the serine or threonine sites in β-catenin, inhibit the degradation of β-catenin, elevating β-catenin protein level. Stabilized β-catenin translocates to the nucleus, binding members of the tcf-lef family, resulting in transcriptional activation

seen in familial adenomatous polyposis, with a prominence of the 3' location in families with familial infiltrating fibromatosis. The different location of the stop codon in familial infiltrating fibromatosis results in an attenuated form of familial adenomatous polyposis, in which a substantially smaller number of colon polyps form, but there is a significantly increased chance of developing a deep fibromatosis. Familial infiltrating fibromatosis is one form of attenuated adenomatous polyposis coli.

The high incidence of this tumor in these conditions gives an important clue to the pathogenesis of the deep fibromatoses. Since these conditions are associated with mutations in the adenomatous polyposis coli gene, tumors have been investigated for abnormalities in this gene. Somatic APC mutations were identified in roughly 10% of sporadic tumors. The APC protein product is part of a multiprotein complex that helps regulate the protein level of beta-catenin in response to Wnt ligand activation. When an appropriate Wnt ligand is present, the multiprotein complex acts to inhibit the phosphorylation of amino-terminal residues in beta-catenin, preventing the degradation of the protein. When beta-catenin protein level rises, it binds to transcription factors in the cell nucleus regulating gene expression (Fig. 8.1). Beta-catenin protein level was investigated in deep fibromatosis, and was found to be elevated, playing a role as an activating gene of transcription. In two-thirds of cases of aggressive fibromatosis, there is a mutation in beta-catenin itself, removing one of the phosphorylation sites, resulting in an elevated intracellular protein level. Thus, beta-catenin protein elevation and transcriptional activation seem to play a cardinal role in the pathogenesis of aggressive fibromatosis (Alman et al. 1997 a, b; Tejpar et al. 1999).

8.2.2 Pathology/Molecular Biology

The fibromatosis is soft tissue tumors that are composed of gray-white colored soft tissue that invades into surrounding tissues. Their histology shows spindle shaped bipolar mesenchymal, fibroblast-like cells encased in a principally collagenous extracellular matrix. There is quite a bit of variability in the cellularity of lesions. In general the mitotic rate is low, but in young infants the mitotic rate may be as high as 10%. The spindle cells may contain proteins indicative of myocytes, such as smooth muscle actin (Flores-Stadler et al. 2000; Oshiro et al. 1994; Stiller and Katenkamp 1975; Weiss 1986). Tumor cells contain high levels of beta-catenin. In the case of deep fibromatosis tumors, in two-thirds of cases there is a mutation in beta-catenin itself, while an additional 10% contain APC mutations. The protein level of beta-catenin cannot be used to distinguish between deep and superficial fibromatosis tumors, as beta-catenin protein elevation is present in both. However, it can be used to distinguish between fibromatosis tumor tissue and normal fibrous tissues. Unlike the deep lesions, superficial lesions have not been found to harbor mutations in either beta-catenin or APC.

Deep fibromatosis consists of clonal lesions (Denys et al. 2004 a, b), and several cytogenetic abnormalities have been identified; however, these are probably related to the clonality of the lesion rather than to a specific causative factor. Since beta-catenin is transcriptionally active in these lesions, a number of target genes are expressed in the lesional tissue. Several studies have examined such genes expressed in this tumor (Clark and Phillips 1996; Rodriguez-Bigas et al. 1994). Although there are a large number of dysregulated genes in this tumor, not enough is known about the profile of gene expression to allow the use of gene profiling as a diagnostic test. Some of the target genes may be able to be modulated using available therapeutic agents, and, as such, this information may be used to identify novel therapeutic approaches (Alman et al. 1997; Denys et al. 2004 a, b; Poon et al. 2001; Tolg et al. 2003).

8.2.3 Clinical Presentation and Diagnosis

The clinical presentation of the fibromatosis depends on the location of the tumor. Superficial lesions present with abnormal pressure superficial to the lesion, or a contracture of a joint. For instance, in the case of plantar fibromatosis this causes pressure on the sole of the feet. The deep fibromatosis presents with a mass the symptoms of which are dependent on their location. In a location in the extremity this causes a mass in a limb. In the thoracic or abdominal cavities

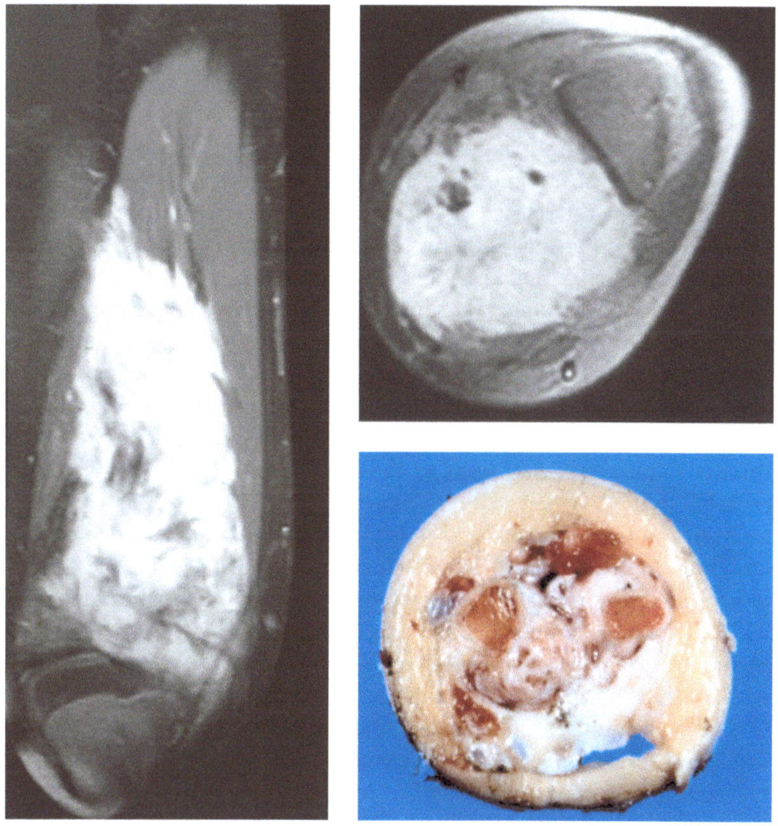

Figure 8.2

MRI and gross appearance of an aggressive fibromatosis. The mass is seen as infiltrating beyond the deep fascia in a lesion of the lower limb on an axial and coronal MR image. A gross axial section from a forearm amputation shows the infiltrating light gray colored tumor

this causes constriction in various organs responsible for the clinical presentation. Contractures of joints are not uncommon due to involvement of major muscle groups.

In the case of superficial lesions, history and physical examination are usually sufficient to make the diagnosis, especially in common locations such as the hands and feet. In other locations, or when a plantar lesion grows in size, an MRI is indicated. If the lesion is located primarily at the fascia, a diagnosis of a superficial lesion can be made. In cases where the lesion seems to be located more deeply, an MRI is needed to determine the anatomic extent of the lesion (Fig. 8.2), and ultimately a biopsy is necessary to make the diagnosis, since it is necessary to rule out other malignant lesions.

8.2.4 Prognostic Factors and Clinical Staging

The overriding prognostic factor is the presence of a superficial or deep lesion. Deep lesions, called aggressive fibromatosis or desmoid tumors, are locally invasive and often recur following local surgical management. An MRI is utilized to determine the anatomic extent of the lesion. This information is used to determine if the lesion can be managed surgically with a wide excision which spares critical structures, or if the lesion is not resectable. There is variability in the behavior of the deep fibromatosis, with some cases growing quite rapidly, others remaining relatively stable in size, and occasionally a case in which the lesion regresses (De Wever et al. 2000; Dormans et al. 2001). There are no factors identified which predict if the lesions will regress, stabilize, or progress.

8.2.4.1 Treatment of Fibrous Tumors

The treatment of superficial lesions is directed at symptomatic management. Depending on the symptoms caused by a given superficial lesion, treatment may range from observation to surgery. Surgery may be indicated for the release of a contracture, or may involve resection of the lesion. In the case of plantar fibromatosis in children, as wide a resection margin as possible, leaving important functional structures, should be performed, to prevent reoccurrence.

The management of deep lesions requires a more aggressive approach. Although most tumors are progressive, a small number of patients will have their tumors stabilize or even regress; therefore it is acceptable to observe selected lesions with serial MRI tests with additional treatments only for progression. Observation should, however, only be used in select lesions which are relatively asymptomatic, and in which growth will not alter the ultimate management. For instance, in a lesion that can be managed with a wide surgical excision without significant functional loss, observation is not indicated.

Several series have shown that surgery with wide margins results in a good chance of long-term cure (Clark and Phillips 1996; Clark et al. 1999; Gurbuz et al. 1994; Jarvinen 1987; Rodriguez-Bigas et al. 1994). However, it is difficult to determine the tumor margins, as it is sometimes hard to determine where the tumor ends and where normal tissue begins. In cases in which curative surgery is possible, the use of MRI to determine the resection margin helps in the surgical planning. Beta-catenin immunohistochemical staining can help in the pathologic assessment to determine if wide margins have indeed been achieved.

In many cases, however, curative surgery will not be possible due to the anatomic location of the tumor. In these cases adjuvant radiotherapy or chemotherapy can be used. Due to the relative rarity of these tumors there are no well controlled studies comparing radiotherapy and chemotherapy, or comparing different chemotherapies. Despite this, there are a large number of case series reporting excellent results with radiation therapy, strongly suggesting that this modality decreases the recurrence rate (Dalen et al. 2003; Merchant et al. 1999; Merchant et al. 2000; O'Dea et al. 2003; Smith et al. 2000; Spiegel et al. 1999). Both pre- and postoperative radiotherapy have been reported. Unfortunately, radiation is associated with a number of side effects, some of which are particularly worrisome in children. For instance, there has been malignant progression reported after radiation therapy. For this reason, radiotherapy has been less popular in children than in adults. A variety of chemotherapeutic regimens have been reported to have moderate activity (Ballo et al. 1998; Ballo et al. 1999; Faulkner et al. 1995; Gronchi et al. 2003; Janinis et al. 2003; Skapek et al. 1998). There are no well controlled studies showing an improved outcome for any one of these regimens.

A subset of deep fibromatosis lesions express estrogen receptors. As such, agents that block these receptors have the potential to be utilized in their management. There is anecdotal evidence that these agents alter tumor growth, but, like all reports of various drugs in this lesion, the numbers of cases reported are small, and there are no trials with matched controls (Janinis et al. 2003).

Since these deep fibromatoses are locally invasive but not metastatic, complete eradication of the tumor may not be necessary. A management that would arrest tumor growth could be used in cases in which the lesion itself does not cause symptoms. A pharmacologic agent with a low toxicity prorate would be preferable to use for this purpose. There are several agents that have been used for this purpose, including cyclo-oxygenase inhibitors, class three tyrosine kinase inhibitors, interferon, and matrix metalloproteinase inhibitors (Fernberg et al. 1999; Kong et al. 2004; Mace et al. 2002).

8.2.4.2 Current Problems and Future Challenges

The rarity of deep fibromatosis and the wide variety of treatment options have made clinical trials with sufficient power to answer important questions about management difficult to design. Some information about potential treatments can be gleaned from animal studies. Genetically engineered mice that develop deep fibromatosis can be used to test potential therapies. Such preclinical trials have been used to identify how downstream target genes regulate neoplastic cell behavior. Ultimately, a multidrug regimen, each of which alters cell behavior in a different way, could be used to slow cell tumor cell growth in a way that the primary lesion could be resected using a local excision, avoiding damage to any important structures, and then additional growth suppressed using such a multidrug regimen. As an alternative, such a multidrug regimen could be used on its own to suppress tumor cell growth. Beta-catenin mediated transcriptional activation is also activated in a variety of neoplastic processes. It is likely that new drugs that act to inhibit beta-catenin mediated transcription may be developed. Such drugs have an excellent potential to be used to treat this tumor.

8.3 Fibrohistiocytic Tumors

The origins of the fibrohistiocytic concept were based on the observation in cell culture that histiocytes could assume fibroblastic properties (Kauffman and Stout 1961). Although the idea of the histiocyte as a facultative fibroblast has long been discredited, the group of known fibrohistiocytic tumors composed of spindled fibroblast-like cells, often with a storiform pattern, rounded histiocyte-like cells and mixtures of giant, foamy and inflammatory cells, has proven to be a valuable concept (Fisher 1996; Kauffman and Stout 1961). While useful for indicating a common pattern, the fibrohistiocytic concept has been challenged over the last decade and is now mostly regarded as a poorly defined descriptor of histiocytic differentiation (De St. Aubain Somerhausen et al. 2002; Fisher 1996). Despite this, there has not been a change in the nomenclature, since a substantially better nomenclature, taking into account the etiology of these tumor types, has not been devised. Most tumors in this group are of mesenchymal derivation and are probably fibroblastic and myofibroblastic in nature (Fisher 1996). For the purposes of this chapter, the benign and intermediate fibrohistiocytic and some fibrous tissue tumors will be discussed.

8.4 So-Called Fibrohistiocytic Tumors

8.4.1 Histologic Classification

In 1994, the fibrohistiocytic tumors of soft tissue were classified by the World Health Organization (WHO) into benign, intermediate, and malignant subgroups based on their combination of clinical features and morphology (Table 8.1) (Weiss 1994). In 2002, the WHO revised its classification (Table 8.2) to omit pleomorphic tumors exhibiting myogenic differentiation; pleomorphic malignant fibrous histiocytoma (MFH) now describes a small group of undifferentiated pleomorphic sarcomas (Daw et al. 2003; De St. Aubain Somerhausen et al. 2002). Myxofibrosarcoma, formerly known as myxoid MFH, and angiomatoid MFH remain as distinctive and discrete

Table 8.1. 1994 WHO Classification of Fibrohistiocytic Tumors (Parc et al. 2004)

Benign

Fibrous histiocytoma
  Cutaneous histiocytoma (dermatofibroma)
  Deep histiocytoma

Juvenile xanthogranuloma
Reticulohistiocytoma
Xanthoma
Intermediate
Atypical fibroxanthoma
Dermatofibrosarcoma protuberans
Pigmented dermatofibrosarcoma protuberans
Giant cell fibroblastoma
Plexiform fibrohistiocytic tumor
Angiomatoid fibrous histiocytoma
Malignant

Malignant fibrous histiocytoma
  Storiform-pleomorphic
  Myxoid
  Giant cell
  Xanthomatous (inflammatory)

Table 8.2. 2002 WHO Classification of Fibrohistiocytic Tumors (Heiskanen and Jarvinen 1996; Jarvinen 1987)

Benign
Giant cell tumor of tendon sheath
Diffuse-type giant cell tumor
Deep benign fibrous histiocytoma
Intermediate (rarely metastasizing)
Plexiform fibrohistiocytic tumor
Giant cell tumor of soft tissues
Malignant
Pleomorphic 'MFH'/undifferentiated pleomorphic sarcoma
Giant cell 'MFH'/undifferentiated pleomorphic sarcoma with giant cells
Inflammatory 'MFH'/undifferentiated pleomorphic sarcoma with prominent inflammation

entities under fibroblastic/myofibroblastic tumors and tumors of uncertain origin, respectively (Bridge et al. 1990). Cutaneous fibrohistiocytic soft tissue tumors are now included in the "Skin" volume of the WHO classification of tumors. In addition, the localized and diffuse forms of giant cell tumor of tendon sheath are now included given that they were descriptively more fibrohistiocytic than synovial (De St. Aubain Somerhausen et al. 2002).

For the purposes of uniformity, the 2002 revised WHO Classification of Tumors of Soft Tissue and Bone will be followed. Cutaneous fibrous histiocytoma, giant cell fibroblastoma and dermatofibrosarcoma protuberans, which are fibroblastic neoplasms included in the WHO volume on skin tumors, are also included in this chapter.

Fibrohistiocytic tumors of bone include benign fibrous histiocytoma and malignant fibrous histiocytoma. Primary bone tumors amount to only 0.2% of the total tumor burden but children are frequently affected and the pathogenesis remains largely unknown (O'Connell et al. 2000). These will be briefly mentioned.

8.4.2 Benign

8.4.2.1 Benign Fibrous Histiocytoma

8.4.2.1.1 Epidemiology/Pathogenesis

Benign fibrous histiocytoma is a common fibrohistiocytic lesion in both children and adults (Meister et al. 1978). There are two categories of benign fibrous histiocytoma: cutaneous and deep. The cutaneous benign fibrous histiocytoma, also known as dermatofibroma, is more common in females and frequently arises in the trunk and extremities (Coffin 1997a; Gonzalez and Duarte 1982; Meister et al. 1978). It may occur in infancy but is mainly seen in the 2nd decade of life and mid adult life. Deep benign fibrous histiocytoma may be congenital but mostly occurs in young adults (Meister et al. 1978). It is seen in noncutaneous soft tissue, such as the upper respiratory tract, mesentery, parenchymal organs, bone, and skeletal muscle (Enzinger and Weiss 1995; Fletcher 1990).

The etiology of benign fibrous histiocytoma remains unknown. Many cases have a history of antecedent trauma possibly suggesting an abnormal response to injury that might be analogous to the increased amount of altered collagen deposition as seen in hypertrophic scar or keloid (Coffin 1997a; Murphy and Mihm 1989). There is also no strong evidence for inheritance; a familial variant of dermatofibroma in one family was seen but the proband died of malignant fibrous histiocytoma (Roberts et al. 1981; Webber and Parham 1996).

Juvenile xanthogranuloma is a nodular cutaneous lesion of infancy and childhood which has two forms: infantile and adolescent/adult. Nearly 20% of cases present congenitally and over 70% occur during the 1st year of life (Seo et al. 1986; Sonoda et al. 1985). For the most part, both sexes seem to be equally affected (Seo et al. 1986; Sonoda et al. 1985). Though it can occur anywhere, it mainly affects the head/neck, upper trunk, and anterior thigh region. It may be multifocal but tends to regress over time and seldom affects the deep soft tissues (Seo et al. 1986; Sonoda et al. 1985; Weiss 1994). Whether it is reactive or neoplastic is unclear but there is speculation that it may be derived from myofibroblasts, dermal histiocytes or dermal dendrocytes (De Graaf et al. 1992; Sonoda et al. 1985).

8.4.2.1.2 Pathology/Molecular Pathology

The mitotic rate in dermatofibroma is quite low or absent. Under microscopy, satellite foci, multinucleated giant cells, foamy macrophages and phagocytosed hemosiderin deposits are typical (Kempson and Hendrickson 1990). It is made up predominantly or exclusively of spindle cells usually with a storiform pattern and is frequently multinodular (Weiss 1994). Deep benign fibrous histiocytoma is not as morphologically varied and is consistently more storiform than dermatofibroma; a hyaline or myxoid stroma is commonly seen and a pericytoma-like pattern, xanthoma cells, and giant cells may be prominent (Fletcher 1990). On gross appearance juvenile xanthogranuloma is a yellowish or light brown plaque or nodule in the dermis which is histologically composed of sheets of histiocytes which have varying numbers of Touton giant cells and eosinophils (Soini 1990; Sonoda et al. 1985; Weiss 1994). Distinction between the fibrohistiocytic form of juvenile xanthogranuloma and fibrous histiocytoma can be problematic and is often resolved by the age and clinical presentation (Coffin 1997a).

8.4.2.1.3 Clinical Presentation and Diagnosis

Dermatofibroma is a solitary, slowly growing nodule. The lesion is usually elevated or pedunculated, with approximately 30% of them occurring as multifocal lesions (Murphy and Mihm 1989). The dermatofibroma lesion is firm and well circumscribed and ranges from being asymptomatic to tender or painful on presentation (Coffin 1997a; Naversen et al. 1993). It is usually less than 2 cm in diameter, but actively growing lesions may reach several centimeters in diameter and often become flattened with time (Murphy and Mihm 1989). They may dimple inward when lateral compression is applied, which aids in distinguishing it from nodular melanomas that protrude outwards with similar palpation (Murphy and Mihm 1989). The deep benign fibrous histiocytomas usually have a larger mass and are more circumscribed than dermatofibroma in appearance (Fletcher 1990). Most lesions present with a painless and slowly enlarging mass.

Juvenile xanthogranuloma has not been associated with abnormal blood lipids but is seen with other conditions such as von Recklinghausen's neurofibromatosis and juvenile chronic myelogenous leukemia (Coffin 1997a; Cooper et al. 1984). In 30–60% of cases in infancy and early childhood, multiple lesions may indicate other unusual sites of involvement, such as the eye and the major organs; hence, a thorough history and physical examination is essential (Seo et al. 1986; Sonoda et al. 1985).

Despite a wide variety of fibrohistiocytic markers which are present in these lesions, including α_1-antitrypsin, α_1-antichymotrypsin, lysozyme, MAC387 and HAM56, their lack of specificity renders them of little diagnostic utility (Marroji et al. 1992; Seo et al. 1986; Soini 1990; Sonoda et al. 1985). CD68 antigen, a commonly used histiocyte/macrophage marker (KP1 is the commercially available monoclonal CD68 antibody), and factor XIIIa (a fibrin stabilizing factor) expression are more useful but not diagnostic (Fisher 1996; Marroji et al. 1992). Immunohistochemistry in the deep lesions shows negativity for epithelial markers, desmin and S100 protein, and CD34 (a vascular progenitor cell marker) is usually negative; if CD34 is positive, solitary fibrous tumor should be considered (De St. Aubain Somerhausen et al. 2002).

In children, these tumors may display varying degrees of cellularity, cytologic atypia and mitotic activity, which causes considerable diagnostic dilemmas (Coffin 1997a; Fisher 1996). Due to the heterogeneity of the group and the overlap with other fibroblastic/myofibroblastic tumors, diagnostic techniques of sensitivity and specificity are limited (Fisher 1996). In dermatofibroma, immunohistochemical results show reactivity for factor XIIIa and focal reactivity for CD34 in a third of cases but are nonspecific in the deep lesions (Fletcher 1990). Dermatofibroma has a low M1B-1 labeling index and p53 staining is absent (Soini 1990).

8.4.2.1.4 Prognostic Factors and Clinical Staging

Though the deep fibrous histiocytoma recurrence rate is 33%, no metastasis has been reported to date. Dermatofibroma seldom recurs after excision (Fletcher 1990). Juvenile xanthogranuloma in infancy or very young children frequently regresses spontaneously even with incomplete excisions; thus, aggressive or cosmetically unsatisfactory surgical procedures should be avoided (Sonoda et al. 1985). However, older children and adults may have persistence of their lesions.

8.4.2.2 Giant Cell Tumor of Tendon Sheath and Diffuse-Type Giant Cell Tumor

8.4.2.2.1 Epidemiology/Pathogenesis

Giant cell tumor of tendon sheath is the most common tumor of synovial tissue. Often referred to as nodular tenosynovitis, this localized form primarily affects the hand, where approximately 85% occur in the digits arising from the synovium of tendon sheath or the region of the interphalangeal joint (De St. Aubain Somerhausen et al. 2002). The wrist, knee, ankle and foot may also be affected and very rarely in the elbow or hip (De St. Aubain Somerhausen et al. 2002; Monaghan et al. 2001). These tumors may occur at any age but usually are seen between 30 and 50 years of age with a 2:1 female preponderance (Ushijima et al. 1989). It is less common in the pediatric population, with approximately 10% of cases occurring in the 2nd decade of life before the age of 20 and as young as 4 years of age (Myers and Masi 1980). This is similar to the diffuse-type giant cell tumor, also known as pigmented villonodular synovitis, which affect patients between 20 and 40 years of age and also has a slight female preponderance (De St. Aubain Somerhausen et al. 2002; Myers and Masi 1980). Rarely there is more than one joint involved. The knee is affected in 75% of cases followed by the hip (15%), ankle, elbow and shoulders; it is much less common in the hand and digits (Myers and Masi 1980).

Both the localized and diffuse-type tumors were initially thought to have an inflammatory basis but the presence of clonal chromosomal abnormalities and the potential for autonomous growth strongly support a neoplastic origin (Monaghan et al. 2001; Myers and Masi 1980; Scoit et al. 1999).

8.4.2.2.2 Pathology/Molecular Pathology

Giant cell tumor of tendon sheath is gray-pink to yellow-brown, is lobulated in appearance with a well defined capsule and is readily excised (De St. Aubain Somerhausen et al. 2002 ; Murphy and Mihm 1989). In children and young adults, the histologic pattern is more cellular (Coffin 1997b). The cells are characterized by a pale cytoplasm and oval nucleus (Coffin 1997b; De St. Aubain Somerhausen et al. 2002). There is a mixture of multinucleated giant cells resembling osteoclasts, lipid-laden macrophages and numerous hemosiderin-laden rounded or spindled cells. Osteoclastic giant cells are less common and may be absent in the diffuse-type giant cell tumor (De St. Aubain Somerhausen et al. 2002). With the diffuse type, there are two histologic components: villous projection of the synovial membrane subsequent to chronic inflammation and numerous pigment and lipid-laden histiocytes (Murphy and Mihm 1989). The villous projections may be several centimeters in length and may have bulbous tips often with evidence of traumatic crushing or fragmentation (Murphy and Mihm 1989). A relatively high mitotic rate is reported in young individuals (Ushijima et al. 1989).

In giant cell tumor of tendon sheath, the region most frequently involved in structural rearrangements is the short arm of chromosome 1 (1p11–13), with chromosome 2 (2q35–36) being the most common translocation partner (Monaghan et al. 2001; Scoit et al. 1999; Ushijima et al. 1989). These and other chromosome abnormalities are similar to those observed in the diffuse-type giant cell tumors. However, one difference between these tumors is that trisomies for chromosomes 5 and 7, which are frequently encountered in the diffuse-type form of the tumor, have not been described for the localized form (De St. Aubain Somerhausen et al. 2002; Scoit et al. 1999).

8.4.2.2.3 Clinical Presentation and Diagnosis

Giant cell tumors of tendon sheath develop gradually often over several years, with the most common presenting complaint being painless swelling. There is usually a history of previous trauma in up to 50% of cases (Monaghan et al. 2001). Radiologically, a well circumscribed soft tissue mass is seen with occasional degenerative or erosive changes in the adjacent joint or bone.

In the diffuse-type tumors, patients complain of pain, swelling and decreased range of motion in the affected joint. Hemorrhagic joint effusions are common and clinically can easily be mistaken for rheumatoid or infective arthritis. It also has a relatively long symptomatic course prior to presentation. Radiographs show an ill-defined periarticular mass usually associated with degenerative changes in the surrounding bone. Magnetic resonance imaging of giant cell tumors shows decreased signal intensity in both the T1- and T2-weighted images.

8.4.2.2.4 Prognostic Factors and Clinical Staging

Although giant cell tumor of tendon sheath is a benign lesion, 4–30 % of cases recur after local excision and may be associated with highly cellular lesions with a high mitotic count and/or incomplete excision (Reilly et al. 1999). Recurrence rates are higher for the diffuse-type giant cell tumors and have been estimated at 18–46 % for intra-articular lesions and 33–50 % for extra-articular lesions (Somerhausen 2000). Recurrence risk does not seem to be related to any histological parameter other than positive excision margins (De St. Aubain Somerhausen et al. 2002).

8.4.3 Intermediate

8.4.3.1 Giant Cell Fibroblastoma and Dermatofibrosarcoma Protuberans

8.4.3.1.1 Epidemiology/Pathogenesis

Giant cell fibroblastoma is a locally recurring childhood tumor of superficial soft tissues. Almost 90 % of cases are diagnosed before 12 years of age and more than 50 % occur prior to 5 years, with some cases presenting in the 1st year of life (Abdul-Karim et al. 1985; Schmookler and Enzinger 1984). Aside from its unusual preference for pediatric patients, it also has a 3:1 male preponderance (De St. Aubain Somerhausen et al. 2002; Schmookler and Enzinger 1984; Webber and Parham 1996). Inheritance has not been documented. Predominant sites of distribution are trunk, thigh, axilla, and distal extremities (Fletcher 1988; Webber and Parham 1996). Dermatofibrosarcoma protuberans has a similar distribution involving mainly the trunk and extremities (Koh and Chung 1995; Rabinowitz et al. 1994). Unlike giant cell fibroblastoma, dermatofibrosarcoma protuberans occurs most frequently in adults. While congenital cases have reported, 10–30 % of pediatric cases are seen in the first 2 decades of life (Koh and Chung 1995; Rabinowitz et al. 1994; Taylor and Helwig 1962). There does not seem to be a firm consensus for predilection in either sex (Fletcher 1988; Fletcher et al.1985; Koh and Chung 1995).

A history of trauma is reported in 16 % of cases of dermatofibrosarcoma protuberans, but the pathogenesis of these tumors remains debatable (Taylor and Helwig 1962). Some cases of dermatofibrosarcoma protuberans have occurred in association with giant cell fibroblastoma and due to their similarity in morphology, it has been suggested that giant cell fibroblastoma is a juvenile form of dermatofibrosarcoma protuberans (Perry et al. 1993; Schmookler et al. 1989). However, though the two lesions are likely related, the hypothesis that giant cell fibroblastoma is a childhood variant of dermatofibrosarcoma protuberans is probably an oversimplification (Beham and Fletcher 1990).

8.4.3.1.2 Pathology/Molecular Pathology

Giant cell fibroblastoma is histologically characterized by an 'angiectoid' component with hyperchromatic mononuclear cells and an incomplete lining of multinucleated giant cells within these pseudovascular sinusoidal spaces (Fletcher and McKee 1990; Schmookler et al. 1989). The solid cellular areas have storiform bundles of stellate or spindle cells randomly arranged in the fibrocollagenous and myxoid stroma (Schmookler et al. 1989). On the other hand, the characteristic histology in dermatofibrosarcoma protuberans consists of a compact, monomorphic storiform dermal proliferation of spindle cells (Fletcher et al. 1985; Taylor and Helwig 1962). The tumor is locally infiltrative and surrounds adnexal structures and blood vessels (Fletcher et al. 1985).

In both of these entities, characteristic chromosome aberrations are documented with t(17;22)(q22;q13) and supernumerary ring chromosomes derived from the t(17;22) (De St. Aubain Somerhausen et al. 2002; Fisher 1996). In 90 % of cases, the translocation causes a rearrangement that fuses the platelet-derived growth factor B-chain (PDGFB) and the collagen type I alpha 1 (COL1A1) genes. PDGFB is a potent mitogen for a number of cell types, and these gene fusions delete exon 1 of PDGFB, and release this growth factor from its normal regulation (Simon et al. 1997, Sirvent et al. 2003). This has implications for treatment, as it is suggested that blocking PDGF-receptor activation by drugs such as imatinib mesylate could be an effective therapy (Greco et al. 2001; Maki et al. 2002). The successful use of imatinib mesylate in treating this tumor has been reported in a patient (Rubin et al. 2002).

8.4.3.1.3 Clinical Presentation and Diagnosis

Giant cell fibroblastoma typically presents as a painless, palpable solitary slow growing nodule in superficial soft tissue and may be adherent to the overlying skin or underlying skeletal muscle (Fletcher and McKee 1990). Initially, dermatofibrosarcoma protuberans has a similar slowly growing period of months to years but differs subsequently by having a rapid growth phase which may be associated with tenderness, pain, red or blue skin discoloration, multinodularity and ulceration (Taylor and Helwig 1962).

Immunohistochemical testing for giant cell fibroblastoma shows consistent reactivity for vimentin and variable reactivity for muscle-specific actin, smooth muscle actin, α_1-antitrypsin and α_1-antichymotrypsin (Fisher 1996; Fletcher 1988). Immunocytochemistry in dermatofibrosarcoma protuberans is positive for actin and CD34 but nonreactive for factor XIIIa, S100 protein, α_1-antichymotrypsin and lysozyme (Fisher 1996; Fletcher et al. 1985).

8.4.3.1.4 Prognostic Factors and Clinical Staging

Giant cell fibroblastoma is prone to recur in up to 47% of cases if incompletely excised but is amenable to reexcision (Abdul-Karim et al. 1985; Schmookler and Enzinger 1984). However, it does not exhibit frankly malignant behavior and metastases have not occurred (Webber and Parham 1996). In contrast, dermatofibrosarcoma protuberans is more difficult to manage due to its potential for destructive recurrence. The incidence of recurrence is usually related to the size of the initial lesion and the extent of the primary excision, but, even following a wide excision with apparent tumor-free margins, recurrence may be still an issue (Coffin 1997b; Fletcher 1988; Kempson and Hendrickson 1990; Taylor and Helwig 1962). Metastases are rare but histologic transformation of dermatofibrosarcoma protuberans to fibrosarcoma or malignant fibrous histiocytoma is documented, mostly in adults (Eisen and Tallini 1993; Fletcher 1988; Fletcher et al. 1985; Koh and Chung 1995).

8.4.3.2 Plexiform Fibrohistiocytic Tumor

8.4.3.2.1 Epidemiology/Pathogenesis

Plexiform fibrohistiocytic tumors commonly affect the deep dermis and subcutaneous tissue of children, adolescents and young adults, predominate in females, and none have known predisposing factors (Enzinger and Zhang 1988). Though the lesion may be congenital, the mean age at presentation is 14.5 years; approximately 30% of cases occur before the age 20 (Enzinger and Zhang 1988; Hollowood et al. 1991). The main sites of involvement include the upper extremities in about 65% of cases, especially the hands and wrist (Enzinger and Zhang 1988; Ramstein et al. 1999). The lower extremities and trunk are less frequently affected and it rarely occurs in the head and neck region (Remstein et al. 1999).

8.4.3.2.2 Pathology/Molecular Pathology

The lesion is usually multinodular, firm and poorly circumscribed and rarely exceeds 3 cm (De St. Aubain Somerhausen et al. 2002). Plexiform fibrohistiocytic tumors have three distinct cell types in varying amounts: mononuclear-histiocyte-like cells, spindle fibroblast-like cells and multinucleate giant cells (De St. Aubain Somerhausen et al. 2002). These are seen in three basic histologic subtypes: a fibrohistiocytic pattern of nodular mononuclear histiocyte-like cells and multinucleated giant cells, a fibroblastic pattern of elongated clusters of short fascicles of fibroblast-like cells and a mixed pattern consisting of both in equal proportion (De St. Aubain Somerhausen et al. 2002; Enzinger and Zhang 1988). Cellular atypia and pleomorphism are minimal with a low mitotic count (De St. Aubain Somerhausen et al. 2002; Enzinger and Zhang 1988). Vascular infiltration is seen in 10–20% of cases (Enzinger and Zhang 1988).

Another two plexiform fibrohistiocytic tumors have been reported to contain chromosomal aberrations, no consistent abnormality has been published to date (Redlich et al. 1999).

8.4.3.2.3 Clinical Presentation and Diagnosis

Plexiform fibrohistiocytic tumors are clinically characterized by slow growth that enlarges over months to years (Enzinger and Zhang 1988; Hollowood et al. 1991). The patient usually presents with an asymptomatic, small and ill-defined mass (Enzinger and Zhang 1988; Hollowood et al. 1991).

With immunohistochemical testing, plexiform fibrohistiocytic tumors display reactivity for vimentin, smooth muscle cell actin and CD68/KP1 (Hollowood et al. 1991; Remstein et al. 1999). It is negative for S100 protein, desmin, cytokeratin and factor XIIIa (Hollowood et al. 1991; Remstein et al. 1999). However, histologically, diagnostic evaluation may be a source of confusion depending on the plexiform fibrohistiocytic tumor subtype that predominates. For instance, a mostly fibroblastic type may resemble a fibromatosis, whereas a predominately fibrohistiocytic type may be mistaken for a dermatofibroma (Enzinger and Zhang 1988). The presence of a plexiform pattern and focal fibrohistiocytic aggregates distinguish a fibroblastic-type plexiform fibrohistiocytic tumor from a fibromatosis and the lack of a storiform pattern in a fibrohistiocytic-type helps distinguish it from dermatofibroma (Enzinger and Zhang 1988).

8.4.3.2.4 Prognostic Factors and Clinical Staging

The local recurrence rate for plexiform fibrohistiocytic tumors ranges from 12.5% (Remstein et al. 1999) to 37.5% (Enzinger and Zhang 1988) and may be related to the incomplete resection of an already poorly defined, infiltrative lesion (Hollowood et al. 1991; Remstein et al. 1999). Regional lymph node metastatic rate is approximately 3%; other metastatic sites have not been reported (Enzinger and Zhang 1988; Remstein et al. 1999). Vascular invasion may play a role in local recurrence. Otherwise, patient prognosis does not seem to be altered by pathologic or cytogenetic factors (Enzinger and Zhang 1988; Remstein et al. 1999).

8.4.3.3 Giant Cell Tumor of Soft Tissue

8.4.3.3.1 Epidemiology/Pathogenesis

Giant cell tumor of soft tissue is a primary neoplasm resembling giant cell tumor of bone both clinically and histologically. It can affect patients between the ages of 5 and 89 years but mostly is seen in the 5th decade of life (O'Connell et al. 2000; Oliveira et al. 2000); it is rare in children. Males and females are equally affected and there does not seem to be any predisposing ethnic factors (O'Connell et al. 2000; Oliveira et al. 2000). Approximately 70% of giant cell tumors of soft tissue occur in the upper and lower extremities and less frequently involving the trunk, head and neck region (Folpe et al. 1999; O'Connell et al. 2000; Oliveira et al. 2000).

The pathogenesis of these lesions remains unknown but it has been associated with Paget's disease or trauma in rare cases (Oliveira et al. 2000).

8.4.3.3.2 Pathology/Molecular Pathology

Giant cell tumor of soft tissue is a well defined, mostly solid, nodule with a fleshy, red-brown or gray cut surface. It has a multinodular structure which is immersed in a heavily vascularized stroma with varying sizes of nodules composed of round to oval mononuclear-type cells and multinucleated, osteoclastic-like giant cells (O'Connell et al. 2000; Oliveira et al. 2000). Mitotic activity is relatively low and generally present but atypia and pleomorphism are absent; necrosis is seen rarely (O'Connell et al. 2000). Metaplastic bone formation, located in the periphery of the lesion, is seen in 50% of tumors, and secondary cystic changes, similar to those seen in aneursymal bone cysts, are present in approximately 30% of tumors (Folpe et al. 1999; O'Connell et al. 2000; Oliveira et al. 2000).

8.4.3.3.3 Clinical Presentation and Diagnosis

Giant cell tumors of soft tissue usually present with a 6-month history of a painless mass (Oliveira et al. 2000). The mass on average is 3 cm in diameter and 70% of them frequently involve the adipose or dermal tissues; only 30% have been deep to the superficial fascia (O'Connell et al. 2000). Radiographically, the tumors have a characteristic appearance of a soft tissue mass with peripheral calcification. Immunohistochemical studies show reactivity for vimentin, CD68 and smooth muscle actin (Folpe et al. 1999; O'-Connell et al. 2000; Oliveira et al. 2000). CD68 stains multinucleated giant cells and smooth muscle actin stains mononuclear cells (Oliveira et al. 2000). Immunoreactivity with keratin and S100 protein is rare (Oliveira et al. 2000).

8.4.3.3.4 Prognostic Factors and Clinical Staging

Giant cell tumor of soft tissue has a local recurrence rate of 12% and is usually secondary to incomplete surgical resection of the lesion (Folpe et al. 1999). In very seldom cases have metastasizes or death occurred (Folpe et al. 1999; O'Connell et al. 2000; Oliveira et al. 2000). At present, no clinical or pathologic factors are predictive of metastatic potential (Folpe et al. 1999; O'Connell et al. 2000; Oliveira et al. 2000).

8.4.3.3.5 Treatment of Fibrohistiocytic Tumors

Surgery is the initial treatment of choice for most soft tissue fibrohistiocytic tumors. Adherence to well-defined surgical principles is a necessity to give the best chance for eradicating local disease. There are four categories of surgical resection for soft tissue tumors in the extremities, which similarly applies to tumors in other locations (Ushijima et al. 1989). As the tumor mass grows, a pseudocapsule is usually formed as it compresses normal surrounding tissue. *Intracapsular* excision resects the tumor mass from within the pseudocapsule by a piecemeal debulking or curettage leaving behind macroscopic disease. *Marginal* local excision, also known as excisional biopsy, resects the tumor mass and pseudocapsule en bloc cutting through the reactive zone, which is a host response to the pseudocapsule consisting of mesenchymal, angiogenic and inflammatory elements; residual microscopic disease often remains. *Wide* local excision resects the tumor mass with a cuff of normal tissue beyond the reactive zone. This procedure is intracompartmental and may still leave the possibility for local recurrence. *Radical* resection gives the best possible chance to remove the tumor mass by resecting the entire muscle compartment, but again does not completely obviate local recurrence (Ushijima et al. 1989).

Nearly all low grade symptomatic benign fibrohistiocytic tumors, except juvenile xanthogranuloma which may regress spontaneously and as such do not always require aggressive surgical intervention, are amenable to complete surgical resection by marginal excision since most benign tumors remain within the pseudocapsule. Local control is usually excellent and the need for additional treatments is rare (Smith et al. 1997).

The standard therapy for all the intermediate grade tumors is wide local surgical excision with tumor-free margins. Surgical reexcision is the mainstay of treatment for local recurrence (Coffin 1997b; Cole et al. 1993; Daw et al. 2003; Smith et al. 1997; Zuppan et al. 1987). Chemotherapy is not generally utilized, but imatinib mesylate may be used for large unresectable giant cell fibroblastomas and dermatofibrosarcoma protuberans (Rubin et al. 2002). Large well controlled series of the use of this agent have not yet been reported.

8.5 Current Problems and Future Challenges

Though significant progress has been made in the diagnosis and treatment of pediatric soft tissue neoplasms, there are substantial gaps in our knowledge and understanding of the pathogenesis and histiogenesis of these tumors. Although the molecular etiology of some of these lesions has been elucidated, in most cases we do not know the molecular genetic cause. Special diagnostic techniques have limited utility in the evaluation of fibrohistiocytic tumors due to their heterogeneity and overlap with other fibroblastic-myofibroblastic tumors, as well as their limitations of sensitivity and specificity (Coffin 1997b; Fisher 1996). Immunohistochemistry has a practical use for excluding other categories of neoplasia but must be considered with care due to its lack of specificity. Similarly, ultrastructural findings also lack specificity and are not very helpful except as a means for cataloguing different cell types in a given tumor (Fisher 1996). Currently, specific cytogenetic and molecular genetic aberrations have not been defined and confirmed for the majority of fibrohistiocytic tumors. The fibrohistiocytic tumours were initially classified together because of cytological similarities. However, as more is learned about their molecular etiology, the traditional classification may be challenged. Once the molecular etiology is understood, it may be possible to develop targeted therapies. This is the case in giant cell fibroblastoma and dermatofibrosarcoma protuberans, where imatinib mesylate holds promise. However, larger scale clinical trials of imatinib mesylate in giant cell fibroblastoma and dermatofibrosarcoma protuberans are needed to more clearly define the indications for use of this agent.

References

Abdul-Karim FW, Evans HL, Silva EG (1985) Giant cell fibroblastoma. A report of three cases. J Clin Pathol 83:165–170

Alman BA, Li C, Pajerski ME, Diaz-Cano S, Wolfe HJ (1997a) Increased beta-catenin protein and somatic APC mutations in sporadic aggressive fibromatoses (desmoid tumors). Am J Pathol 151(2):329–334

Alman BA, Pajerski ME, Diaz-Cano S, Corboy K, Wolfe HJ (1997b) Aggressive fibromatosis (desmoid tumor) is a monoclonal disorder. Diagn Mol Pathol 6(2):98–101

Anthony T, Rodriguez-Bigas MA, Weber TK, Petrelli NJ (1996) Desmoid tumors. Am Coll Surg 182(4):369–377

Ballo MT, Zagars GK, Pollack A (1998) Radiation therapy in the management of desmoid tumors. Int J Radiat Oncol Biol Phys 42(5):1007–1014

Ballo MT, Zagars GK, Pollack A, Pisters PW, Pollack RA (1999) Desmoid tumor: prognostic factors and outcome after surgery, radiation therapy, or combined surgery and radiation therapy. J Clin Oncol 17(1):158–167

Beham A, Fletcher CDM (1990) Dermatofibrosarcoma protuberans with areas resembling giant cell fibroblastoma: report of two cases. Histopathology 17:165–167

Berner JM, Forus A, Elkahloun A et al. (1997) HMGIC, the gene for architectural transcription factor, is amplified and rearranged in a subset of human sarcomas. Oncogene 14: 2935–2941

Bridge JA, Neff JR, Sandberg AA (1990) Cytogenetic analysis of dermatofibrosarcoma protuberans. Cancer Genet Cytogenet 49:199–202

Chew C, Reid R, O'Dwyer PJ (2004) Evaluation of the long term outcome of patients with extremity desmoids. Eur J Surg Oncol 30(4):428–432

Clark SK, Phillips RK (1996) Desmoids in familial adenomatous polyposis. Br J Surg 83(11):1494–1504

Clark SK, Neale KF, Landgrebe JC, Phillips RK (1999) Desmoid tumours complicating familial adenomatous polyposis. Br J Surg 86(9):1185–1189

Coffin CM (1997a) Fibrohistiocytic tumors. In: Coffin CM, Dehner LP, O'Shea PA (eds) Pediatric soft tissue tumors. Williams and Wilkins, Baltimore, pp 179–213

Coffin CM (1997b) Synovial-based tumors and synovial sarcoma. In: Coffin CM, Dehner LP, O'Shea PA (eds) Pediatric soft tissue tumors. Williams and Wilkins, Baltimore, pp 295–310

Coffin CM, Dehner LP (1992) The soft tissues. In: Stocker JT, Dehner LP (eds) Pediatric pathology. JB Lippincott, Philadelphia, pp 1091–1132

Cole CH, Magee JF, Gianoulis M et al. (1993) Malignant fibrous histiocytoma in childhood. Cancer 71:4077–4083

Cooper PH, Frierson HF, Kayne AL et al. (1984) Association of juvenile xanthogranuloma with juvenile chronic myeloid leukemia. Arch Dermatol 120:371–375

Corpron CA, Black CT, Raney RB et al. (1996) Malignant fibrous histiocytoma in children. J Pediatr Surg 31:1080–1083

Craver RD, Correa H, Kao YS et al. (1995) Aggressive giant cell fibroblastoma with a balanced 17;22 translocation. Cancer Genet Cytogenet 80:20–22

Dalen BP, Bergh PM, Gunterberg BU (2003) Desmoid tumors: a clinical review of 30 patients with more than 20 years' follow-up. Acta Orthop Scand 74(4):455–459

Daw NC, Billups CA, Pappo AS, Jenkins, JJ, Mahmoud HH, Krasin MJ, Rao BN (2003) Malignant fibrous histiocytoma and other fibrohistiocytic tumors in pediatric patients. Cancer 97:2839–2847

De Graaf JH, Timens W, Tamminga RYJ et al. (1992) Deep juvenile xanthogranuloma: a lesion related to dermal indeterminate cells. Human Pathol 23:905–910

De St. Aubain Somerhausen N, Dal Cin P, Fletcher CDM et al. (2002) So-called fibrohistiocytic tumors. In: Fletcher CDM, Unni KK, Mertens K (eds) World Health Organization classification of tumors of soft tissue and bone. IARC Press, Washington, DC, pp 109–126

De Wever I, Dal Cin P, Fletcher CD, Mandahl N, Mertens F, Mitelman F, Rosai J, Rydholm A, Sciot R, Tallini G, Van Den Berghe H, Vanni R, Willen H (2000) Cytogenetic, clinical, and morphologic correlations in 78 cases of fibromatosis: a report from the CHAMP Study Group. Chromosomes and morphology. Mod Pathol 13(10):1080–1085

Denys H, De Wever O, Nusgens B, Kong Y, Sciot R, Le AT, Van Dam K, Jadidizadeh A, Tejpar S, Mareel M, Alman B, Cassiman JJ (2004a) Invasion and MMP expression profile in desmoid tumours. Br J Cancer 90(7):1443–1449

Denys H, Jadidizadeh A, Amini Nik S, Van Dam K, Aerts S, Alman BA, Cassiman JJ, Tejpar S (2004b) Identification of IGFBP-6 as a significantly downregulated gene by beta-catenin in desmoid tumors. Oncogene 23(3):654–664

Dormans JP, Spiegel D, Meyer J, Asada N, Alman BA, Pill SG, Himelstein B, Womer R (2001a) Fibromatoses in childhood: the desmoid/fibromatosis complex. Med Pediatr Oncol 37:126–131

Dormans JP, Spiegel D, Meyer J, Asada N, Alman BA, Pill SG, Himelstein B, Womer R (2001b) Fibromatoses in childhood: the desmoid/fibromatosis complex. Med Pediatr Oncol 37(2):126–131
Dreinhofer KE, Akerman M, Willen H et al. (1994) Proliferating cell nuclear antigen (PCNA) in high-grade malignant fibrous histiocytoma: prognostic value in 48 patients. Int J Cancer 59:379–382
Eccles DM, van der Luijt R, Breukel C, Bullman H, Bunyan D, Fisher A, Barber J, du Boulay C, Primrose J, Burn J, Fodde R (1996) Hereditary desmoid disease due to a frameshift mutation at codon 1924 of the APC gene. Am J Hum Genet 59(6):1193–1201
Eisen RN, Tallini G (1993) Metastatic dematofibrosarcoma protuberans with fibrosarcomatous change in the absence of local recurrence. Cancer 72:462–468
Enneking WF (1983) Musculoskeletal tumor surgery. Churchill Livingstone, New York, pp 839–122
Enzinger FM, Weiss SW (1995) Benign fibrohistiocytic tumors. In: Enzinger FM, Weiss SW (eds) Soft tissue tumors, 3rd edn. Mosby-Year Book, St. Louis, pp 293–323
Enzinger FM, Zhang R (1988) Plexiform fibrohistiocytic tumor presenting in children and young adults: an analysis of 65 cases. Am J Surg Pathol 12:818–826
Faulkner LB, Hajdu SI, Kher U, La Quaglia M, Exelby PR, Heller G, Wollner N (1995) Pediatric desmoid tumor: retrospective analysis of 63 cases. J Clin Oncol 13(11):2813–2818
Fernberg JO, Brosjo O, Larsson O, Soderlund V, Strander H (1999) Interferon-induced remission in aggressive fibromatosis of the lower extremity. Acta Oncol 38(7):971–972
Fisher C (1996) Fibrohistiocytic tumors. In: Weiss SW, Brooks JSJ (eds) Soft tissue tumors. Williams and Wilkins, Baltimore, pp 62–180
Fletcher CDM (1988) Giant cell fibroblastoma of soft tissue: a clinicopathological and immunohistochemical study. Histopathology 13:499–508
Fletcher CDM (1990) Benign fibrous histiocytoma of subcutaneous and deep soft tissue: a clinicopathologic analysis of 21 cases. Am J Surg Pathol 14:801–809
Fletcher CDM, McKee PH (1990) Progress in benign soft tissue tumors. In: Fletcher CDM, McKee PH (eds) Pathobiology of soft tissue tumors. Churchill Livingstone, London, pp 239–264
Fletcher CDM, Evans BJ, Macartney JC et al. (1985) Dermatofibrosarcsoma protuberans: a clinicopathological and immunohistochemical study with a review of the literature. Histopathology 9:921–938
Flores-Stadler EM, Chou PM, Barquin N, Thangavelu M, Gonzalez-Crussi F (2000) Fibrous tumors in children – a morphologic and interphase cytogenetic analysis of problematic cases. Int J Oncol 17(3):433–437
Folpe AL, Morris RJ, Weiss SW (1999) Soft tissue giant cell tumor of low malignant potential: a proposal for the reclassification of malignant giant cell tumor of soft parts. Mod Pathol 12:894–902
Gonzalez S, Duarte I (1982) Benign fibrous histiocytoma of the skin: a morphologic study of 290 cases. Pathol Res Pract 174:370–391
Greco A, Roccato E, Miranda C, Cleris L, Formelli F, Pierotti MA (2001) Growth-inhibitory effect of STI571 on cells transformed by the COL1A1/PDGFB rearrangement. Int J Cancer 92(3):354–360
Groden J, Thliveris A, Samowitz W, Carlson M, Gelbert L, Albertsen H, Joslyn G, Stevens J, Spirio L, Robertson M (1991) Identification and characterization of the familial adenomatous polyposis coli gene. Cell 66(3):589–600
Gronchi A, Casali PG, Mariani L, Lo Vullo S, Colecchia M, Lozza L, Bertulli R, Fiore M, Olmi P, Santinami M, Rosai J (2003) Quality of surgery and outcome in extra-abdominal aggressive fibromatosis: a series of patients surgically treated at a single institution. J Clin Oncol 21(7):1390–1397
Gurbuz AK, Giardiello FM, Petersen GM, Krush AJ, Offerhaus GJ, Booker SV, Kerr MC, Hamilton SR (1994) Desmoid tumours in familial adenomatous polyposis. Gut 35(3):377–381
Hansmann A, Adolph C, Vogel T, Unger A, Moeslein G (2004) High-dose tamoxifen and sulindac as first-line treatment for desmoid tumors. Cancer 100(3):612–620
Heiskanen I, Jarvinen HJ (1996) Occurrence of desmoid tumours in familial adenomatous polyposis and results of treatment. Int J Colorectal Dis 11(4):157–162
Herbert S, Corn B, Solin L et al. (1993) Limb-preserving treatment for soft tissue sarcomas of the extremities. Cancer 72:1230–1238
Hollowood K, Holley MP, Fletcher CDM (1991) Plexiform fibrohistiocytic tumor: clinicopathological, immunohistochemical and ultrastructural analysis in favour of a myofibroblastic lesion. Histopathology 19:503–513
Ilhan I, Arikan U, Buyukpamukcu M (1995) Rothmund-Thomson syndrome and malignant fibrous histiocytoma: a case report. Pediatr Hematol Oncol 12:103–105
International Union Against Cancer (UICC) (1992) Soft tissue sarcomas: paediatric. In: Hermanek P, Sogin LH (eds) TNM classification of malignant tumors, 4th edn. Springer-Verlag, Berlin, pp 213–217
Janinis J, Patriki M, Vini L, Aravantinos G, Whelan JS (2003) The pharmacological treatment of aggressive fibromatosis: a systematic review. Ann Oncol 14(2):181–190
Jarvinen HJ (1987) Desmoid disease as a part of familial adenomatous polyposis coli. Acta Chir Scand 153(5–6): 379–383
Jelinek JS, Kransdorf MJ, Shmookler BM et al. (1994) Giant cell tumor of tendon sheath: MR findings in nine cases. AJR Am J Roentgenol 162:919–922
Kauffman SL, Stout AP (1961) Histiocytic tumors (fibrous xanthoma and histiocytoma) in children. Cancer 14:469–482
Kempson RL, Hendrickson MR (1990) What is a fibrohistiocytic tumor? In: Fletcher CDM, McKee PH (eds) Pathobiology of soft tissue tumors. Churchill Livingstone, London, pp 105–140

Kinzler KW, Nilbert MC, Su LK, Vogelstein B, Bryan TM, Levy DB, Smith KJ, Preisinger AC, Hedge P, McKechnie D (1991) Identification of FAP locus genes from chromosome 5q21. Science 253(5020):661–665

Koh CK, Chung BK (1995) Dermatofibrosarcoma protuberans. Int J Dermatol 34:256–260

Kong Y, Poon R, Nadesan P, Di Muccio T, Fodde R, Khokha R, Alman BA (2004) Matrix metalloproteinase activity modulates tumor size, cell motility, and cell invasiveness in murine aggressive fibromatosis. Cancer Res 64(16):5795–5803

Laskin WB, Silverman TA, Enzinger FM (1988) Postradiation soft tissue sarcomas. An analysis of 53 cases. Cancer 62:2330–2340

Le Doussal V, Coindre JM, Leroux A et al. (1996) Prognostic factors for patients with localized primary malignant fibrous histiocytoma: a multicenter study of 216 patients with multivariate analysis. Cancer 77:1823–1830

Leithner A, Gapp M, Leithner K, Radl R, Krippl P, Beham A, Windhager R (2004) Margins in extra-abdominal desmoid tumors: a comparative analysis. J Surg Oncol 86(3):152–156

Mace J, Sybil Biermann J, Sondak V, McGinn C, Hayes C, Thomas D, Baker L (2002) Response of extraabdominal desmoid tumors to therapy with imatinib mesylate. Cancer 95(11):2373–2379

Maki RG, Awan RA, Dixon RH, Jhanwar S, Antonescu CR (2002) Differential sensitivity to imatinib of 2 patients with metastatic sarcoma arising from dermatofibrosarcoma protuberans. Int J Cancer 100(6):623–626

Marroji AJ, Dehner LP, Coffin CM et al. (1992) Benign cutaneous histiocytic tumors in childhood and adolescence, excluding Langerhans' cell proliferations: a clinicopathologic and immunohistochemical analysis. Am J Dermatopathol 14:8–18

Meister P, Konrad E, Kyriakos M (1978) Fibrous histiocytoma: a histological and statistical analysis of 155 cases. Pathol Res Pract 162:361–379

Melhem MF, Meisler AI, Saito R et al. (1993) Cytokines in inflammatory malignant fibrous histiocytoma presenting with leukemoid reaction. Blood 82:2038–2044

Merchant NB, Lewis JJ, Woodruff JM, Leung DH, Brennan MF (1999) Extremity and trunk desmoid tumors: a multifactorial analysis of outcome. Cancer 86(10):2045–2052

Merchant TE, Nguyen D, Walter AW, Pappo AS, Kun LE, Rao BN (2000) Long-term results with radiation therapy for pediatric desmoid tumors. Int J Radiat Oncol Biol Phys 47(5): 1267–1271

Mitelman (2002) Database of chromosome aberrations in cancer. http://cgap nci nih gov/Chromosomes/Mitelman

Monaghan H, Salter DM, Al Nafussi A (2001) Giant cell tumor of tendon sheath (localized nodular synovitis): clinicopathological features in 71 cases. J Clin Pathol 54:404–407

Montgomery E, Lee JH, Abraham SC, Wu TT (2001) Superficial fibromatoses are genetically distinct from deep fibromatoses. Mod Pathol 14(7):695–701

Murphy GF, Mihm MC (1989) The skin. In: Cotran RS, Kumar V, Robbins SL (eds) Robbins pathologic basis of disease. WB Saunders, Philadelphia, pp 1290–1291

Myers BW, Masi AT (1980) Pigmented villonodular synovitis and tenosynovitis: a clinical epidemiologic study of 166 cases and literature review. Medicine 59:223–238

Naversen DN, Trask DM, Watson FH et al. (1993) Painful tumors of the skin: "LEND AN EGG." J Am Acad Dermatol 28:298–300

O'Connell JX, Wehrli BM, Nielsen GP, Rosenberg AE (2000) Giant cell tumors of soft tissue: a clinicopathologic study of 18 benign and malignant tumors. Am J Surg Pathol 24:386–395

O'Dea FJ, Wunder J, Bell RS, Griffin AM, Catton C, O'Sullivan B (2003) Preoperative radiotherapy is effective in the treatment of fibromatosis. Clin Orthop (415):19–24

Oliveira AM, Dei Tos AP, Fletcher CD, Nascimento AG (2000) Primary giant cell tumor of soft tissues: a study of 22 cases. Am J Surg Pathol 24:248–256

Oshiro Y, Fukuda T, Tsuneyoshi M (1994) Fibrosarcoma versus fibromatoses and cellular nodular fasciitis. A comparative study of their proliferative activity using proliferating cell nuclear antigen, DNA flow cytometry, and p53. Am J Surg Pathol 18(7):712–719

Parc Y, Piquard A, Dozois RR, Parc R, Tiret E (2004) Long-term outcome of familial adenomatous polyposis patients after restorative coloproctectomy. Ann Surg 239(3):378–382

Perry DA, Schultz LR, Dehner LP (1993) Giant cell fibroblastoma and dermatofibrosarcoma protuberans-like transformation. J Cutan Pathol 20:451–454

Pezzi CM, Rawlings MS, Esgro JJ et al. (1992) Prognostic factors in 227 patients with malignant fibrous histiocytoma. Cancer 69:2098–2103

Poon R, Smits R, Li C, Jagmohan-Changur S, Kong M, Cheon S, Yu C, Fodde R, Alman BA (2001) Cyclooxygenase-two (COX-2) modulates proliferation in aggressive fibromatosis (desmoid tumor). Oncogene 20(4):451–460

Rabinowitz LG, Luchetti ME, Segura AD et al. (1994) Acrally occurring dermatofibrosarcoma protuberans in children and adults. J Dermatol Surg Oncol 20:655–659

Raney RB, Allen A, O'Neill J et al. (1986) Malignant fibrous histiocytoma of soft tissue in childhood. Cancer 57:198–201

Redlich GC, Montgomery KD, Allgood GA, Joste NE (1999) Plexiform fibrohistiocytic tumor with a clonal cytogenetic anomaly. Cancer Genet Cytogenet 108:141–143

Reid AH, Tsai MM, Venzon DJ et al. (1996) MDM2 amplification, P53 gene mutation, and accumulation of the P53 gene product in malignant fibrous histiocytoma. Diagn Mol Pathol 5:65–73

Reilly KE, Stern PJ, Dale JA (1999) Recurrent giant cell tumors of tendon sheath. J Hand Surg Am 24:1298–1302

Remstein ED, Arndt CA, Nascimento AG (1999) Plexiform fibrohistiocytic tumor: clinicopathologic analysis of 22 cases. Am J Surg Pathol 23:662–670

Roberts JT, Byrne EH, Rosenthal D (1981) Familial variant of dermatofibroma with malignancy in the proband. Arch Dermatol 117:12–15

Rodriguez-Bigas MA, Mahoney MC, Karakousis CP, Petrelli NJ (1994) Desmoid tumors in patients with familial adenomatous polyposis. Cancer 74(4):1270–1274

Rubin BP, Schuetze SM, Eary JF, Norwood TH, Mirza S, Conrad EU, Bruckner JD (2002) Molecular targeting of platelet-derived growth factor B by imatinib mesylate in a patient with metastatic dermatofibrosarcoma protuberans. J Clin Oncol 20(17):3586–3591

Schmookler BM, Enzinger FM (1984) Giant cell fibroblastoma. Anat Pathol 8:1–4

Schmookler BM, Enzinger FM, Weiss SW (1989) Giant cell fibroblastoma. A juvenile form of dermatofibrosarcoma protuberans. Cancer 64:2154–2161

Scoit R, Rosai J, Dal Cin P et al. (1999) Analysis of 35 cases of localized and diffuse tenosynovial giant cell tumor: a report from the chromosomes and morphology. Mod Pathol 12:576–579

Sen-Gupta S, Van der Luijt RB, Bowles LV, Meera Khan P, Delhanty JD (1993) Somatic mutation of APC gene in desmoid tumour in familial adenomatous polyposis. Lancet 342(8870):552–553

Seo IS, Min KW, Mirkin LD (1986) Juvenile xanthogranuloma ultrastructural and immunohistochemical studies. Arch Pathol Lab Med 110:911–915

Simon MP, Pedeutour F, Sirvent N, Grosgeorge J, Minoletti F, Coindre JM, Terrier-Lacombe MJ, Mandahl N, Craver RD, Blin N, Sozzi G, Turc-Carel C, O'Brien KP, Kedra D, Fransson I, Guilbaud C, Dumanski JP (1997) Deregulation of the platelet-derived growth factor B-chain gene via fusion with collagen gene COL1A1 in dermatofibrosarcoma protuberans and giant-cell fibroblastoma. Nat Genet 15(1):95–98

Simons A, Schepens M, Jeuken J et al. (2000) Frequent loss of 9p21 (p16INK4A) and other genomic imbalances in malignant fibrous histiocytoma. Cancer Genet Cytogenet 118:89–98

Sirvent N, Maire G, Pedeutour F (2003) Genetics of dermatofibrosarcoma protuberans family of tumors: from ring chromosomes to tyrosine kinase inhibitor treatment. Genes Chromosomes Cancer 37(1):1–19

Skapek SX, Hawk BJ, Hoffer FA, Dahl GV, Granowetter L, Gebhardt MC, Ferguson WS, Grier HE (1998) Combination chemotherapy using vinblastine and methotrexate for the treatment of progressive desmoid tumor in children. J Clin Oncol 16(9):3021–3027

Smith AJ, Lewis JJ, Merchant NB, Leung DH, Woodruff JM, Brennan MF (2000) Surgical management of intra-abdominal desmoid tumours. Br J Surg 87(5):608–613

Smith L, Watterson J, Scott SM, Priest JR (1997) Medical and surgical management of pediatric soft tissue tumors. In: Coffin CM, Dehner LP, O'Shea PA (eds) Pediatric soft tissue tumors. Williams and Wilkins, Baltimore, pp 360–371

Soini Y (1990) Cell differentiation in benign cutaneous fibrous histiocytomas. An immunohistochemical study with antibodies to histiomonocytic cells and intermediate filament proteins. Am J Dermatopathol 12:134–140

Somerhausen NS, Fletcher CD (2000) Diffuse-type giant cell tumor: clinicopathologic and immunohistochemical analysis of 50 cases with extraarticular disease. Am J Surg Pathol 24:479–492

Sonoda T, Hashimoto H, Enjoji M (1985) Juvenile xanthogranuloma: clinicopathologic analysis and immunohistochemical study of 57 patients. Cancer 56:2280–2286

Spiegel DA, Dormans JP, Meyer JS, Himelstein B, Mathur S, Asada N, Womer RB (1999) Aggressive fibromatosis from infancy to adolescence. J Pediatr Orthop 19(6):776–784

Stiller D, Katenkamp D (1975) Cellular features in desmoid fibromatosis and well-differentiated fibrosarcomas: an electron microscopic study. Virchows Arch A Pathol Anat Histol 369(2):155–164

Taylor HB, Helwig EB (1962) Dermatofibrosarcoma protuberans: a study of 115 cases. Cancer 15:717–725

Tejpar S, Nollet F, Li C, Wunder JS, Michils G, dal Cin P, Van Cutsem E, Bapat B, van Roy F, Cassiman JJ, Alman BA (1999) Predominance of beta-catenin mutations and beta-catenin dysregulation in sporadic aggressive fibromatosis (desmoid tumor). Oncogene 18(47):6615–6620

Tolg C, Poon R, Fodde R, Turley EA, Alman BA (2003) Genetic deletion of receptor for hyaluronan-mediated motility (Rhamm) attenuates the formation of aggressive fibromatosis (desmoid tumor). Oncogene 22(44):6873–6882

Ushijima M, Hashimoto H, Tsuneyoshi M, Enjoji M (1989) Giant cell tumor of tendon sheath (nodular tenosynovitis). A study of 207 cases to compare the large joint group with the common digit group. Cancer 57:875–884

Webber BL, Parham DM (1996) Soft tissue tumors other than rhabdomyosarcoma and peripheral neuroepithelioma. In: Parham DM (ed) Pediatric neoplasia morphology and biology. Lippincott-Raven, Philadelphia, pp 205–257

Weiss SW (1986) Proliferative fibroblastic lesions. From hyperplasia to neoplasia. Am J Surg Pathol 10 Suppl 1:14–25

Weiss SW (1994) Fibrohistiocytic tumors. In: Sobin LH (ed) World Health Organization international histological classification of tumors: histological typing of soft tissue tumors, 2nd edn. Springer-Verlag, Berlin, pp 19–22

Zuppan CW, Mierau GW, Wilson HL (1987) Malignant fibrous histiocytoma in childhood: a report of two cases and review of the literature. Pediatr Pathol 7:303–318

Ewing Sarcoma Family of Tumors

Carlos Rodriguez-Galindo, Fariba Navid, Joseph Khoury, Matthew Krasin

Contents

9.1 Introduction

The term Ewing sarcoma family of tumors (ESFT) defines a group of small round cell neoplasms of neuroectodermal origin, which manifests as a continuum of neurogenic differentiation, with Ewing sarcoma of bone representing the least differentiated and primitive neuroectodermal tumor and peripheral neuroepithelioma the most differentiated forms. The ESFT comprise 3% of all pediatric malignancies, and are rare in the non-white population (Gurney et al. 1999).

The histogenesis of ESFT has been a source of controversy since its first description in 1921. Various hypotheses have been proposed in an attempt to identify the possible cell of origin; among these, cells of endothelial, pericytic, myeloid, mesenchymal, and neuroectodermal origin have all been suggested (Dehner 1993). The existence of either a mesenchymal stem cell or an early primitive neuroectodermal cell that has retained its ability for multilineage differentiation is the currently accepted hypothesis. It is now well accepted that the ESFT constitute a single group of neurally derived neoplasms that share unique immunocytochemical, cytogenetic, and molecular markers (de Alava and Gerald 2000; Dehner 1993). Despite aggressive treatment, 30–40% of patients with localized disease and 80% of patients with metastatic disease die due to disease progression (Coterill et al. 2000).

9.2 Epidemiology

ESFT of bone is the second most common bone malignancy in children, accounting for approximately 40% of all bone cancers (Gurney et al. 1999). Its average annual incidence rate is 2.9 per million; it peaks in the 2nd decade of life (5 per million), and it is extremely rare during the first 5 years of age (0.6 per million) (Gurney et al. 1999).

Approximately 200–250 new cases of ESFT are diagnosed in the United States each year, including a small percentage of tumors that arise in the soft tissue (extraosseous Ewing sarcoma). The disease occurs slightly more commonly in males than females with a ratio of 1.3:1. ESFT is predominantly seen in Caucasians, and is rarely diagnosed in African-Americans (Gurney et al. 1999). The protective etiology of this phenomenon has yet to be elucidated. In several African countries, the ratio of ESFT to osteosarcoma is very similar to that of US blacks. The incidence of ESFT is also lower in Hispanic and Asian populations (Parkin et al. 1993).

A number of studies have evaluated predisposing factors in ESFT. Parental farming exposure, history of inguinal hernia, and family history of gastric cancer or melanoma have been reported as associated with increased risk of developing ESFT (Gurney et al. 1999). These findings have been based on retrospective analysis, small sample size and selection bias, and have not been reproducible in all studies. Therefore, at this time, there is no convincing evidence that ESFT is associated with any disease, familial predisposition syndrome, or environmental factors. However, ESFT has been observed as second malignancy in irradiated and non-irradiated sites in a rare number of patients. Most of these cases were associated with retinoblastoma, but also have been reported in non-Hodgkin's lymphoma, leukemia, Hodgkin's disease and Wilms' tumor (Spunt et al. 2004).

Table 9.1. Chromosomal translocations in ESFT

Translocation	Gene fusion	Incidence (%)
t(11;22)(q24;q12)	EWS-FLI1	80–95%
t(21;22)(q22;q12)	EWS-ERG	5–10%
t(7:22)(p22;q12)	EWS-ETV1	Rare
t(17;22)(q12;q12)	EWS-EIAF	Rare
t(2;22)(q33;q12)	EWS-FEV	Rare

9.3 Pathogenesis

Understanding the pathogenesis of ESFT has been hampered by the still unknown cell of origin of this tumor. A variable expression of neuronal immunohistochemical markers and ultrastructural features, and the ability of ESFT cells to differentiate along a neural pathway in vitro, point to a neuroectodermal origin (Dehner 1993). However, since ESFT can arise in bone and soft tissue, and these tumors can also show mesenchymal and epithelial features, it has been postulated that the cell of origin for ESFT is more likely to be a primitive cell that has the capacity to differentiate along a number of cell types. Torchia et al. (2003) recently demonstrated in an experimental system that bone marrow-derived stromal cells transduced with EWS/ETS fusion proteins (described below) recapitulate some of the features of ESFT, namely they exhibit a block in osteogenic and adipogenic differentiation and express neural markers.

Despite the limitation of not knowing the cell of origin, a number of advances in our understanding of the basic biology of ESFT have been made over the last few years. This progress can be attributed to the identification of recurring chromosomal translocations in this tumor type involving the N-terminus transactivation domain of the EWS gene on chromosome 22 band q12 with the C-terminus DNA-binding domain of an ETS family of transcription factors. The ETS family fusion partner most commonly detected is FLI-1 on chromosome 11 band q24 followed by ERG on chromosome 21 band q22 and less commonly FEV, ETV1 and E1AF (Table 9.1) (de Alava and Ger-

Table 9.2. Proteins regulated by EWS-FLI1

Protein	Classification	Function	Reference
↑ Manic fringe	Glycosyltransferase	Cell transformation	May et al. 1997
↓ Transforming growth factor β II receptor (TGFβIIR)	Tumor suppressor gene	Cell transformation	Hahm et al. 1999; Im et al. 2000
↑ c-myc	Transcription factor	Cell proliferation	Dauphinot et al. 2001; Tanaka et al. 1997
↑ Platelet derived growth factor C (PDGFC)	Growth factor	Cell transformation	Zwerner and May 2001, 2002
↑ Stromelysin (MMP-3)	Matrix metalloproteinase	Invasion and metastasis	Braun et al. 1995
↑ EWS-FLI1-activated transcript (EAT2)	Signaling protein	Cell transformation	Thompson et al. 1996
↑ E2-C/UbcH10	Cyclin-specific ubiquitin-conjugating enzyme	Cell proliferation	Arvand et al. 1998
↑ ERK1 and ↑ ERK2	MAPK signaling proteins	Cell transformation	Silvany et al. 2000
↑ Id2	Helix-loop-helix protein	Cell proliferation and block differentiation	Fukuma et al. 2003; Nishimori et al. 2002
↓ $p57^{KIP}$	G1 cyclin-dependent kinase inhibitor	Cell proliferation	Dauphinot et al. 2001
↓ Insulin-like growth factor binding protein-3 (IGFBP-3)	Growth factor modulator	Cell proliferation and prevent apoptosis	Prieur et al. 2004

ald 2000; Delattre et al. 1994). The resulting fusion protein from the rearrangement of these genes has been implicated in the tumorigenesis of ESFT.

The best characterized of the fusion proteins is EWS-FLI1. EWS is an RNA-binding protein whose function is unclear. FLI1 is a transcription factor and contains a sequence specific DNA binding domain, GGA(A/T). FLI1 plays a role in embryonic development, hematopoiesis, cell growth and differentiation, as well as tumorigenesis. The fusion product of these two genes, EWS and FLI-1, can cause neoplastic transformation in a number of in vitro and in vivo experimental systems (May et al. 1993a). Furthermore, ESFT cell lines transduced with anti-sense oligonucleotides, small interfering RNAs (siRNA) or competitive inhibitors to EWS-FLI1 demonstrate growth inhibition as well as increased susceptibility to chemotherapy induced apoptosis in culture and in mice (Prieur et al. 2004; Tanaka et al. 1997).

Although the mechanism by which EWS-FLI-1 contributes to the pathogenesis of ESFT is not completely understood, this fusion protein does bind to target genes in a sequence specific manner determined by FLI-1, but these genes are controlled by EWS regulatory domains, a more potent transcriptional activator than FLI-1 (May et al. 1993b). This aberrant gene regulation appears to result in the transforming properties of EWS-FLI1. Overexpression of FLI-1 and mutations in the DNA-binding domain of FLI1 do not recapitulate the transforming properties of EWS-FLI1, suggesting that the EWS-FLI-1 chimeric protein may also affect different target genes (May et al. 1993b). The critical genes modulated by EWS-FLI1 that contribute to the oncogenesis are not known. Some candidate genes and their potential role in the pathogenesis of ESFT are listed in Table 9.2.

At the molecular level, there are several in-frame EWS-FLI1 chimeric transcripts. The most common fusions involve fusion of EWS exon 7 with FLI1 exon 6 (type 1) and fusion of EWS exon 7 with FLI1 exon 5 (type 2) with a relative frequency of 60% and 25%, respectively (Zucman et al. 1993). All chimeric products include the DNA-binding domain of FLI1 and the transactivation domain of EWS. Lin et al. (Lin et al. 1999) compared the transactivation potential of the type 1 fusion product with six other fusion types in vitro and showed that the type 1 fusion was a weaker transactivator than the other fusion types. This finding may in part explain the better outcome in patients whose tumors contain the type 1 translocation (de Alava et al. 1998; Zoubek et al. 1996).

The karyotype of ESFT cells is not restricted to the rearrangement involving chromosome 22. Using conventional cytogenetics and comparative genomic hybridization, trisomies in chromosome 8 and 12 as well as an unbalanced translocation have been repeatedly observed in ESFT (de Alava et al. 1998; Brisset et al. 2001; Gurney et al. 1999; Hattinger et al. 1999; Ozaki et al. 2001). The biologic and clinical significance of these abnormalities remains to be fully explored in a large group of patients. Individual genes frequently altered in human cancer and those that typically regulate cell proliferation and apoptosis have also been evaluated in ESFT. Of these genes, alterations in p53, primarily missense mutations, and alterations in INK4A, primarily homozygous deletions often associated with loss of p15 and ARF genes, have been detected in 7–15% and 18–30% of primary tumor samples from patients with ESFT, respectively (Kovar et al. 1993). Aberrations in either one of these genes have been correlated with poor overall survival (Abudu et al. 1999; Tsuchiya et al. 2000). Rarely have abnormalities in MDM2, RB or CDK4 been detected in ESFT.

In addition to genetic aberrations, dysregulation of growth factor and apoptotic pathways have also been implicated in the pathogenesis of ESFT. The best studied of these in ESFT is the insulin-like growth factor (IGF) signaling pathway. Insulin-like growth factors, IGFI and IGFII, primarily mediate their effects through the insulin-like growth factor I receptor (IGFIR). IGFIR are found on the surface of most, if not all, ESFT that have been studied to date (Scotlandi et al. 1996). Activated IGFIR results in a number of different responses that are mediated by two primary pathways, mitogen-activated protein kinase (MAPK) and phosphatidylinositol-3-kinase (PI3-K) (Benini et al. 2004). Impairment of IGFIR function by antisense strategies, antibodies, or dominant negative constructs ameliorates its effects on proliferation, migration, angiogenesis, metastasis, and transformation as well as enhancing chemosensitivity of ESFT cells to conventional cytotoxic drugs (Scotlandi et al. 1996, 2002; Toretsky et al. 1999). These observations would suggest that IGF signaling plays a central role in the tumorigenesis of ESFT. The dominant role of this pathway is further substantiated by the fact that the presence of IGFIR is necessary for the transforming ability of EWS/ETS fusion proteins (Toretsky et al. 1997). Furthermore, Prieur et al. (2004) have recently shown that EWS/FLI1 binds to the promoter region of insulin-like growth factor binding protein-3 (IGF-BP-3), a negative regulator of IGF-I signaling, and causes repression of its activity, demonstrating a direct link between IGF-1 signaling and EWS-FLI1.

Basic fibroblast growth factor (bFGF) and its receptors are also expressed in ESFT. bFGF belongs to a family of heparin-binding polypeptide growth factors that are important in neuronal development. The role of this growth factor in ESFT remains to be determined. One group of investigators has shown that both in vivo and vitro, the proliferation of ESFT cell lines can be inhibited by exogenous bFGF (Sturla et al. 2000). However, other investigators have shown the opposite effect, bFGF-induced cell proliferation (Girnita et al. 2000).

The recent development of molecular targeted therapy in cancer has led to the investigation of specific pathways for which these therapies exist. Imatinib mesylate is an inhibitor of structurally related tyrosine kinases including c-KIT, platelet-derived growth factor receptors (PDGFR) α and β, c-ABL, BCR-ABL, v-ABL and ABL-related gene (ARG). Chronic myelogenous leukemia (CML) cells, which express BCR-ABL tyrosine kinase, and gastrointestinal stromal tumor (GIST) cells, which have activating mutations in c-KIT, are highly sensitive to imatinib mesylate. These observations prompted an evaluation of c-KIT and PDGFR expression in ESFT. c-KIT and its ligand, stem cell factor (SCF), as well as PDGFRβ are expressed in some ESFT (Smithey et al. 2002; Scotlandi et al. 2003). In vitro experiments suggest that the c-KIT/SCF and PDGF pathways play a role in cell proliferation, transformation and motility of ESFT and may serve as novel targets for therapy (Scotlandi et al. 2003; Uren et al. 2003). Whether the presence of these pathways is critical for the survival of ESFT cells remains to be determined.

Another promising target for cancer chemotherapy that has shed light on the biology of ESFT is the activation of death receptors of the TNF-receptor superfamily resulting in activation of effector caspases and ultimately apoptosis. Death inducing ligands for these receptors include TNF-related apoptosis-inducing ligand (TRAIL), Fas ligand, and tumor necrosis factor (TNF). Of these, TRAIL is the most potent inducer of apoptosis in ESFT (Kontny et al. 2001). However, not all ESFT that express death receptors are sensitive to TRAIL. Absence or downregulation of caspase 8 by hypermethylation of promoter region of this gene appears to be a frequent mechanism of TRAIL resistance. Fulda et al. (2001) have demonstrated that in the presence of a DNA demethylating agent, apoptosis can be induced in TRAIL insensitive ESFT cells. DNA demethylating agents and TRAIL are currently in clinical development (see Sect. 9.7, below, "Future Developments").

In summary, genetic alterations, growth factor and apoptotic signaling pathways have been shown to play a role in the pathogenesis of ESFT. EWS/ETS fusion proteins have been recognized as playing a central role in this process. Several downstream targets of these fusion proteins have been identified. The contribution of each of these proteins and their targets, as well as their mechanism of action, requires further investigation. Using oligonucleotide or DNA microarrays and proteomics, it will be possible to begin to map out a signature gene/protein profile for ESFT. These techniques will be useful in validating existing hypotheses as well as identifying yet unrecognized signaling pathways in this tumor.

9.4 Pathology

9.4.1 Microscopic Features

As a group, ESFT exhibit a wide spectrum of cellular morphologic features. Tumors arising in bone (Ewing sarcoma) are usually composed of uniform small round cells with round nuclei containing fine chromatin and small nucleoli, scant clear or eosinophilic cytoplasm, and indistinct cytoplasmic membranes (Fig. 9.1). True rosette structures may be identified occasionally. Mitotic figures and necrosis are variable in frequency. A small subset of tumors is composed of

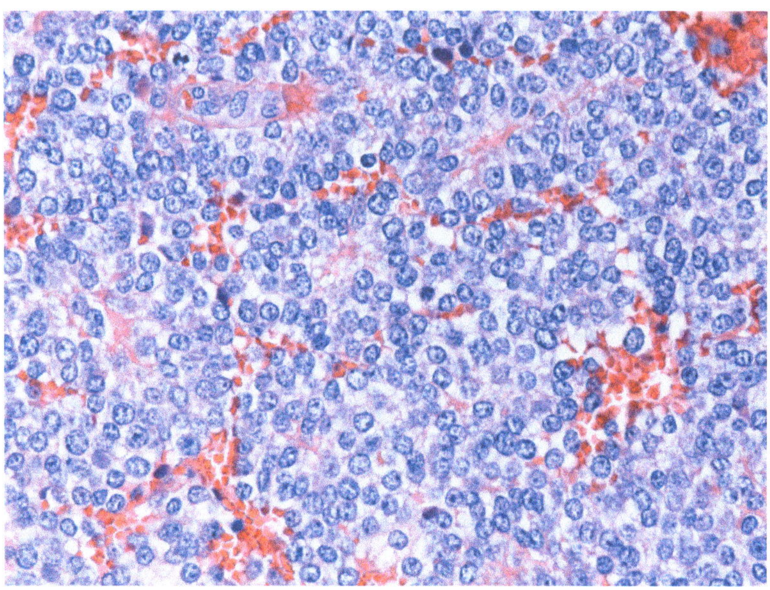

Figure 9.1

Ewing sarcoma composed of small round neoplastic cells arranged in vague nests. H&E stain, ×200

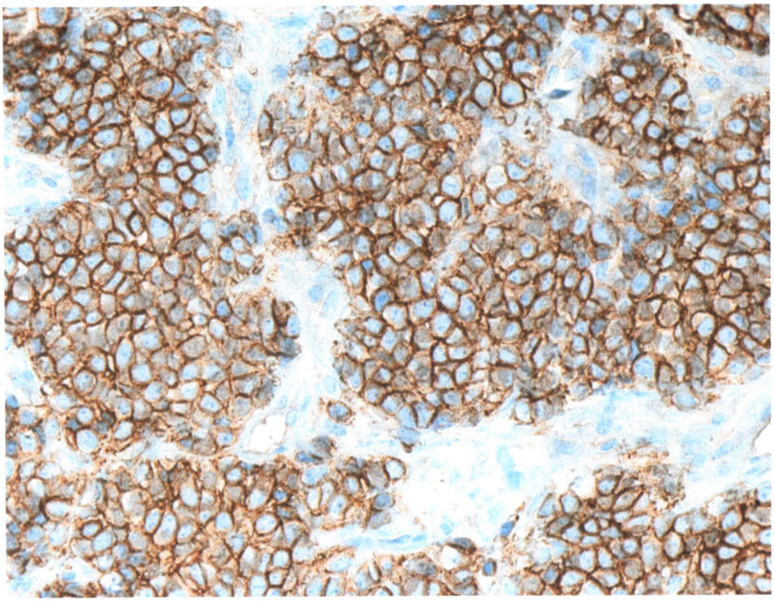

Figure 9.2

Characteristic intense membranous CD99 immunostaining in Ewing sarcoma family of tumors

relatively larger cells with irregular nuclear contours and prominent nucleoli.

Intracytoplasmic glycogen within neoplastic cells may be demonstrated using PAS staining and diastase digestion. While of historical value, this technique lacks specificity and is not recommended currently for the diagnostic workup for ESFT. Primitive intercellular junctions, indicating epithelial differentiation, and dense core granules, indicating neural differentiation, may be identified by electron microscopy.

Most ESFT express CD99 (Fig. 9.2), which is a cell membrane protein encoded by the MIC2 gene located in the pseudoautosomal region at the end of the short arms of the X and Y chromosomes (Ambros et al. 1991). CD99 is a 32-kDa cell surface antigen with broad cellular expression whose function remains incompletely understood but is believed to be involved in T-cell regulation (Wingett et al. 1999). While expressed by most ESFT, CD99 expression is not specific for ESFT and may be detected in lymphoblastic lymphoma, embryonal rhabdomyosarcoma, and other soft tissue sarcomas (Perlman et al. 1994). Nevertheless, in the absence of conclusive molecular data, strong diffuse CD99 immunostaining constitutes a useful marker for ESFT in tumors lacking features suggestive of other round cell malignancies. CD99 is most useful as part of a panel of immunostains that also includes Myo-D1, TdT, and synaptophysin, which are helpful in ruling out the major differential diagnostic considerations of rhabdomyosarcoma, lymphoblastic lymphoma, and neuroblastoma, respectively. Distinction between ESFT and small cell osteosarcoma rests on the absence of CD99 expression and identification of osteoid deposition in the latter and on identification of ESFT-specific translocations in the former.

9.4.2 Molecular Pathology

Translocations involving the EWS gene are detected in the vast majority of ESFT, most commonly using reverse transcriptase polymerase chain reaction (RT-PCR) and fluorescence in situ hybridization (FISH). Up to 18 types of in-frame EWS-FLI1 chimeric transcripts are possible and, of note, all contain the transactivating amino-terminal domain of EWS (exons 1–7) and the ETS-type DNA-binding domain of FLI1 (exon 9) (Fig. 9.3) (Zucman et al. 1993). The portion of the chimeric protein between these two domains is

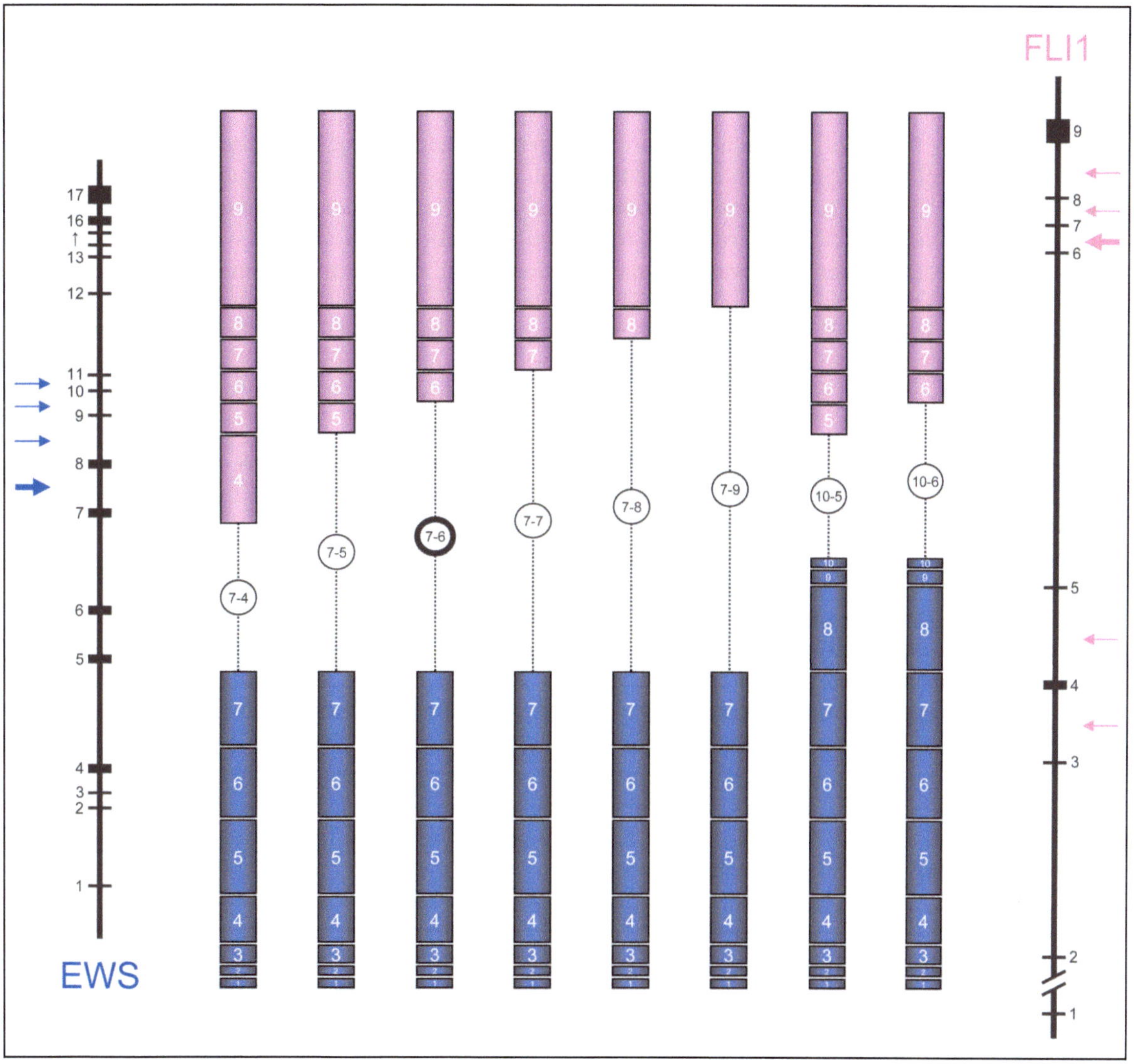

Figure 9.3

Types of EWS/FLI-1 chimeric transcripts

variable in size and composition, reflecting genomic breaks in one of four EWS introns and one of six FLI1 introns. The two main fusion types, fusion of EWS exon 7 to FLI1 exon 6 (so-called type 1) and fusion of EWS exon 7 to FLI1 exon 5 (so-called type 2), account for about 85% of EWS-FLI1 fusions (Zoubek et al. 1994, 1996). All other EWS-FLI1 fusion types are designated by the exons involved, by convention.

EWS exon 7 forward and FLI1 exon 9 reverse primers should amplify all forms of EWS-FLI1, with potential amplification products of variable sizes. However, using this approach may result in false negative results in tumors harboring large fusions such as types 9–4 or 10–5, especially if sample RNA is partially degraded. An alternative approach entails using initially a FLI1 exon 6 reverse primer in combination with an EWS exon 7 forward primer. Such a primer pair will yield small RT-PCR products in more than 85% of cases with EWS-FLI1. To ensure detection of a minority of false-negative cases, a second-line reaction in which the EWS exon 7 forward primer is paired with a FLI1 exon 9 reverse primer and an ERG reverse primer is performed. Because of their frequency, type 1 and type 2 EWS-FLI1 products can be recognized by their size identity with an appropriate normal control.

Approximately 5% of ESFT harbor a complex or cryptic t(21;22)(q22;q12) that rearranges EWS with another ETS family gene, ERG. With an exon structure highly analogous to FLI1, several translocation variants of EWS-ERG have been noted (Zucman et al. 1993). It is noteworthy that enough molecular homology exists between FLI1, ERG, and FEV to allow the design of consensus reverse primers that could detect all the corresponding translocations using one assay.

Detection of translocations in ESFT using formalin-fixed paraffin-embedded tissue is possible using RT-PCR or a variety of FISH methods. A highly sensitive FISH assay utilizing a dual-color break-apart DNA probe flanking the EWS-R1 breakpoint region on chromosome 22 is commonly utilized. An intact DNA target is indicated by juxtaposition of the DNA probes whereas rearrangements of the EWS gene lead to separation of hybridization signals. Using this approach, all translocations involving EWS may be detected regardless of the translocation partner or fusion type. While sensitive, this approach lacks high specificity since it may detect other tumors that may harbor translocations involving the EWS gene (Fuller et al. 2004).

Genomic breakpoints in EWS are clustered within a 7-kb region, making Southern blotting useful in some circumstances. Although requiring a significant amount of tissue for DNA extraction, this technique can reliably detect EWS rearrangements regardless of the translocation partner or molecular variation in the fusion gene.

Common additional chromosomal abnormalities in ESFT include both numerical and structural findings. Most common are gains of chromosomes 8, 12, 20, and 1q and losses of 16q and 19q and der(16)t(1;16)(q12;q11.2) (Brisset et al. 2001; Ozaki et al. 2001). It appears that the presence and frequency of secondary chromosomal changes may be associated with worse clinical outcome. In one study, deletions at the short arm of chromosome 1 were associated with an unfavorable outcome in patients with localized disease (Hattinger et al. 1999). In another study, loss of 16q was an independent prognostic factor by multivariate analysis (Ozaki et al. 2001).

9.5 Clinical Features

Patients with ESFT commonly present during the 2nd decade of life; 80% of patients are younger than 18 years of age, and the median age at diagnosis is 14 years (Cotterill et al. 2000; Grier et al. 2003; Gurney et al. 1999). Males are more commonly affected than females, and the disease is very rare in African-Americans (Gurney et al. 1999).

ESFT has a tendency to involve the shaft of long tubular bones, pelvis, and ribs but practically every bone can be affected (Table 9.3). More than 50% of

Table 9.3. Primary sites of ESFT of bone (Cotterill et al. 2000; Grier et al. 2003; Paulussen et al. 2001a)

Site	Frequency
Central axis	52–55%
Skull	2–6%
Clavicle/scapula	4–6%
Ribs	12–13%
Spine	6–8%
Pelvis	23–27%
Extremities	41–47%
Humerus	5–7%
Radius/ulna	1–3%
Hand	<1%
Femur	16–19%
Tibia	7–10%
Fibula	6–9%
Foot	2–3%

the tumors arise from axial bones, with the pelvis being the most commonly involved (23–27%); one-third of the tumors originate in the lower extremities, and less than 10% in the upper extremities (Cotterill et al. 2000; Grier et al. 2003; Gurney et al. 1999; Paulussen et al. 2001a). In the long bones, diaphyseal involvement predominates over metaphyseal disease. ESFT usually presents with localized pain and a visible palpable mass, and almost one-half of patients have symptoms referable to their primary tumor for more than 3 months prior to the diagnosis. Older patients have a higher proportion of pelvic primaries and larger tumors. Pathologic fractures may be present in up to 15% of cases (Cotterill et al. 2000).

ESFT are aggressive neoplasms; systemic manifestations such as fever or anemia are present in 10–15% of the patients (Bacci et al. 2000), and approximately 20–25% of cases have clinically apparent metastatic disease at the time of diagnosis (Craft et al. 1998; Miser et al. 2004; Sandoval et al. 1996). Metastatic disease appears to be associated with older age (Kolb et al. 2003) and large tumors (Kolb et al. 2003; Paulussen et al. 1998a; Spunt et al. 2001) or pelvic primaries (Miser et al. 2004; Paulussen et al. 1998a; Sandoval et al. 1996). Isolated lung disease, usually bilateral, occurs in 25–45% of metastate cases; the majority of patients (50–60%) have extrapulmonary disease (usually bone and bone marrow) (Cotterill et al. 2000; Craft et al. 1998; Miser et al. 2004; Paulussen et al. 1998b; Sandoval et al. 1996).

9.5.1 Extraosseous ESFT

ESFT have been described in many different extraosseous locations, such as soft tissues (Raney et al. 1997), skin and subcutaneous tissue (Chow et al. 2000), gastrointestinal tract (Shek et al. 2001), kidney (Parham et al. 2001), or genitourinary tract (Gaona-Luviano et al. 2003).

In the past, ESFT of the soft tissues have been classified as undifferentiated sarcomas, and may account for 5–10% of the cases enrolled in the cooperative Intergroup Rhabdomyosarcoma Study Group trials. The most common locations are the paraspinal and retroperitoneal soft tissues (35%), followed by extremities (26%), head and neck (18%), chest wall (10%), and abdominal wall (3%). Age and racial distributions, and outcome do not seem to differ from ESFT arising in bone (Raney et al. 1997).

Neuroectodermal tumors of the kidney appear to encompass a group of primitive, highly malignant neoplasms that histologically and clinically are not well characterized. They may occur at any age, but the peak occurs during the 2nd and 3rd decades. Histologically, they are defined as primitive neural tumors, with varying amounts of rosettes and neuropil. Approximately half of the tumors have the histological appearance typical of ESFT, whereas atypical features are present in the remainder. The vast majority of tumors express CD99, but molecular confirmation of ESFT only occurs in one-third of them (Parham et al. 2001).

Cutaneous and subcutaneous ESFT appear to have an indolent course and an excellent outcome (Chow et al. 2000). Finally, an interesting association is the development of ESFT in the genitourinary tract after kidney transplant (Gaona-Luviano et al. 2003).

A small proportion of ESFT arise in the face. In this location, ESFT should be distinguished from esthesioneuroblastoma, an uncommon malignant neoplasm of the nasal vault, believed to arise from the olfactory epithelium. The exact cell of origin is controversial, but neuronal or neural crest origin is supported by the presence of neurofilaments. Inclusion within the ESFT has been proposed; however, these tumors do not express CD99, and molecular studies have not confirmed the presence of the typical fusion transcript, and therefore should be considered a different entity (Dulguerov et al. 2001).

9.5.2 Laboratory and Radiologic Evaluation

Patients with suspected ESFT should be thoroughly evaluated to define the extent of local disease and the presence of metastases. Elevations of the erythrocyte sedimentation rate and serum lactate dehydrogenase (LDH) are not uncommon. Bilateral bone marrow aspirates and biopsies should also be performed, and evaluation using molecular techniques such as RT-PCR is recommended. Important imaging studies included in the evaluation are chest radiograph, plain radiographs of primary and metastatic sites, bone scintigraphy, CT of the chest, and MRI of the primary site with T_1- and T_2-weighted sequences.

Plain radiographs in ESFT typically show an ill-defined, permeative or focally moth-eaten, destructive intramedullary lesion. An ill-defined soft tissue mass adjacent to the primary bone lesion is very common. The lesion is often accompanied by a prominent multilayered periosteal reaction ("onion skin"); the perpendicular "sunburst" type of periosteal new bone formation can be present but is less common than in osteosarcoma. MRI is better than CT to define the intramedullary component of the primary tumor and the extent of soft tissue mass. In contrast to osteosarcoma, dynamic contrast-enhanced MRI is not a very reliable prognostic indicator (Miller et al. 2001). However, newer techniques such as positron emission tomography may be useful in the non-invasive evaluation of chemotherapy response.

9.5.3 Prognostic Factors

For patients with localized disease, large tumor size, trunk and pelvic primaries, older age, elevated LDH, and poor response to induction chemotherapy have been typically associated with worse outcome (Bacci et al. 2000; Cotterill et al. 2000; Grier et al. 2003). However, the relative importance of some of these factors may diminish as treatments evolve and improved regimens, with better systemic and local control rates, are being developed. Recent studies have shown that the use of more intensive chemotherapy, with the incorporation of ifosfamide and etoposide, for example, tend to decrease the adverse effect on outcome associated with large size and pelvic location (Grier et al. 2003; Marina et al. 1999). Nevertheless, high disease burden, as indicated by tumor volume or LDH, continues to be associated with an adverse prognosis, although this may be limited to patients treated without surgery (Oberlin et al. 2001). Older age is consistently associated with a worse outcome (Bacci et al. 2000; Cotterill et al. 2000; Grier et al. 2003; Kolb et al. 2003). Patients older than 14 years have a higher proportion of large tumors and pelvic primaries (Cotterill et al. 2000) and metastatic disease (Kolb et al. 2003). In contrast to other factors, the benefit of the addition of ifosfamide and etoposide is not seen in older patients (Grier et al. 2003).

The degree of histologic response appears to be one of the most relevant prognostic factors, on which future studies should build. Recent studies consistently have shown the prognostic value of a histologic response to induction chemotherapy, the significance of which applies across protocols and appears to be independent of the drugs used. Patients with good histologic responses had a significantly better outcome than those with poor responses in the consecutive REN-1, 2 and 3 Italian trials (Bacci et al. 2000; Picci et al. 1997) and in the CESS-81 (Jürgens et al. 1988) and CESS-86 (Paulussen et al. 2001a) German trials. Contrary to the above prognostic factors, treatment intensification may not have a major impact in increasing the proportion of patients with a favorable histologic response, probably because biologic factors influence the response to treatment. Despite the strong association between histologic response and outcome, there is no evidence to suggest that this phenomenon of resistance is mediated by expression of multidrug resistance proteins; 50–60 % of ESFT express p-glycoprotein, but this expression does not seem to correlate with outcome (Hijazi et al. 1994). However, the role of other members of the ATP binding cassette (ABC) family of membrane transporters in drug resistance in ESFT has yet to be elucidated.

The type of fusion transcript also seems to influence the clinical behavior of ESFT. Although the biological behavior of tumors with the fusions EWS-FLI1 and EWS-ERG do not seem to differ (Ginsberg et al. 1999), the type of EWS-FLI1 fusion may affect prognosis. The hybrid transcripts resulting from the fusion of exons 7 and 6 of the EWS and FLI1 genes, respectively (type 1 fusion), seem to result in sarcomas of a less aggressive behavior than other fusion types (de Alava et al. 1998; Lin et al. 1999; Zoubek et al. 1996). Because ESFT manifests a continuum of neuroectodermal differentiation, the histological diversity could reflect different biological behaviors. However, there is no evidence to suggest that the degree of neuroectodermal differentiation in ESFT correlates with prognosis (Terrier et al. 1995).

The most important prognostic factor remains the presence of metastatic disease at diagnosis (Fig. 9.4)

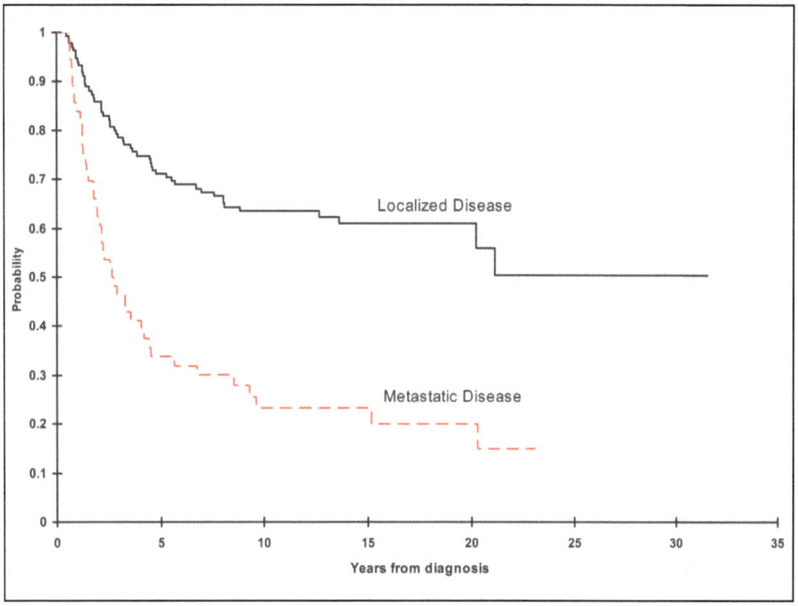

Figure 9.4

Outcome for 191 patients with ESFT treated in the St. Jude Children's Research Hospital studies ES-79, EW-87, and EW-92. The 5- and 10-year survival estimates for patients with localized disease were 71.1±3.9% and 63.5±4.6%, respectively. The 5- and 10-year survival estimates for patients with metastatic disease were 33.9±6.2% and 23.3±6.2%, respectively ($p<0.001$)

(Cotterill et al. 2000). Advances in the treatment of ESFT have only resulted in a very modest improvement in the outcome of patients with metastases (Cotterill et al. 2000; Marina et al. 1999; Sandoval et al. 1996). However, even among patients with metastatic disease, there is some heterogeneity. With an appropriately intensive treatment that includes bilateral lung radiation, the EICESS studies have shown that patients with isolated lung metastases may have a better prognosis, albeit still worse than patients with localized disease, while patients with extrapulmonary metastases have a worse prognosis (Paulussen et al. 1998a, b).

With the use of molecular techniques in the staging of ESFT, it is evident that a significant proportion of patients with localized ESFT (20–40%) have micrometastatic disease, measured as molecular detection of tumor cells by RT-PCR in peripheral blood or bone marrow (Fagnou et al. 1998; Schleiermacher et al. 2003; West et al. 1997; Zoubek et al. 1998). This proportion is higher among patients with clinically detectable metastases (Schleiermacher et al. 2003; Zoubek et al. 1998), and seems to correlate with the pattern of metastatic spread; 90% with isolated lung metastases have a lower incidence at RT-PCR detected metastases than patients with bone or bone marrow desease (Zoubek et al. 1998, Schleiermacher 2003). The prognostic significance of molecular microstaging for patients with localized disease is still unclear. However, recent studies suggest that the detection of circulating tumor cells or bone marrow micrometastases by molecular techniques may predict unfavorable outcome (Schleiermacher et al. 2003). In a large series of 172 patients, the detection of occult tumor cells was significantly associated with a worse outcome; the 2-year DFS estimates for patients with presence versus absence of bone marrow micrometastases were 43±18.4% and 76±9.2%, respectively ($p=0.007$) (Schleiermacher et al. 2003). In this same study, patients with localized disease and bone marrow micrometastases or circulating tumor cells were comparable to patients with metastases in terms of the location of the primary tumor, outcome, and pattern of relapse (Schleiermacher et al. 2003). These data suggest that the use of molecular techniques may further define clinically relevant distinct groups of patients at diagnosis.

In the future, risk definitions will likely be based on: (1) "tumor load," as defined by the volume of the primary tumor (>200 cm^3), the metastatic pattern (pulmonary vs. extrapulmonary), or the presence of micrometastatic disease detected by molecular techniques; and (2) "biologic factors," defined by biological features, grade of histologic response, or type of fusion transcript (Rodriguez-Galindo et al. 2003).

9.6 Treatment

As defined by current imaging techniques, approximately 80% of patients with ESFT have localized disease at diagnosis (Cotterill et al. 2000). However, treatment with local control measures alone can cure less than 10% of the patients, suggesting that most patients have disseminated disease at diagnosis that is not detected with conventional methods. Thus, treatment of ESFT ought to achieve two major goals, local control and eradication of the systemic disease. These two components of therapy are staged in three phases: (a) induction chemotherapy, the goal of which is to achieve rapid initial cytoreduction and facilitate local control; (b) local control, using surgery, irradiation, or both, usually after 10–12 weeks of chemotherapy; and (c) continuation therapy, with the same (or similar) chemotherapy used for induction therapy.

9.6.1 Treatment of Patients with Localized Disease

The last 3 decades have witnessed a major improvement in the outcome of patients with ESFT. These advances in the treatment of ESFT derive largely from the cooperative trials, which have defined the active agents and their optimal schedules and combinations, and have explored treatment intensification and risk-stratification approaches (Rodriguez-Galindo et al. 2003).

9.6.1.1 Four-Drug Regimens

Following the early reports documenting improved outcomes for patients with ESFT receiving adjuvant chemotherapy (Jaffe et al. 1976), several prospective studies documented the efficacy of a four-drug regimen with vincristine, actinomycin D, cyclophosphamide, and doxorubicin (VACD) as well as the need to perform early aggressive cytoreduction with higher doses of alkylators, and early dose-intensification of doxorubicin (Table 9.4). Using different variants of the VACD regimen, along with local control measures, survival rates improved from less than 20% to 40–60% (Bacci et al. 1989; Burgert et al. 1990; Craft et al. 1997; Donaldson et al. 1998; Evans et al. 1991; Hayes et al. 1989; Jürgens et al. 1988; Nesbit et al. 1990; Razek et al. 1980; Oberlin et al. 2001). These early studies defined that large tumors [defined as >8 cm (Hayes et al. 1989) or >100 cm^3 (Jürgens et al. 1988)], pelvic (and axial) locations, and poor histologic response to preoperative chemotherapy were strong prognostic indicators of outcome. Surgery for local control was seldom used, and radiation therapy alone was used in more than 75% of the patients (Burgert et al. 1990; Craft et al. 1997; Donaldson et al. 1998; Evans et al. 1991; Nesbit et al. 1990; Razek et al. 1980). In these studies, local control was suboptimal (particularly in pelvic primaries), 20–30% of patients developed local recurrences, and distant metastases occurred in 30–40% of patients. However, it soon became clear that with improvements in radiation planning (Jürgens et al. 1988; Burgert et al. 1990), and more aggressive local measures (Bacci et al. 1989), local control could be improved.

9.6.1.2 Role of Ifosfamide and Etoposide

The next generation of studies evaluated the incorporation of ifosfamide and etoposide (Table 9.5). In the CESS-86 study, patients with small extremity tumors continued to receive the VACD regimen, whereas ifosfamide replaced cyclophosphamide (VAID) in the treatment of patients with high risk disease (defined as >100 ml or axial location). Using the VAID regimen, the CESS-86 and the ET-2 studies obtained a modest improvement in the outcome for patients with high-risk disease (Craft et al. 1998; Paulussen et al. 2001a), establishing the VAID regimen as the standard for patients with localized ESFT. However, considering the nephrotoxicity associated with the high cumulative doses of ifosfamide, patients with standard risk disease may require less intensive therapies.

Table 9.4. Treatment of localized ESFT with VACD (*V* vincristine, *A* actinomycin D, *C* cyclophosphamide, *D* doxorubicin, *Sx* surgery, *RT* radiation therapy, *NR* not reported, *LRT* lung irradiation, *DFS* disease-free survival, *OS* overall survival)

Study	N	Regimen	Local control (% patients)	Outcome	Failures	Poor prognostic factors
IESS-I (1973–1978) (Nesbit et al. 1990; Razek et al. 1980)	342	VAC VAC+lung RT VAC+D	Sx (3%) Sx+RT (NR) RT (NR): whole bone 45–55 Gy; boost 5–10 Gy	5-year DFS VAC: 24% VAC+LRT: 44% VAC+D: 60%	Local: 6% Local+distant: 22% Distant: 41%	Site (pelvis) Size
IESS-II (1978–1982) (Burgert et al. 1990; Evans et al. 1991)	273	VACD – intense VACD – moderate	Sx (21%) Sx+RT (NR) RT (NR): whole bone 45–55 Gy; boost 5–10 Gy	5-year DFS VACD (I): Non-pelvic: 68% Pelvic: 55% VACD (M): Non-pelvic: 48% Pelvic: 23%	Local: 3% Local+distant: 8% Distant: 29%	Site (pelvis)
ES-79 (1978–1986) (Hayes et al. 1989)	52	VACD	Sx (21%) Sx+RT (35 Gy) (NR) RT (NR): 35 Gy (good responders) – 55 Gy (poor responders)	5-year DFS: <8 cm: 82% >8 cm: 64%	Local: 19% Local+distant: 8% Distant: 6%	Leukocytosis Size >8 cm
CESS 81 (1981–1985) (Jürgens et al. 1988)	93	VACD	Sx (33%) Sx+RT (36 Gy) (31%) RT: 46–60 Gy (34%)	5-year DFS: 55%	Local: 23% Local+distant: 10% Distant: 19%	Volume (>100 cm^3) Site (axial) Poor histologic response
ET-1 (1978–1986) (Hayes et al. 1989)	120	VACD	Sx (5%) Sx+RT (18%) RT (77%): long bones: 55–60 Gy Ribs: 35–40 Gy Pelvis: 40–45 Gy	5-year DFS: 41%	Local: 18% Local+distant: 7% Distant: 37%	Site (pelvis)
REA-2 (1979–1982) (Bacci et al. 1989)	59	VACD	Sx (NR) Sx+RT (35–45 Gy) (NR) RT: 40–60 Gy (NR)	5-year DFS: 54%	Local: 5% Local+distant: 14% Distant: 25%	Site (axial)
POG 8346 (1983–1988) (Donaldson et al. 1998)	141	VACD	Sx (15%) Sx+RT (55.8 Gy) (11%) RT: 55.8 Gy (74%)	5-year DFS: 51%	Local: 23% Distant: 40%	Site (pelvis)
SFOP EW84 (Oberlin et al. 2001)	141	VACD	Sx (40%) Sx+RT (40 Gy) (38%) RT: (60 Gy) (22%)	5-year DFS: 58% 5-year OS: 66%	Local: 13% Local+distant: 6% Distant: 20%	Poor histologic response

Table 9.5. Treatment of localized ESFT with ifosfamide and etoposide (*V* vincristine, *A* actinomycin D, *C* cyclophosphamide, *D* doxorubicin, *I* ifosfamide, *E* etoposide, *Sx* surgery, *RT* radiation therapy, *LRT* lung irradiation, *DFS* disease-free survival, *OS* overall survival)

Study	N	Regimen	Local control (% patients)	Outcome	Failures	Poor prognostic factors
CESS-86 (1986–1991) (Paulussen et al. 2001a)	301	SR[a]: VACD	Sx (23%)	10-year EFS	Local: 7%	Tumor volume (>200 ml)
		HR[a]: VAID	Sx+RT (44.8 Gy) (49%)	VACD: 52%	Local+distant: 4%	Poor histologic responders
			RT (60 Gy) (28%)	VAID: 51%	Distant: 35%	
ET-2 (1987–1993) (Craft et al. 1998)	201	VAID	Sx (58%)	5-year DFS: 62%	Local: 11%	Site (pelvis)
			Sx+RT (45 Gy) (9%) RT (55 Gy) (31%)			Older age
REN-2 (1988–1991) (Bacci et al. 1998)	82	VAID+IE	Sx (27%)	5-year DFS: 51%	Local: 1%	Elevated LDH
			Sx+RT (40–45 Gy) (27%) RT (55–60 Gy) (46%)		Local+distant: 5% Distant: 41%	
INT-0091 (1988–1992) (Grier et al. 2003)	398	Randomized VACD vs. VACD +IE	Sx (38%)	5-year EFS:	VACD / VACD/IE	
			Sx+RT (45 Gy) (23%)	VACD: 54%	L: 15% / L: 5%	Size (>8 cm) Site (pelvis)
			RT (55.8 Gy) (39%)	VACD/IE: 69%	L+D: 5%, D: 21% / L+D: 2%, D: 20%	Older age
EICESS-92 (1992–1999)	470	Randomized SR[b]: VAID vs. VAID/VACD HR[b]: VAID vs. EVAID		3-year DFS: SR: VAID 79%; VAID/VACD: 71% HR: VAID 54%; EVAID 62%	Local 3.6%	

[a] SR (standard risk): small extremity tumors; HR (high risk): >100 ml or central axis tumors
[b] SR: <200 ml; HR: >200 ml

The EICESS-92 study randomized patients with small primaries (<200 ml) to receive VAID or a combination of VAID and VACD, where cyclophosphamide replaced ifosfamide for the last half of the treatment. The 3-year DFS was 79% and 71%, respectively, showing that less intensive therapy may be equally effective for a selected group of patients (Craft et al. 2000).

Subsequent studies built on these findings and investigated the addition of etoposide to the VAID regimen. Preclinical and clinical evidence indicates that the combined administration of etoposide and alkylators has a synergistic antitumor effect, and that the efficacy of both agents improves with fractionated administration. The combined administration of ifosfamide and etoposide (IE) proved to be very active in patients with recurrent ESFT (Miser et al. 1987), and the response rate in untreated patients was 96% (Meyer et al. 1992). Two multi-institutional randomized studies investigated the impact of adding etoposide to the VACD and VAID regimens (Craft et al. 2000; Grier et al. 2003). In the European EICESS-92 study, patients with localized high-risk disease (>200 ml) were randomized to the addition of etoposide (VAID vs. EVAID). The early results of this study showed a modest (but not significant) benefit from the addition of etoposide (3-year DFS 62% vs. 54%, p=0.6) (Craft et al. 2000). The first American Intergroup Ewing trial (INT-0091 – POG-8850/CCG-7881) investigated the incorporation of the ifosfamide-etoposide combination in the front line treatment of ESFT, and all patients were randomized to receive VACD with or without IE (Grier et al. 2003). In both the standard and the experimental treatment regimens, the planned courses of standard therapy (VACD) consisted of vincristine (2 mg/m^2, with maximal dose of 2 mg), cyclophosphamide (1.2 g/m^2 as a single dose), and doxorubicin (75 mg/m^2 as a bolus); actinomycin D (1.25 mg/m^2) was substituted for doxorubicin after the cumulative dose of doxorubicin had reached 375 mg/m^2. In the experimental arm, standard therapy courses were alternated with ifosfamide and etoposide (ifosfamide 1.8 g/m^2/day for 5 consecutive days, etoposide 100 mg/m^2/day for 5 consecutive days). Among patients with metastatic disease, the addition of ifosfamide and etoposide did not prove to be advantageous; 5-year EFS were 22±5% and 22±6% for the experimental and standard arms, respectively. For patients with non-metastatic disease, however, the VACD/IE regimen was superior to the standard VACD (5-year EFS 69±3% vs. 54±4% respectively, p=0.005) (Grier et al. 2003). The beneficial effect of the incorporation of the IE pair was more pronounced for patients with large tumors and patients with pelvic primaries.

Overall, this generation of studies resulted in a marked improvement in the outcome for patients with localized disease. However, advances in surgery and radiation techniques were factored into these developments. In contrast to earlier studies, more aggressive measures for local control were taken (radiation therapy alone was used in less than 50% of the patients), and the local failure rate decreased significantly, usually to less than 15% (Table 9.5) (Bacci et al. 1998; Craft et al. 1998; Grier et al. 2003; Paulussen et al. 2001a). An important contribution of the INT-0091 study was that it demonstrated that the benefit of more intensive chemotherapy was not limited to its systemic effects, but also to its effect on local control. Patients treated on the VACD/IE arm had fewer local failures than patients on the VACD arm (7% vs. 20%) (Grier et al. 2003).

9.6.1.3 Increasing Dose Intensity

In recent years, chemotherapy treatment for many solid malignancies has relied on increasing the total cumulative doses of the active agents, as well as intensifying therapy by increasing the doses per cycle (and per unit of time) (Table 9.6). The incorporation of granulocyte colony-stimulating factor (G-CSF) into treatment regimens has allowed modest dose intensification of multiagent chemotherapy by increasing the total dose per cycle (Granowetter et al. 2001; Kolb et al. 2003; Marina et al. 1999) or shortening the interval of time between treatments (Womer et al. 2000). ESFT are very sensitive to alkylating agents, which have a very steep dose-response curve. Based on this evidence, a rational approach to the treatment of ESFT has been to use treatment intensification, by which high doses of different non-cross-resistant agents, primarily alkylating agents and topoisomerase-II inhibitors, are administered at maximum frequency. This approach has been evaluated by three groups (Table 9.7) (Kolb et al. 2003; Granowetter et al. 2001; Marina et al. 1999).

St. Jude Children's Research Hospital's EWI-92 protocol evaluated the feasibility of an aggressive early induction with three courses of VCDIE (vincristine 1.5 mg/m^2, cyclophosphamide 1.5 g/m^2, doxorubicin 45 mg/m^2, ifosfamide 2 g/m^2 × 3, and etoposide 150 mg/m^2 × 3), followed by a prolonged maintenance therapy with intensification of alkylating agents and etoposide, including four courses of VDC (vincristine 1.5 mg/m^2, cyclophosphamide 1–1.5 g/m^2, and doxorubicin 60 mg/m^2) and four courses of IE (ifosfamide 2 g/m^2 × 5, etoposide 150 mg/m^2 × 5). The 3-year EFS and OS for patients with localized disease were 78% and 90%, respectively. However, an important finding was that only 66% of patients completed therapy, and that intensification was feasible only in 25% of the patients (Marina et al. 1999).

The importance of dose intensification in the treatment of ESFT has also been evaluated in the second American Intergroup POG-CCG Ewing trial (POG-9354/CCG-7942), in which patients were

Table 9.6. Cumulative doses per protocol

Study	Doxorubicin		Cyclophosphamide		Etoposide		Ifosfamide	
	mg/m^2	mg/m^2/week	g/m^2	g/m^2/week	mg/m^2	mg/m^2/week	g/m^2	g/m^2/week
St. Jude studies								
ES79 (Hayes et al. 1989)	385	9.6	11.6	0.029	–	–	–	–
EW87 (Meyer et al. 1992)	315	5	95	0.15	3,000	48.3	48	0.77
EW92 (Marina et al. 1999)	375	8.15	12.5–16.5	0.24–0.36	4,350	98.8	58	1.3
CESS studies								
CESS-81 (Jürgens et al. 1988)	480	12	14.4	0.36	–	–	–	–
CESS-86 (Paulussen et al. 2001a)	480	12	–	–	–	–	72	1.8
EICESS-92 Arm A (Paulussen et al. 2001b) VACA/VAIA	420	10	12	0.28	–	–	24	0.57
EICESS-92 Arm B (Paulussen et al. 2001b) VAIA	420	10	–	–	–	–	84	2
EICESS-92 Arm C (Paulussen et al. 2001b) EVAIA	420	10	–	–	6,300	150	84	2
POG-CCG studies								
INT 0091 Reg A (Grier et al. 2003)	375	7.6	20.4	0.41	–	–	–	–
INT0091 Reg B (Grier et al. 2003)	375	7.6	9.6	0.19	5,000	102	90	1.8
INT00 Reg C (Miser et al. 1996)	450	8.3	17.6	0.32	5,000	92.6	140	2.6
POG9354 Reg A (Granowetter et al. 2001)	375	7.8	10.8	0.23	4,000	83.3	72	1.5
POG9354 Reg B (Granowetter et al. 2001)	375	12.5	12	0.4	3,000	100	72	2.4
MSKCC studies								
P-6 (Kolb et al. 2003)	300	14.2	16.8	0.8	1,500	71	27	1.28

Table 9.7. Intensification regimens for treatment of ESFT (*V* vincristine, *C* cyclophosphamide, *D* doxorubicin, *I* ifosfamide, *E* etoposide, *Sx* surgery, *RT* radiation therapy, *EFS* event-free survival, *OS* overall survival)

Study	N	Regimen	Local control	Outcome	Failures	Poor prognostic factors
EWI-92 (1991–1996) (Marina et al. 1999)	53 (19 met)	Induction: VCDIE ×3	(Localized only) Sx	Localized: 3-year EFS: 78%	Local: 6% Local +distant: 6%	Metastatic disease only prognostic factor
		Maintenance:	Sx+RT (36 Gy)	3-year OS: 90%	Distant: 16%	Size and site no prognostic value
		IE ×4	RT (60–68.4 Gy)	Metastatic:		
		VCD ×4		3-year EFS: 27% 3-year OS: 35%		
P-6 (1991–2001) (Kolb et al. 2003)	68 (24 mets)	HD-VCD ×4	(Localized only)	Localized:	Local: 2%	Metastatic disease only prognostic factor
		IE ×3	Sx	4-year EFS: 82%	Local +distant: 0%	Site, size, age, histologic response no prognostic value
			Sx+RT (45–50 Gy)	4-year OS: 89%	Distant: 9%	
			RT (55.8 Gy)	Metastatic: 4-year EFS: 12% 4-year OS: 18%		
POG-9354/CCG-7942 (1995–1998) (Granowetter et al. 2001)	492	Reg A: VCD/IE (48 weeks)	Sx	3-year EFS	Local	
		Reg B: VCD/IE (30 weeks)	Sx+RT (45 Gy)	Reg A: 76%	Local+distant	
			RT (55.8 Gy)	Reg B: 74%	Distant	

randomized to receive alternating courses of VCD (vincristine 1.5 mg/m^2, cyclophosphamide 1.2 g/m^2, doxorubicin 75 mg/m^2) and IE (ifosfamide 1.8 g/m^2 × 5, and etoposide 100 mg/m^2 × 5) over either 48 or 30 weeks. The cumulative doses of agents were similar in both arms, but in the 30-week arm higher doses per cycle were given (Tables 9.6, 9.7). The early results of this randomized trial demonstrate no difference in outcome between the standard and the dose-intensified arms (3-year EFS 76±4% vs. 74±4%, respectively, p=0.57) (Granowetter et al. 2001).

An alternative approach to long-term intensification is the use of high-dose, short-term regimens. This is the approach evaluated by investigators at the Memorial Sloan Kettering Cancer Center with the P6 protocol, in a group of 68 patients (44 localized) with ESFT. The P6 protocol consists of four courses of high-dose CDV (cyclophosphamide 4.2 g/m^2, doxorubicin 75 mg/m^2, vincristine 2 mg/m^2) alternated with three courses of IE (ifosfamide 1.8 g/m^2 and etoposide 100 mg/m^2, both given daily for 5 days). The 4-year EFS and OS for patients with localized disease were 82% and 89%, respectively (Kolb et al. 2003).

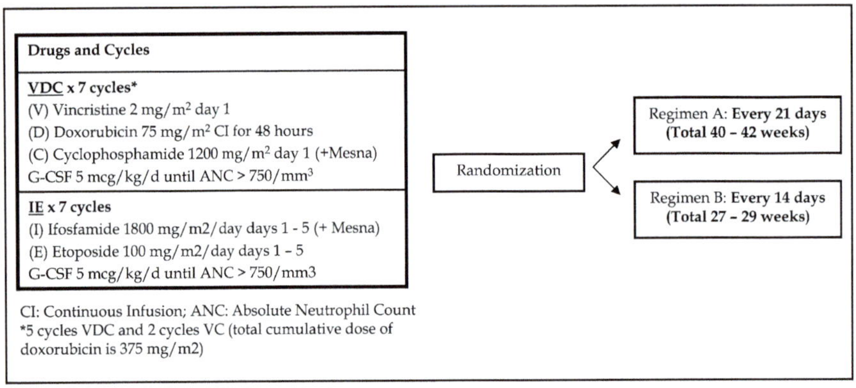

Figure 9.5

COG AEWS0031 Protocol for Localized ESFT

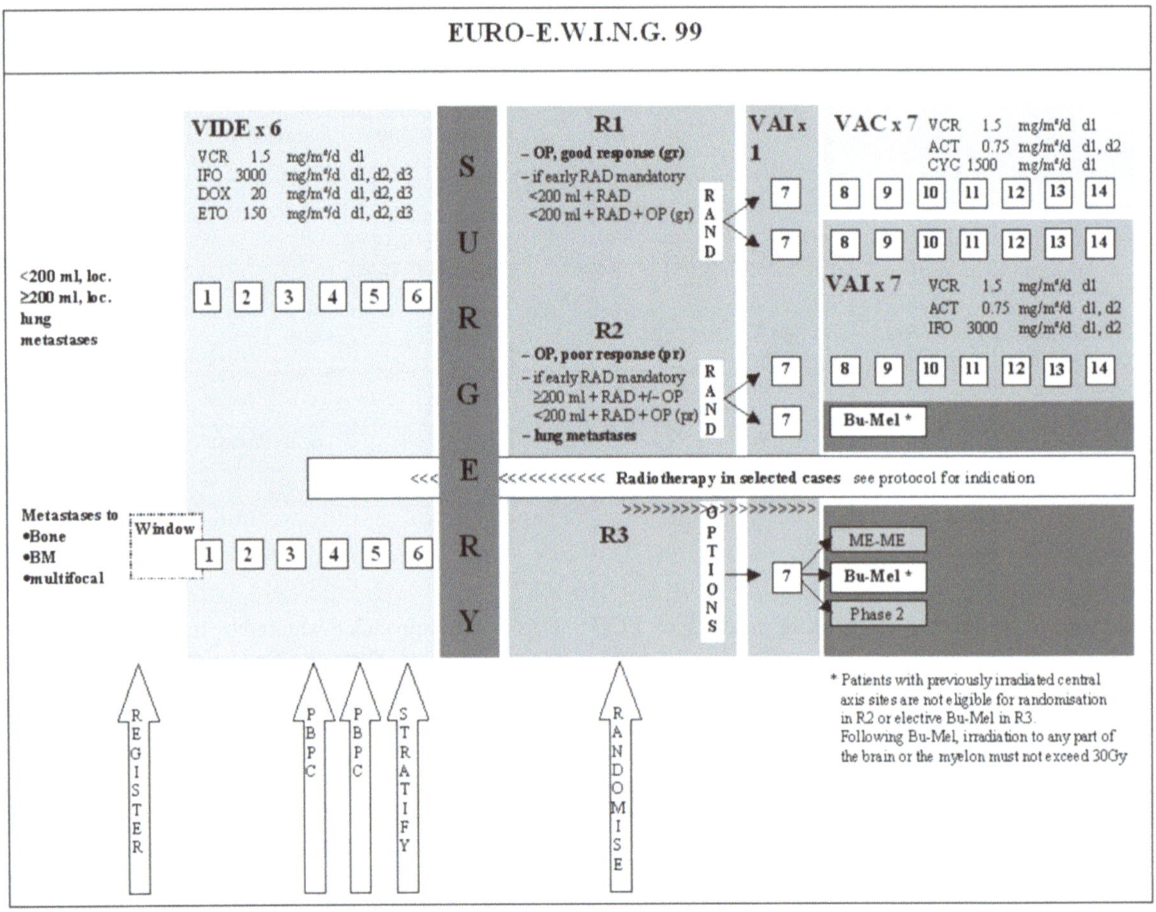

Figure 9.6

EURO-EWING 99 Protocol

9.6.1.4 Current Studies

An alternative to increasing dose intensity is decreasing the intervals between cycles while maintaining the same dose-per-cycle with the use of G-CSF. This interval compression has the potential advantages of allowing dose intensification of all agents (without apparent increases in toxicity), and limiting the time of recovery of partially resistant cells (Womer et al. 2000). In the United States, this is the approach taken by the current Children's Oncology Group AEWS-0031 study (www.cancer.gov/clinicaltrials/cog-aews 0031#studyidnro_cdr000006823), in which patients are randomized to receive alternating cycles VDC and IE every 3 weeks (standard arm) or 2 weeks (dose-compression arm), which results in 33% dose intensification (Fig. 9.5).

It is important to consider that not all patients require the same intensified approach. Risk factors such as age, tumor size and site, pattern of metastatic disease, histologic response to preoperative chemotherapy, and presence of micrometastatic disease may be combined to define risk categories that will allow risk-adapted therapies, by which the cumulative doses of alkylating agents and etoposide can be tailored. This is the approach taken by the European EURO-EWING 99 protocol, a randomized, prospective study that incorporates several cooperative groups. In this European study, all patients receive induction chemotherapy with six cycles of VIDE (vincristine, ifosfamide, doxorubicin, and etoposide), after which they are stratified into three risk groups based on tumor volume, presence and pattern of metastatic disease, and histologic response to induction therapy (Fig. 9.6). This study has been designed to provide answers to very relevant questions: (1) patients with small (<200 ml) or chemoresponsive, localized tumors are randomized to receive consolidation with VAI or VAC, in an attempt to better define the least toxic regimen for low-risk patients; (2) non-metastatic high-risk patients [defined as large (>200 ml) tumors treated with radiation only, or tumors with poor histologic response] are randomized to receive consolidation with high-dose chemotherapy with autologous stem cell rescue, or VAI; (3) patients with pulmonary metastases are randomized to VAI consolidation therapy and whole lung radiation, or high-dose chemotherapy and autologous stem cell rescue. In addition to these important therapeutic questions, this study will also evaluate in a prospective manner the incidence and prognostic significance of detection of micrometastatic disease with molecular methods.

9.6.2 Local Control in ESFT (Fig. 9.7)

The local management of pediatric and young adult patients diagnosed with ESFT continues to be an important but controversial subject. Patients with ESFT require local therapy for cure but no randomized clinical trials are available to define the most appropriate local therapy modality for specific patient

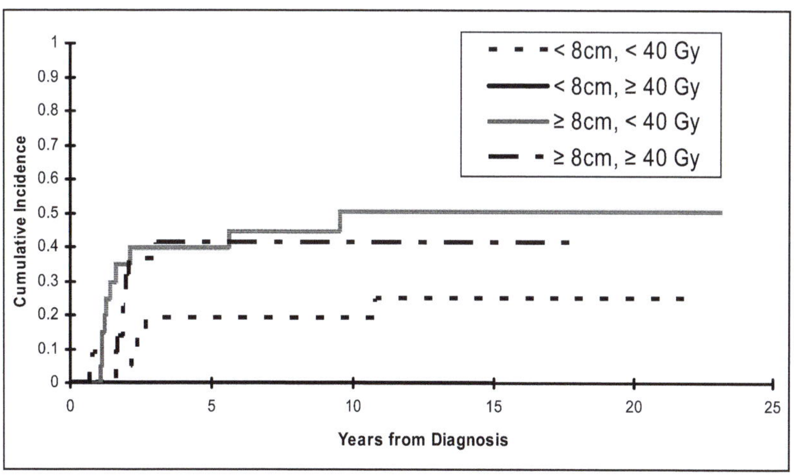

Figure 9.7

Local failure by tumor size and radiation dose for patients with localized ESFT treated with definitive radiation therapy at St. Jude Children's Research Hospital

groups. In the absence of randomized studies to guide treatment, local therapy has been delivered based on information from prospective studies as well as historic series that have gradually incorporated the changes in treatment techniques that have evolved over time for both surgical therapy and radiation therapy. Approximately 150–200 cases of ESFT are diagnosed annually in the United States. This small group of patients may be subdivided into three general subgroups when considering selection of a local therapy modality. The most favorable group of patients has small localized tumors that are amenable to surgical resection or local radiation therapy. The overall outcome for this group of patients is good with high local tumor control rates and favorable overall survival. A less favorable group of patients with localized disease exists that often have large tumors, or tumors that are not amenable to surgical resection. These patients are often managed with radiation therapy alone, though multimodal local therapy incorporating both surgery and radiation may also be appropriate. Patients in this group experience local tumor control rates between 50% and 75% and also have comparatively worse overall survival rates. The most unfavorable patients with ESFT are those that present with overt metastatic disease at diagnosis. The majority of these patients receive local radiation therapy as definitive local therapy though surgical therapy may be employed in select cases. In this group of patients, local therapy still plays an important role though controlling metastatic disease now becomes a primary issue and overall disease-control rates are less than 40%. Though this classification overly simplifies the approach to local therapy, it highlights the need for a multimodal approach to patient evaluation involving the pediatric oncologist, orthopedic oncologist, pediatric surgeon, and radiation oncologist at the time of diagnosis. This allows full evaluation of disease extent including local disease involvement, which facilitates selection of the most appropriate local therapy at the time for local tumor control. Local therapy may be classified by the individual modalities employed. Evaluation of outcome in this fashion allows a more detailed analysis of prognostic factors that vary depending upon the approach to local tumor control.

9.6.2.1 Surgical Therapy

Available local tumor control data suggest a superior outcome with wide local surgical excision, defining wide local excision as removal of all gross tumor with a margin of normal surrounding tissue. Though bias exists in selecting smaller, more peripheral tumors for definitive surgical resection and no randomized study is available to guide selection of a local modality, concerns regarding late effects including secondary malignancies and loss of growth have moved oncologists to a primary surgical approach for local therapy. Cooperative group studies approach the dilemma of local control with treatment guidelines based on resectability of the primary lesion in the context of known clinical prognostic factors. With careful selection for surgical therapy, the local control results are favorable for this group of tumors, with 5-year local failure rate of less than 10% (Table 9.8). Volume or size of tumor has been noted as a prognostic factor for event free survival in multiple series (Grier et al. 2003; Hayes et al. 1989; Oberlin et al. 2001; Paulussen et al. 2001a). The effect of tumor size on local failure is less clear. The combined Cooperative Ewing's Sarcoma Studies (CESS) and European Intergroup Cooperative Ewing's Sarcoma Studies (EICESS) did not demonstrate a difference in local failure for patients treated with surgery with tumors <100 cc vs. ≥100 cc (6.1% vs. 5.6%, respectively) (Schuck et al. 2003). Patients undergoing wide local excision at St. Jude Children's Research Hospital had no difference in local failure based on tumor size <8 cm or ≥8 cm (16.7% vs. 13.3%, respectively) (Krasin et al. 2004a). Histologic response to induction chemotherapy may play a role in predicting local outcome with surgical therapy. Patients that achieved a favorable histologic response (≥90% necrosis) had a 2% incidence of local failure in the EICESS experience while patients with poor histologic response may benefit from adjuvant radiation therapy (Krasin et al., in press; Schuck et al. 2003). The group of patients classified as extraosseous ESFT present another local challenge. Though treated with ESFT- or rhabdomyosarcoma-specific systemic therapy (Krasin et al., in press; Raney et al. 1997), appropriate local therapy for this group of patients is less clear. Patients

Table 9.8. Local failure rates according to treatment modality

Study	Local treatment modality	Local failure rate
EI/CESS (Schuck et al. 2003)	Surgery	4.7%
	Surgery+radiation	11.0%
	Radiation	29.3%
Rizzoli (Bacci et al. 2004)	Surgery	8.8%
	Surgery+radiation	8.9%
	Radiation	29.3%
Italian Cooperative (SE-91) (Rosito et al. 1999)	Surgery	7.1%
	Surgery+radiation	6.5%
	Radiation	6.7%
POG 8346 (Donaldson et al. 1998)	Surgery±radiation	12%
	Radiation	35%
St. Jude (Krasin et al. 2004a, b; Krasin et al., in press)	Surgery	12.5%
	Surgery+radiation	10.8%
	Radiation	30.4%

with extraosseous ESFT treated with postoperative radiotherapy at St. Jude Children's Research Hospital had an 8-year local failure rate of 8% when adjuvant radiation was delivered postoperatively. In patients managed with surgery without radiation, the cumulative incidence of local failure and event free survival appear to be inferior compared to ESFT arising in bone (Krasin et al. 2004a; Krasin et al., in press). The ability to achieve a complete surgical resection for patients with ESFT clearly predicts a favorable outcome. With modern surgical techniques this approach will likely remain a favored local approach if a non-morbid procedure is readily achievable.

9.6.2.2 Surgery and Adjuvant Radiation Therapy

Postoperative and, more recently, preoperative irradiation have been systematically applied to patients with marginally resected or poorly responding tumors. Despite the selection bias of unfavorable patients (positive surgical margins, large tumor size and poor histologic response to neoadjuvant chemotherapy) treated with combined local therapy, the available literature suggests that there is equivalent local control compared to surgery alone (Carrie et al. 1999; Rosito et al. 1999; Schuck et al. 2003; Shankar et al. 1999). The rationale for combining radiation therapy and surgical resection is based on the belief that high local tumor control rates can be achieved with limited resection and adjuvant radiation therapy. Specific rates of local tumor control are shown in Table 9.8. Prognostic factors are similar to those of patients managed with surgery alone though the effect of surgical margins and poor histologic response appear to be nullified by the addition of adjuvant radiation therapy (Schuck et al. 2003). The incidence of positive surgical resection margins appears to relate to the timing of surgical resection; upfront resection results in more frequent positive surgical margins, noted in an analysis of chest wall ESFT treated in cooperative group studies (77% vs. 50%) (Shamberger et al. 2003) and at St. Jude Children's Research Hospital (59% vs. 18%) (Krasin et al. 2004a; Krasin et al., in press). The role of preoperative radiation is under evaluation in the current European Intergroup study (EURO-EWING 99) as well as the previous European Intergroup Cooperative Ewing's Sarcoma Study (EICESS 92) (Schuck et al. 2003). The results from that study indicate that despite selection of a higher proportion of patients with large, central tumors the local failure rate for patients receiving preoperative radiation was 5.1% compared to 9.2% for those receiving postoperative radiation.

Several studies have evaluated the efficacy of low-dose adjuvant radiation therapy (<40 Gy) for resected ESFT (Arai et al. 1991; Dunst et al. 1991; Krasin et al., in press; Merchant et al. 1999). Selection of low dose irradiation has usually been based on young age, limited tolerance of surrounding tissues to irradiation or favorable tumor characteristics such as small primary size and response to chemotherapy. Even in institutions with large numbers of pediatric cancer patients it is difficult to draw statistically supported conclusions for this rare tumor and limited experience with low-dose adjuvant irradiation. Local failure rates with low-dose adjuvant radiation are reported as 0%, 15% and 17% from Memorial Sloan-Kettering Cancer Center, St. Jude Children's Research Hospital, and the CESS 81 study respectively (Dunst et al. 1991; Krasin et al., in press; Schuck et al. 2003). Patients treated with standard doses of adjuvant radiation therapy at St. Jude Children's Research Hospital have a local failure rate of 0% at 8 years. Results from contemporary prospective studies of patients with ESFT indicate that local tumor control following a complete surgery with either a wide local excision or marginal excision should result in a local tumor control rate of approximately 90% at 5 years (Dunst et al. 1991; Schuck et al. 2003). The excellent results obtained in modern surgical series as well as our results with standard dose adjuvant irradiation suggest that radiation therapy at a dose below 40 Gy is inadequate to provide the high rates of local tumor control (Krasin et al., in press).

9.6.2.3 Definitive Radiation Therapy

Selection of definitive irradiation as a local management approach for ESFT requires weighing the associated surgical morbidities against the efficacy and treatment effects of irradiation. Overall local failure rates for patients managed with radiation therapy are consistently higher than those in patients undergoing surgery, with recurrence rates of nearly 30% (Table 9.8). The previously noted biases in selecting a more favorable patient population for surgical resection may explain some of these differences. The patient and treatment variables that affect the local outcome of those treated with radiation are similar to those noted above but also include patient age ≥14 years and the quality of radiation planning and delivery. Local outcomes for patients treated at St. Jude Children's Research Hospital were positively influenced by age <14 years, tumor size <8 cm and radiation dose ≥40 Gy. Local failure rates at 10 years for patients with tumors <8 cm were only 11% compared to 46% for those with larger tumor size. Age also played a role in predicting local failure, particularly for patients with tumors of 8 cm whose risk of local failure doubled from 31% for patients <14 years of age to 60% for those patients 14 years of age (p=0.035) (Krasin et al. 2004b). The role for definitive low-dose irradiation is limited and appeared to result in inferior rates of local tumor control even for tumors <8 cm (p=0.010) (Fig. 9.6) (Krasin et al. 2004b).

The role of the quality of radiation planning and delivery cannot be overstated. Three cooperative group studies have demonstrated the importance of quality radiation therapy (CESS 81 and 86 and POG 8346). Central treatment plan review was instituted in CESS 86 following a local failure rate of 50% in CESS 81 for patients undergoing definitive irradiation; subsequent patients treated with definitive radiation therapy on CESS 86 had a local failure rate of only 13% (Dunst et al. 1991). Patients undergoing definitive irradiation on POG 8346 had an 84% incidence of local failure if a major deviation in dose or volume of treatment was noted. Even patients with a minor deviation experienced a 52% local failure rate compared to 20% for those with no deviation (p=0.005) (Donaldson et al. 1998). In light of the limited number of patients diagnosed with ESFT each year, great care must be given to ensure adequate targeting and dose delivery for this readily curable malignancy.

9.6.2.4 Role of Systemic Chemotherapy in Local Control

Clinical trials that have investigated the incorporation of new agents such as doxorubicin (Razek et al. 1980) or ifosfamide and etoposide (Grier et al. 2003), and the use of treatment intensification (Craft et al. 1998), have shown that systemic chemotherapy also contributes to local tumor control. The best example of this impact was recently provided by the results of the American Intergroup Ewing trial (INT-0091 – POG-8850/CCG-7881), which randomized patients to receive VACD or VACD/IE (Grier et al. 2003). As discussed above, this study demonstrated that the benefit of more intensive chemotherapy was also due to its improvement on local control. Using the same local control guidelines, the 5-year cumulative incidence of local progression was 15% and 5% for the control VACD arm and the experimental VACD/IE arm, respectively ($p<0.001$) (Grier et al. 2003).

In summary, management of localized ESFT mandates a multidisciplinary approach to selection of local tumor control. With a limited number of cases annually patients should either be treated at specialized treatment centers or in cooperative group studies to ensure quality and consistency in the treatment approach. Based on current prognostic factors, appropriate local treatment may be selected for favorable patient groups to maximize local tumor control and minimize late effects. Patients with adverse prognostic factors may require intensification of systemic therapy as well as aggressive combined local therapy to maximize cure.

9.6.3 Treatment of Metastatic ESFT

The advances experienced in the treatment of patients with localized ESFT have not impacted the outcome of patients with metastases; using conventional treatment only 20–25% of patients can be cured (Fig. 9.4) (Table 9.9) (Cangir et al. 1990; Craft et al. 1997, 1998; Miser et al. 2004; Paulussen et al. 1998b; Sandoval et al. 1996; Rodriguez-Galindo et al. 2003).

Table 9.9. Treatment of metastatic ESFT with conventional regimens (*V* vincristine, *A* actinomycin D, *C* cyclophosphamide, *D* doxorubicin, *I* ifosfamide, *E* etoposide, *Sx* surgery, *DFS* disease-free survival, *EFS* event-free survival, *OS* overall survival, *t-AML* therapy-related acute myeloid leukemia)

Study	Patients	Regimen	Outcome	Comments
IESS I-II (Cangir et al. 1990) 1975–1983	122	VACD	5-year DFS: 30%	
First POG-CCG 1988–1993 (Miser et al. 1996, 2004)	120	Randomization:	8-year OS	Addition of IE or dose intensification does not improve results
		Reg. A: VACD	Reg. A: 32%	Better outcome for isolated lung disease:
		Reg. B: VACD+IE Single arm: Reg. C: VACDIE (intensified)	Reg. B: 29% 4-year EFS: Reg. C: 26%	8-year OS: 41% vs. 28%
ET-1 (Craft et al. 1997) 1978–1986	22	VACD	5-year OS: 9%	
ET-2 (Craft et al. 1998) 1987–1993	42	VAID	5-year OS: 23%	
EICESS (Paulussen et al. 1998b) 1990–1995	171	VAID±E	4-year OS: 27%	Better outcome for isolated lung disease: Lungs: 34% Bone/bone marrow: 28% Combined: 14%
EW-92 (Marina et al. 1999)	19	VCDIE ×3	3-year OS: 35%	Intensification does not improve results
		VCD/IE		High toxicity Incidence t-AML: 8%

Table 9.10. Intensive, short-term regimens for high-risk ESFT

Author	Regimen	Agents
Strauss et al. (2003)	VIDE ×6	VCR 1.4 mg/m² day 1 DOX 20 mg/m² day 1–3 IFO 3 g/m² day 1–3 ETO 150 mg/m² day 1–3
Felgenhauer et al. (2000)	VACIME ×8	VCR 2 mg/m² day 1 DOX 20 mg/m² day 1–4 CYC 360 mg/m² day 1–5 IFO 1.8 g/m² day 1–5 ETO 100 mg/m² day 1–5
Kolb et al. (2003)	P6	Cycles 1, 2, 3, 6: VCR 0.67 mg/m² day 1–3 CYC 2.1 g/m² day 1–2 DOX 25 mg/m² day 1–3 Cycles 4, 5, 7: IFO 1.8 g/m² day 1–5 ETO 100 mg/m² day 1–5

Several institutions have explored the impact of maximum treatment intensification in metastatic ESFT. This approach explores the administration of very high doses of non-cross-resistant agents in a short period of time. Different regimens have been explored (Table 9.10) (Felgenhauer et al. 2000; Kolb et al. 2003; Strauss et al. 2003; Miser et al. 1996). Short and intensive therapy is feasible, and toxicity is substantial but manageable. Although the majority of patients with metastatic disease treated using these regimens have good clinical and histological responses, the final results are not better than those obtained with conventional therapy (Felgenhauer et al. 2000; Kolb et al. 2003; Strauss et al. 2003).

However, even among patients with metastatic disease, there is some heterogeneity. Patients with isolated lung metastases may have a better prognosis than patients with extrapulmonary metastases (Table 9.9), with long term survival rates approaching 40–45% (Miser et al. 2004; Paulussen et al. 1998b; Spunt et al. 2001). Among patients with lung metastases, those with unilateral disease (Paulussen et al. 1998a; Spunt et al. 2001) and those with good histologic response to induction chemotherapy (Paulussen et al. 1998a) appear to have a survival advantage. However, a complete radiological response to induction chemotherapy does not seem to correlate with outcome (Paulussen et al. 1998a; Spunt et al. 2001).

In approximately 50% of patients with isolated lung metastases, failures to therapy occur as isolated pulmonary disease again (Paulussen et al. 1998a; Spunt et al. 2001), suggesting that further response consolidation could potentially improve the outcome of these patients. In this regard, whole lung radiation (15–18 Gy) seems to provide a modest survival advantage (Paulussen et al. 1998a). Preliminary data of the European Bone Marrow Transplant Registry (EBMTR) (Ladenstein et al. 1999) (see below) suggest that an alternative approach to the treatment of patients with isolated lung metastases may be the use of consolidation with high-dose chemotherapy using a busulfan-based regimen, and autologous stem cell rescue. As discussed above, these two approaches are compared in a randomized manner in the current EURO-EWING 99 protocol.

Table 9.11. Treatment of metastatic extrapulmonary ESFT with hematopoietic stem cell transplant (*V* vincristine, *A* actinomycin D, *C* cyclophosphamide, *D* doxorubicin, *I* ifosfamide, *E* etoposide, *MEL* melphalan, *ETO* etoposide, *CBP* carboplatin, *TBI* total body irradiation, *DFS* disease free survival, *HSCT* hematopoietic stem cell transplant, *OS* overall survival, *t-AML* therapy-related acute myeloid leukemia, *TT* thiotepa, *BUS* busulfan, *NR* not reported)

Author	Patients	Induction	Megatherapy	Results	Comments
Paulussen (1998b) EICESS 1990–95	36	VAID	MEL/ETO ±CBP±TBI	4-year DFS 23%	No benefit of HSCT No influence of conditioning regimen
Burdach (2000) EICESS 1986–94	17	VACD VAID EVAID	MEL+ETO+TBI ±CBP	5-year DFS 24%	High incidence of t-AML
Ladenstein (1996) Austria 1984–1996	18	VACD VAID	MEL/ETO ±CBP±TBI	4-year OS 26%	OS 3/6 of patients undergoing allo-HSCT
Meyers (2001) CCG	23	P6	MEL+ETO +TBI	2-year DFS 24%	No benefit of HSCT High toxicity
Kolb (2003) MSKCC 1990–2001	24	P6	MEL+TBI TT+CBP	4-year EFS 12%	No benefit of HSCT High toxicity
Ladenstein (1995) EBMTR 1982–1992	22	VAC VACD VAID	MEL± BCNU± ETO±BUS ±TBI	5-year DFS 21%	TBI: inferior results? MEL+BUS: best results?
Ladenstein (1999) EBMTR 1978–1997	111	N.R.	+BUS –BUS	5-year OS 44% 5-year OS 23%	BUS: best results
Burdach (2003) EICESS 1986–2000	54 Hyper ME: MEL+ETO+TBI	EVAIA 5-year EFS: VIDE	Toxic deaths: Tandem ME: MEL+ETO ×2	Hyper ME: 22% Tandem ME: 29%	Hyper ME: 23% Tandem ME: 4%

9.6.4 Myeloablative Therapy with Hematopoietic Stem Cell Rescue for Metastatic ESFT

The results of treatment with megatherapy and HSCT for patients with high-risk ESFT must be analyzed considering the absence of randomized studies and the heterogeneity of the patients studied. The role of and indications for HSCT in ESFT have been reviewed by Kushner and Meyers (2001). Very few studies have evaluated the response of ESFT to the agents used in many megatherapy regimens. In general, the alkylating agents thiotepa, busulfan and melphalan have shown good responses in phase I and phase II studies (Schiffman et al. 1996), and most regimens use different combinations of these agents.

The experience of the European Cooperative Ewing Sarcoma Group (EICESS) has been reported recently in three studies by Paulussen et al. (1998b) and Burdach et al. (2000, 2003) (Table 9.11). In the first two studies, initial treatment was based on the CESS 81 and 86 protocols, and the megatherapy regimen was with melphalan and etoposide, with the addition of carboplatin and total body irradiation (TBI) for a subset of patients. The results were poor, with DFS rates of 23–24% for patients with metastatic disease to bone or bone marrow. More recently, the results of two sequential studies exploring high-dose therapy for patients with primary metastatic (multifocal bone) or recurrent disease have been reported (Burdach et al. 2003). In the first study, patients received treatment consolidation with total body irradiation, melphalan and etoposide (HyperME); in the second study, total body irradiation was not given, and patients underwent two courses of melphalan/etoposide and HSCT (TandemME). The EFS rate was 22±8% and 29±9% for the HyperME and TandemME protocols, respectively. Of note, the HyperME regimen resulted in a significantly higher incidence of toxic deaths (23% vs. 4%) (Burdach et al. 2003). In vitro studies have suggested a possible benefit of the administration of IL-2 after high-dose chemotherapy and autologous rescue; however, treatment with IL-2 does not seem to provide any beneficial antitumor effect in vivo (Burdach et al. 2003).

In the United States, Meyers et al. (2001) and Kushner and Meyers (2001) have reported the experience using the intensive P6 therapy (Kushner and Meyers 2001) or a similar intensive approach (Meyers et al. 2001), as induction, followed by similar consolidation with HSCT. In both studies, melphalan and TBI were used. The results were very poor, with DFS rates of less than 25% (Table 9.11).

As for any megatherapy approach, the agents used for myeloablation and eradication of residual disease have to be considered. Ladenstein et al. (1995, 1999) reported the results of the EBMTR for a selected series of patients in two consecutive studies. In a first review of the patients that underwent a HSCT between 1982 and 1992, the DFS rate for the group of 22 patients with metastatic disease to bone and bone marrow was 21% (Ladenstein et al. 1995). However, when analyzing in detail the different megatherapy regimens for the whole group of 63 patients receiving a HSCT, the results were superior for the group of patients that received the combination melphalan-busulfan, and for the patients that did not receive TBI. In a more updated review that included 111 patients with ESFT with bone and bone marrow metastases who underwent HSCT between 1978 and 1997, the advantage of the regimens that included busulfan was confirmed (Ladenstein et al. 1999). The overall survival at 5 years was 44% for the group of 18 patients that received busulfan, and only 23% for the group of 93 patients that were treated with regimens without busulfan. The use of busulfan provided a survival advantage also for patients with pulmonary disease alone (66% vs. 39%) and for patients with localized high-risk disease (75% vs. 38%) (Table 9.11). In summary, in these retrospective studies there appears to be an advantage for regimens that incorporate high doses of alkylating agents, generally busulfan and melphalan (Ladenstein et al. 1995, 1999). The administration of TBI does not seem to provide any additional benefit, and may only add toxicity (Burdach et al. 2003; Kushner and Meyers 2001; Ladenstein et al. 1995). It is still not clear whether this approach is beneficial for patients with bone/bone marrow metastases, and such an approach should be undertaken only in the context of an investigational study, preferably randomized.

Studies performed in children with advanced neuroblastoma and medulloblastoma have shown the feasibility and efficacy of the use of repeat cycles of high-dose chemotherapy with autologous HSCT. However, available data suggest that this approach may not be advantageous for patients with metastatic ESFT (Burdach et al. 2003).

Gene marking studies in patients with neuroblastoma that received an autologous HSCT have shown that the stem cell graft has tumor cells that may contribute to disease recurrence after HSCT (Rill et al. 1994). Although there are no similar studies in ESFT, several investigators have shown that ESFT cells are detectable by PCR in stem cell grafts, even after positive selection for CD34+ cells. As for other pediatric solid malignancies, the value of purging the stem cell harvest (and by which method) has not been clearly established (Ladenstein et al. 1997). Negative selection methodologies using pharmacological agents or antibodies have historically been the most commonly used methods to remove tumor cells from grafts. The efficacy of pharmacological agents depends on the differential sensitivity of tumor cells and normal hematopoietic progenitors to cytotoxic agents. However, interpatient variability and excessive toxicity to normal progenitors may result in significant delays in hematopoietic reconstitution. Furthermore, these methods have a suboptimal therapeutic ration in solid tumors. In contrast to the negative selection strategies, positive selection methods are designed to attain a highly purified hematopoietic cell population. The most commonly used positive selection systems use the $CD34^+$ antigen, which is expressed on primitive hematopoietic progenitors that have the ability to reconstitute hematopoiesis.

In recent years, some institutions have performed allogeneic HSCT in patients with ESFT. The number of patients is low, and the results are contradictory (Burdach et al. 2000; Ladenstein et al. 1996). Nevertheless, with refinements in the conditioning techniques and immune manipulation, allogeneic HSCT may be a valid alternative for patients with solid tumors, and in particular ESFT (Koscielniak et al. 2005). These tumors are characterized by the expression of surface proteins derived from the characteristic gene fusion. These chimeric oncoproteins may attach to the HLA molecules and induce antitumor immune responses. It is therefore conceivable that there a clinically significant graft versus tumor effect could occur. Moreover, the immune response may not be restricted to the MHC molecules. Some tumor cells express low levels of class I molecules, and there may be an antitumor effect through the lytic function of NK cells. The main problem with allogeneic HSCT is its greater toxicity. A good alternative would be the induction of a mixed chimerism state that would result in a bidirectional immune tolerance. The induction of mixed chimerism has several advantages. First, the conditioning is less toxic and should result in less toxicity. Second, the development of host tolerance toward the graft is the first step towards adoptive immunotherapy with the infusion of immunocompetent cells of the donor that could maximize the graft versus tumor effect. Finally, mixed chimerism may help decrease the incidence and severity of graft versus host disease.

9.6.5 Second Malignancies

Classically, the incidence of second cancers in survivors of ESFT has not been higher than in other childhood cancers. The cumulative incidence of second neoplasms in most large series is not higher than 2% (Grier et al. 2003; Paulussen et al. 2001b), and sarcomas arising in the radiation field represent more than 75% of the cases (Bacci et al. 2004; Kuttesch et al. 1996). The development of radiation-induced sarcomas has a latency of several years, and it is dose dependent, with very low risk below 48 Gy and very high cumulative incidence (CI at 10 years of 35%) in patients receiving doses >60 Gy (Kuttesch et al. 1996; Tucker et al. 1987a). The use of alkylating agents appears to increase the risk of radiation-induced sarcomas (Tucker et al. 1987a).

In recent years, the use of protocols that include intensification of alkylators and topoisomerase-II inhibitors has resulted in a significant increase in the incidence of treatment-related leukemia and myelodysplastic syndromes (t-AML/MDS). This therapeutic strategy appears to be leukemogenic, and patients are at increased risk of developing both alkylator-related and etoposide-related t-AML/MDS (Kolb et al. 2003; Kushner et al. 1998; Miser et al. 1996; Rodriguez-Galindo et al. 2000a). The cumulative incidence of t-AML/MDS at 40 months was 8% in survivors of the P6 protocol (Kushner et al. 1998). Likewise, in the St. Jude EW92 protocol, the cumulative incidence of t-AML/MDS was 8%, compared to 0% in patients treated on the ES87 protocol, in which the same drugs were used, but much less intensively, and in which no G-CSF was given (Rodriguez-Galindo et al. 2000a) (Table 9.12). Compared to the low incidence of t-AML/MDS traditionally observed in less intensive protocols for non-metastatic patients, the risks seen in the high-dose studies represent major increases. This increased risk for t-AML/MDS appears to be related to both the increase in the total cumulative doses and dose intensification of alkylating agents and topoisomerase-II inhibitors, and growth factors may also play a role. Combinations of alkylators and topoisomerase-II inhibitors appear to be associated with a greater risk of t-MDS and t-AML than either class of drugs administered alone (Tucker et al. 1987b; Pedersen-Bjergaard et al. 1993). Moreover, even the addition of small doses of etoposide to an alkylator-based regimen can significantly increase the incidence of t-MDS and t-AML (Heyn et al. 1994). Although the risk for anthracycline-associated t-MDS/t-AML is generally low because of dose limitations imposed to circumvent cardiotoxicity, use of these agents with DNA-damaging drugs such as cisplatin or alkylators clearly increases the probability of leukemia induction (Pedersen-Bjergaard et al. 1992; Sandoval et al. 1993). Topoisomerase-II inhibitors have a synergistic effect when administered with

Table 9.12. Incidence of therapy-related leukemia as a function of the total cumulative doses and treatment intensification

Protocol	Doxorubicin (mg/m^2)		Cyclophosphamide (g/m^2)		Etoposide (mg/m^2)		Ifosfamide (g/m^2)		Incidence t-AML/MDS
	Total	Per week	Total	Per week	Total	Per week	Total	Per week	
ES-87 (Meyer et al. 1992)	315	5	9.5	0.15	3,000	48.3	48	0.77	0%
EW-92 (Marina et al. 1999)	375	8.15	12.5–16.5	0.24–0.36	4,350	98.8	58	1.3	8%
P-6 (Kolb et al. 2003)	300	14.2	16.8	0.8	1,500	71	27	1.28	8%
First POG-CCG Regimen C (Miser et al. 1996)	450	8.3	17.6	0.32	5,000	92.6	140	2.6	22.7%

drugs that interact with DNA (Pedersen-Bjergaard et al. 1993). The role of G-CSF has not been defined, but may provide a survival advantage to genetically damaged stem cells that otherwise would undergo apoptosis, thus preventing the elimination of the genetic damage.

9.6.6 Recurrent ESFT

Although improved local control therapy and the development of new and more intensive chemotherapy combinations have reduced the failure rates, a large proportion of patients continue to experience relapse. Recurrences can be local, distant, or combined (Rodriguez-Galindo et al. 2002). During the earlier years of multimodal therapy, approximately 25% of all patients experienced local treatment failure, and another 20–40% experienced distant treatment failure (Bacci et al. 1989; Craft et al. 1997; Jürgens et al. 1988; Nesbit et al. 1990; Razek et al. 1980). The patterns of relapse have evolved over the past 3 decades, reflecting the effect of improvements in the multimodal treatment. A significant proportion of recurrences in the early studies were local or combined local and distant (Table 9.4) (Razek et al. 1980; Burgert et al. 1990; Craft et al. 1997; Nesbit et al. 1990; Jürgens et al. 1988). Improvements in the multidisciplinary approach have decreased the local recurrence rates to less than 10%.

Outcome after recurrence is very poor; the probability of survival at 5 years is less than 20% (Bacci et al. 2003; Rodriguez-Galindo et al. 2002; Shankar et al. 2003). However, patients experiencing late recurrences, patients with isolated local recurrences amenable to radical surgery, and patients with isolated lung recurrences appear to have a survival advantage (Bacci et al. 2003; Rodriguez-Galindo et al. 2002; Shankar et al. 2003).

9.7 Future Developments

Intensification of therapy has proven to have a limited role, and patients with high-risk disease continue to have a poor outcome. New agents and therapeutic approaches are still needed for ESFT (Rodriguez-Galindo 2004). Preclinical and clinical studies have shown that the camptothecin derivatives are among the most effective compounds for treating pediatric malignancies (Rodriguez-Galindo et al. 2000b), and their role in the treatment of ESFT is being investigated. Although phase I and II studies of topotecan and irinotecan as single agents have shown little or no activity in patients with refractory disease, recent studies suggest that their combination with alkylating agents may be more promising. Phase II studies of the combination of topotecan (0.75 mg/m^2/day × 5 days) with cyclophosphamide (250 mg/m^2/day ×

5 days) resulted in responses in 36% of patients with recurrent disease (Saylors et al. 2001), and in 56% of patients with untreated metastatic disease (Bernstein et al. 2001). In a recently reported phase I study, irinotecan was administered on a protracted schedule (10–15 mg/m^2/day for 5 days in two consecutive weeks) in combination with temozolomide (100 mg/m^2/day for 5 days) to children with refractory solid tumors. In this population of heavily pretreated patients, three responses were observed among the seven patients with refractory ESFT (Wagner et al. 2004). The use of topoisomerase-I inhibitors in combination with alkylating agents thus deserves further evaluation in ESFT.

Our better understanding of the molecular pathogenesis and biology of ESFT is leading to a new definition of potential targets for antitumor therapy. The tyrosine kinase inhibitor STI-571 (imatinib mesylate) has shown in preclinical models a high degree of specificity for BCR-ABL, the receptor for platelet-derived growth factor (PDGFR), and c-kit tyrosine kinases. The stem cell factor receptor c-kit is also expressed in ESFT cells, and its activation appears to be involved in cell survival. Ewing sarcoma cell lines express several imatinib mesylate-sensitive tyrosine kinases, including c-kit and PDGFR (Scotlandi et al. 2003; Uren et al. 2003). Immunohistochemical studies performed in primary ESFT tumors have shown that approximately 70% of tumors express c-kit, although the staining is strong and diffuse only in 30% of the cases (Scotlandi et al. 2003; Smithey et al. 2002), but there appears to be no association with outcome (Scotlandi et al. 2003). Despite these interesting preliminary data, in vitro studies have shown a modest effect of imatinib mesylate on the growth and proliferation of Ewing sarcoma cell lines. A phase II study of imatinib mesylate is currently being performed in the United States by the Children's Oncology Group in children with recurrent ESFT.

Another promising agent in the treatment of sarcomas is ecteinascidin-743 (ET-743). This novel compound is a minor groove binding, guanine-specific alkylating agent which also interacts with the microtubule network and blocks cell cycle progression at late S/G2. ET-743 has shown antitumoral activity in adults with advanced, pretreated soft tissue sarcomas (Yovine et al. 2004). In a recently completed phase I study in children, a complete response was observed in a patient with metastatic ESFT (Lau et al. 2005). A phase II study in children with recurrent sarcomas, including ESFT, is under development by the Children's Oncology Group.

The tumor necrosis factor (TNF) receptor superfamily is a main regulator of apoptosis, and in recent years members of this family have shown to have a pivotal role in inducing apoptosis of ESFT cells. The TNF-related apoptosis-inducing ligand (TRAIL) induces apoptosis by binding to two members of this family, the death receptor (DR) 4 and DR5. ESFT cells are exquisitely sensitive to TRAIL (Mitsaides et al. 2001; van Valen et al. 2003), and in this in vitro model sensitivity is dependent on the presence of DR4 and DR5 (Mitsaides et al. 2001). Interestingly, both death receptors are detected by immunohistochemistry in over 70% of tumor samples (Mitsaides et al. 2001). Therefore, the wide expression of DR4/DR5 in ESFT in vivo and the high sensitivity to TRAIL in vitro would suggest that further exploration of the TRAIL pathway as a therapeutic tool would be indicated. The tumoricidal activity of TRAIL in animal models of cancer is well documented (Walczak et al. 1999). However, TRAIL is expressed in a wide range of normal tissues. Although early reports suggested that TRAIL would induce apoptosis only in transformed and malignant cells, recent reports have demonstrated that TRAIL can elicit apoptosis in normal tissues as well, such as hepatocytes and brain tissue (Jo et al. 2000; Nitsch et al. 2000), a finding that limits its therapeutic use. However, further investigation of this pathway is under way. It has been shown that interferons can induce expression of TRAIL (Fanger et al. 1999), and recent studies have documented strong synergistic in vitro and in vivo antitumor effect when type I interferons (α or β) are given with ifosfamide (Sanceau et al. 2002) or with type II interferon (γ) (Abadie et al. 2004). Furthermore, in these preclinical models, the antitumor effect correlates with TRAIL induction, which would suggest that TRAIL contributes to the triggering of apoptosis in ESFT cells in an autocrine or paracrine manner.

Inhibition of histone deacetylation has proven to result in a significant antitumor effect in preclinical and clinical models. Acetylation and deacetylation of histones alter higher order chromatin structure by influencing histone interaction with DNA. Deacetylated histones are associated with cell growth, whereas acetylated histones are associated with cell growth arrest, differentiation, and apoptosis (Peart et al. 2003). Transcription factors may also be acetylated, and the acetylation status influences their interaction with DNA. In this regard, chimeric transcription factors present in a variety of tumor systems might cause transcriptional repression of growth regulatory target genes by recruitment of transcriptional corepressors and their associated histone deacetylase (HDAC) activity (Peart et al. 2003). This is particularly relevant in ESFT, since it has been shown that the EWS-FLI1 chimeric transcription factor suppresses transforming growth factor β type II receptor (TGF-βR-II) transcription (Hahm et al. 1999). This is important, since studies indicate that restoration of TGFβ pathway in ESFT cells inhibits their growth (Hahm et al. 1999). In the xenograft model, the HDAC inhibitor MS-27–275 was able to induce an increase in TGFβR-II mRNA and restore TGFβ signaling, and this correlated with growth inhibition (Jaboin et al. 2002). Moreover, in this same model, $p21^{WAF/CIP1}$ was induced in most cell lines irrespective of the p53 status (Jaboin et al. 2002). Finally, HDAC inhibitors appear to interfere with angiogenesis, an effect that deserves further investigation (Jaboin et al. 2002). The HDAC inhibitor depsipeptide is currently under phase I investigation by the Children's Oncology Group in children with refractory solid tumors.

The insulin-like growth factor-I pathway (IGF-1/IGF-1R) is actively involved in the cell transformation induced by EWS-FLI1 and inhibition of apoptosis induced by chemotherapy (Benini et al. 2004; Toretsky et al. 1999). Studies have shown that the inhibition of the IGF-1R or of some downstream elements such as MAPK, PI3-K or Akt may provide effective antitumor activity and potentiate the effects of chemotherapeutic agents (Benini et al. 2004; Toretsky et al. 1999). Inhibition of the activation of downstream elements of PI3-K, such as mTOR, is also a rational target for antitumor therapy. Rapamycin and its derivatives such as CCI-779 might have a role in the treatment of ESFT; in vitro studies have shown that rapamycin may block cell line proliferation by promoting cell cycle arrest at the G_1 phase, downregulation of EWS-FLI-1 proteins, and concomitant restoration of expression of TGFβ R-II in ESFT cells (Mateo-Lozano et al. 2003).

EWS-FLI-1 may promote cell cycle progression accompanied by the suppression of the expression of cyclin-dependent kinase inhibitor $p27^{kip1}$ in ESFT cells (Matsumoto et al. 2001). Matsunobu et al. analyzed the prognostic relevance of $p27^{kip1}$ in patients with ESFT, and found that low expression levels of p27 protein correlated with poor outcome (Matsunobu et al. 2004). In the in vitro model, overexpression of p27 using an adenoviral vector inhibited cell growth and induced apoptosis, and treatment of mice bearing ESFT xenografts with intratumoral injections of p27-expressing adenovirus resulted in significant growth inhibition (Matsunobu et al. 2004). Therefore, mechanisms of increasing expression of p27 could potentially have a role in the treatment of ESFT. In this regard, it is well known that the level of p27 expression is regulated at the post-translational level, and the ubiquitin-proteasome pathway is the principal mechanism regulating p27 protein degradation (Pagano et al. 1995). In ESFT, data suggest that the EWS-FLI1 chimeric transcript might attenuate p27 protein level via activation of the proteasome-mediated degradation pathway (Matsunobu et al. 2004). Treatment of ESFT cells with a proteasome inhibitor resulted in increased expression of the p27 protein (Matsunobu et al. 2004). Proteasome inhibitors are in different phases of clinical development, and a phase I trial of the proteasome in inhibitor bortezomib (PS-341) in children with refractory solid tumors has been recently completed by the Children's Oncology Group.

Resistance of tumors to chemotherapy is often due to abnormalities in the apoptotic pathways. Caspase-8 expression is pivotal in chemotherapy-induced apoptosis in a variety of tumor systems, and decreased expression is associated with chemoresistance (Fulda et al. 2001). Decreased expression of caspase-8 protein may occur as a result of hypermethylation of caspase-8 regulatory sequences (Fulda et al. 2001). In ESFT, treatment of tumor cell lines with low caspase-8 expression with the demethylation agent

5-aza-2'-deoxycytidine reversed hypermethylation of caspase-8, resulting in restoration of caspase-8 expression and restitution of drug-induced apoptosis (Fulda et al. 2001).

Because the EWS-FLI-1 fusion product that characterizes ESFT may induce a cytotoxic T lymphocyte response, the generation of specific cytotoxic T lymphocytes is currently under investigation (Mackall et al. 2000). Enhancement of the immune response in vivo has also been explored. However, the use IL-2 after HSCT has failed to show any advantage (Burdach et al. 2003). Finally, because the formation of the chimeric *EWS-FLI-1* gene is one of the initial transforming events in ESFT, the use of antisense oligonucleotides targeting the fusion is an attractive approach. In fact, this method has shown to be able to inhibit the growth of xenografted ESFT into nude mice (Maksimenko et al. 2003).

References

Abadie A, Besancon F, Wietzerbin J (2004) Type I interferon and TNFa cooperate with type II interferon for TRAIL induction and triggering of apoptosis in SK-N-MC EWING tumor cells. Oncogene 23:4911–4920

Abudu A, Mangham DC, Reynolds GM et al. (1999) Overexpression of p53 protein in primary Ewing's sarcoma of bone: relationship to tumour stage, response and prognosis. Br J Cancer 79:1185–1189

Ambros IM, Ambros PF, Strehl S, Kovar H, Gadner H, Salzer-Kuntschik M (1991) MIC2 is a specific marker for Ewing's sarcoma and peripheral primitive neuroectodermal tumors. Evidence for a common histogenesis of Ewing's sarcoma and peripheral primitive neuroectodermal tumors from MIC2 expression and specific chromosomal aberration. Cancer 67:1886–1893

Arai Y, Kun LE, Brooks T, Fairclough DL, Fontanesi J, Meyer WH et al. (1991) Ewing's sarcoma: Local tumor control and patterns of failure following limited-volume radiation therapy. Int J Radiat Oncol Biol Phys 21:1501–1508

Arvand A, Bastians H, Welford SM, Thompson AD, Ruderman JV, Denny CT (1998) EWS/FLI1 upregulates mE2-C, a cyclin-selective ubiquitin conjugating enzyme involved in cyclin B destruction. Oncogene 17:2039–2045

Bacci G, Toni A, Avella M, Manfrini M, Sudanese A, Ciaroni D et al. (1989) Long-term results in 144 localized Ewing's sarcoma patients treated with combined therapy. Cancer 63: 1477–1486

Bacci G, Picci P, Ferrari S, Mercuri M, Brach del Prever A, Rosito P et al. (1998) Neoadjuvant chemotherapy for Ewing's sarcoma of bone. No benefit observed after adding ifosfamide and etoposide to vincristine, actinomycin, cyclophosphamide, and doxorubicin in the maintenance phase. Results of two sequential studies. Cancer 82:1174–1183

Bacci G, Ferrari S, Bertoni F, Rimondini S, Longhi A, Bacchini P et al. (2000) Prognostic factors in nonmetastatic Ewing's sarcoma of bone treated with adjuvant chemotherapy: Analysis of 359 patients at the Istituto Ostopedico Rizzoli. J Clin Oncol 18:4–11

Bacci G, Ferrari S, Longhi A, Donati D, De Paolis M, Forni C et al. (2003) Therapy and survival after recurrence of Ewing's tumors: the Rizzoli experience in 195 patients treated with adjuvant and neoadjuvant chemotherapy from 1979 to 1997. Ann Oncol 14:1654–1659

Bacci G, Forni C, Longhi A, Ferrari S, Donati D, De Paolis M et al. (2004) Long-term outcome for patients with non-metastatic Ewing's sarcoma treated with adjuvant and neoadjuvant chemotherapies. 402 patients treated at Rizzoli between 1972 and 1992. Eur J Cancer 40:73–83

Benini S, Manara MC, Cerisano V, Perdichizzi S, Strammiello R, Serra M et al. (2004) Contribution of MEK/MAPK and PI3-K signaling pathway to the malignant behavior of Ewing's sarcoma cells: therapeutic prospects. Int J Cancer 108:358–366

Bernstein ML, Goorin A, Devidas M, Lafreniere D, Stine K, Meyers P et al. (2001) Topotecan and topotecan, cyclophosphamide window therapy in patients (pts) with Ewing sarcoma (EWS) metastatic at diagnosis: an Intergroup Pediatric Oncology Group (POG) study (P-9457). Med Pediatr Oncol 37:176 (abstract)

Braun BS, Frieden R, Lessnick SL, May WA, Denny CT (1995) Identification of target genes for the Ewing's sarcoma EWS/FLI fusion protein by representational difference analysis. Mol Cell Biol 15:4623–4630

Brisset S, Schleiremacher G, Peter M et al. (2001) Analysis of secondary genetic changes in Ewing tumors: correlation with metastatic disease in a series of 43 cases. Cancer Genet Cytogenet 130:57–61

Burdach S, van Kaick B, Laws HJ, Ahrens S, Haase R, Korholz D et al. (2000) Allogeneic and autologous stem-cell transplantation in advanced Ewing tumors. An update after long-term follow-up from two centers of the European Intergroup Study EICESS. Ann Oncol 11:1451–1462

Burdach S, Meyer-Bahlurg A, Laws HJ, Haase R, van Kaik B, Metzner B et al. (2003) High-dose therapy for patients with primary multifocal and early relapsed Ewing's tumors: results of two consecutive regimens assessing the role of total-body irradiation. J Clin Oncol 21:3072–3078

Burgert EO, Nesbit ME, Garnsey LA, Gehan EA, Herrmann J, Vietti TJ et al. (1990) Multimodal therapy for the management of nonpelvic, localized Ewing's sarcoma of bone: Intergroup Study IESS-II. J Clin Oncol 8:1514–1524

Cangir A, Vietti TJ, Gehan EA, Burgert EO, Thomas P, Tefft M et al. (1990) Ewing's sarcoma metastatic at diagnosis. Results and comparisons of two Intergroup Ewing's Sarcoma Studies. Cancer 66:887–893

Carrie C, Mascard E, Gomez F, Habrand J-L, Alapetite C, Oberlin O et al. (1999) Nonmetastatic pelvis Ewing sarcoma: Report of the French Society of Pediatric Oncology. Med Pediatr Oncol 33:444–449

Chow E, Merchant TE, Pappo A, Jenkins JJ, Shah AB, Kun LE (2000) Cutaneous and subcutaneous Ewing's sarcoma: An indolent disease. Int J Radiat Oncol Biol Phys 46:433–438

Cotterill SJ, Ahrens S, Paulussen M, Jürgens HF, Voûte PA, Gadner H et al. (2000) Prognostic factors in Ewing's tumor of bone: Analysis of 975 patients from the European Intergroup Cooperative Ewing's Sarcoma Study Group. J Clin Oncol 18:3108–3114

Craft AW, Cotterill SJ, Bullimore JA, Pearson D (1997) Long-term results from the first UKCCSG Ewing's tumour study (ET-1). Eur J Cancer 33:1061–1069

Craft A, Cotterill S, Malcolm A, Spooner D, Grimer R, Souhami R et al. (1998) Ifosfamide-containing chemotherapy in Ewing's sarcoma: The second United Kingdom Children's Cancer Study Group and the Medical Research Council Ewing's Tumor Study. J Clin Oncol 16:3628–3633

Craft AW, Paulussen M, Douglas C, Mapp T, Lewis IB, Jurgens H (2000) EICESS 92 – Early results of an international Ewing's tumour study. Med Pediatr Oncol 35:191 (abstract)

Dauphinot L, De Oliveira C, Melot T et al. (2001) Analysis of the expression of cell cycle regulators in Ewing cell lines: EWS-FLI-1 modulates p57KIP2 and c-Myc expression. Oncogene 20:3258–3265

de Alava E, Gerald WL (2000) Molecular biology of the Ewing's sarcoma/primitive neuroectodermal tumor family. J Clin Oncol 18:204–213

de Alava E, Kawai A, Healey JH, Fligman I, Meyers PA, Huvos AG et al. (1998) EWS-FLI1 fusion transcript structure is an independent determinant of prognosis in Ewing's sarcoma. J Clin Oncol 16:1248–1255

Dehner LP (1993) Primitive neuroectodermal tumor and Ewing's sarcoma. Am J Surg Pathol 17:1–13

Delattre O, Zucman J, Melot T, Sastre Garau X, Zucker J-M, Lenoir GM et al. (1994) The Ewing family of tumors: A subgroup of small-round-cell tumors defined by specific chimeric transcripts. N Engl J Med 331:294–299

Donaldson SS, Torrey M, Link MP, Glicksman A, Gilula L, Laurie F et al. (1998) A multidisciplinary study investigating radiotherapy in Ewing's sarcoma: end results of POG #8346. Int J Radiat Oncol Biol Phys 42:125–135

Dulguerov P, Allal AS, Calcaterra TC (2001) Esthesioneuroblastoma: A meta-analysis and review. Lancet Oncol 2:683–690

Dunst J, Sauer R, Burgers JM et al. (1991) Radiation therapy as local treatment in Ewing's sarcoma. Results of the Cooperative Ewing's Sarcoma Studies CESS 81 and CESS 86. Cancer 67:2818–2825

Evans RG, Nesbit ME, Gehan EA, Garnsey LA, Burgert O, Vietti TJ et al. (1991) Multimodal therapy for the management of localized Ewing's sarcoma of pelvic and sacral bones: A report from the Second Intergroup Study. J Clin Oncol 9:1173–1180

Fagnou C, Michon J, Peter M, Bernoux A, Oberlin O, Zucker J-M et al. (1998) Presence of tumor cells in bone marrow but not in blood is associated with adverse prognosis in patients with Ewing's tumor. J Clin Oncol 16:1707–1711

Fanger NA, Maliszewski CR, Schooley K, Griffith TS (1999) Human dendritic cells mediate cellular apoptosis via tumor necrosis factor-related apoptosis-inducing ligand (TRAIL). J Exp Med 190:1155–1164

Felgenhauer J, Hawkins D, Pendergrass T, Lindsley K, Conrad EU, Miser JS (2000) Very intensive, short-term chemotherapy for children and adolescents with metastatic sarcomas. Med Pediatr Oncol 34:29–38

Fukuma M, Okita H, Hata J, Umezawa A (2003) Upregulation of Id2, an oncogenic helix-loop-helix protein, is mediated by the chimeric EWS/ets protein in Ewing sarcoma. Oncogene 22:1–9

Fulda S, Kufer MU, Meyer E, van Valen F, Dockhorn-Dworniczak B, Debatin K-M (2001) Sensitization for death receptor- or drug-induced apoptosis by re-expression of caspase-8 through demethylation or gene transfer. Oncogene 20:5865–5877

Fuller CE, Dalton J, Jenkins JJ, Shurtleff S (2004) Detection of translocations involving the EWS gene locus in Ewing sarcoma/primitive neuroectodermal tumor and desmoplastic small round cell tumor by dual color break-apart probe FISH assay. Mod Pathol 17:329 (abstract)

Gaona-Luviano P, Unda-Franco E, Gonzalez-Jara L, Romero P, Medina-Franco H (2003) Primitive neuroectodermal tumor of the vagina. Gynecol Oncol 91:456–458

Ginsberg JP, de Alava E, Ladanyi M, Wexler LH, Kovar H, Paulussen M et al. (1999) *EWS-FLI1* and *EWS-ERG* gene fusions are associated with similar clinical phenotypes in Ewing's sarcoma. J Clin Oncol 17:1809–1814

Girnita L, Girnita A, Wang M, Meis-Kindblom JM, Kindblom LG, Larsson O (2000) A link between basic fibroblast growth factor (bFGF) and EWS/FLI-1 in Ewing's sarcoma cells. Oncogene 19:4298–4301

Granowetter L, Womer R, Devidas M, Perlman E, Shamberger R, Link M et al. (2001) Comparison of dose intensified and standard dose chemotherapy for the treatment of non-metastatic Ewing's sarcoma (ES) and primitive neuroectodermal tumor (PNET) of bone and soft tissue: a Pediatric Oncology Group-Children's Cancer Group phase III trial. Med Pediatr Oncol 37:172 (abstract)

Grier HE, Krailo MD, Tarbell NJ, Link MP, Fryer CJH, Pritchard DJ et al. (2003) Addition of ifosfamide and etoposide to standard chemotherapy for Ewing's sarcoma and primitive neuroectodermal tumor of bone. N Engl J Med 348:694–701

Gurney JG, Swensen AR, Bulterys M (1999) Malignant bone tumors. In: Ries LAG et al. (ed) Cancer incidence and survival among children and adolescents: United States SEER program 1975–1995, National Cancer Institute, SEER Program. NIH Pub. No. 99-4649. Bethesda, MD

Hahm KB, Cho K, Lee C, Im YH, Chang J, Choi SG et al. (1999) Repression of the gene encoding the TGF-b type II receptor is a major target of the EWING's SARCOMA-FLI1 oncoprotein. Nat Genet 23:222–227

Hattinger CM, Rumpler S, Strehl S et al. (1999) Prognostic impact of deletions at 1p36 and numerical aberrations in Ewing tumors. Genes Chromosomes Cancer 24:243–254

Hayes FA, Thompson EI, Meyer WH, Kun L, Parham D, Rao B et al. (1989) Therapy for localized Ewing's sarcoma of bone. J Clin Oncol 7:208–213

Heyn R, Khan F, Ensign LG et al. (1994) Acute myeloid leukemia in patients treated for rhabdomyosarcoma with cyclophosphamide and low-dose etoposide on Intergroup Rhabdomyosarcoma Study III. Med Pediatr Oncol 23: 99–106

Hijazi Y, Axiotis CA, Navarro S, Steinberg SM, Horowitz ME, Tsokos M (1994) Immunohistochemical detection of P-glycoprotein in Ewing's sarcoma and peripheral primitive neuroectodermal tumors before and after chemotherapy. Am J Clin Pathol 102:61–67

Im YH, Kim HT, Lee C et al. (2000) EWS-FLI1, EWS-ERG, and EWS-ETV1 oncoproteins of Ewing tumor family all suppress transcription of transforming growth factor beta type II receptor gene. Cancer Res 60:1536–1540

Jaboin J, Wild J, Hamidi H, Khanna C, Kim CJ, Robey R et al. (2002) MS-27-275, an inhibitor of histone deacetylase, has marked in vitro and in vivo antitumor activity against pediatric solid tumors. Cancer Res 62:6108–6115

Jaffe N, Traggis D, Salian S, Cassady JR (1976) Improved outlook for Ewing's sarcoma with combination chemotherapy (vincristine, actinomycin D and cuclophosphamide) and radiation therapy. Cancer 38:1925–1930

Jo M, Kim TH, Seol DW, Esplen JE, Dorko K, Billiar TR et al. (2000) Apoptosis induced in normal human hepatocytes by tumor necrosis factor-related apoptosis-inducing ligand. Nat Med 6:564–567

Jürgens H, Exner U, Gadner H, Harms D, Michaelis J, Sauer R et al. (1988) Multidisciplinary treatment of primary Ewing's sarcoma of bone. Cancer 61:23–32

Kolb EA, Kushner BH, Gorlick R, Laverdiere C, Healey JH, LaQuaglia MP et al. (2003) Long-term event-free survival after intensive chemotherapy for Ewing's family of tumors in children and young adults. J Clin Oncol 21:3423–3430

Kontny HU, Hammerle K, Klein R, Shayan P, Mackall CL, Niemeyer CM (2001) Sensitivity of Ewing's sarcoma to TRAIL-induced apoptosis. Cell Death Differ 8:506–514

Koscielniak E, Gross-Wieltsch U, Treuner J, Winkler P, Klingebiel T, Lang P et al. (2005) Graft-versus-Ewing sarcoma effect and long-term remission induced by haploidentical stem-cell transplantation in a patient with relapse of metastatic disease. J Clin Oncol 23:242–244

Kovar H, Auinger A, Jug G et al. (1993) Narrow spectrum of infrequent p53 mutations and absence of MDM2 amplification in Ewing tumours. Oncogene 8:2683–2690

Krasin MJ, Rodriguez-Galindo C, Davidoff AM, Billups CA, Fuller CE, Neel MD et al. (2004a) Efficacy of combined surgery and irradiation for localized Ewing's sarcoma family of tumors. Pediatr Blood Cancer 43:229–236

Krasin MJ, Rodriguez-Galindo C, Billups CA, Davidoff AM, Neel MD, Merchant TE et al. (2004b) Definitive irradiation in multidisciplinary management of localized Ewing sarcoma family of tumors in pediatric patients: outcome and prognostic factors. Int J Radiat Oncol Biol Phys 60:830–838

Krasin MJ, Davidoff AM, Rodriguez-Galindo C et al. (2005) Definitive surgery and multiagent systemic therapy for patients with localized Ewing sarcoma family of tumors: Local outcome and prognostic factors. Cancer in press

Kushner BH, Meyers PA (2001) How effective is dose-intensive/myeloablative therapy against Ewing's sarcoma/primitive neuroectodermal tumor metastatic to bone or bone marrow? The Memorial Sloan-Kettering Experience and a literature review. J Clin Oncol 19:870–880

Kushner BH, Heller G, Cheung NK, Wollner N, Kramer K, Bajorin D et al. (1998) High risk of leukemia after short-term dose-intensive chemotherapy in young patients with solid tumors. J Clin Oncol 16:3016–3020

Kuttesch JF, Wexler LH, Marcus RB, Fairclough D, Weaver-McClure L, White M et al. (1996) Second malignancies after Ewing's sarcoma: radiation dose-dependency of secondary sarcomas. J Clin Oncol 14:2818–2825

Ladenstein R, Lasset C, Pinkerton R, Zucker J-M, Peters C, Burdach S et al. (1995) Impact of megatherapy in children with high-risk Ewing's tumours in complete remission: a report from the EBMT solid tumour registry. Bone Marrow Transpl 15:697–705

Ladenstein R, Peters C, Zoubek A, Mann G, Kronberger M, Hocker H et al. (1996) The role of megatherapy (MGT) followed by stem cell rescue (SCR) in high risk Ewing tumors (ET). 11 years single center experience. Med Pediatr Oncol 27:237 (abstract)

Ladenstein R, Philip T, Gardner H (1997) Autologous stem cell transplantation for solid tumors in children. Curr Opin Pediatr 9:55–69

Ladenstein R, Hartmann O, Pinkerton R, Dallorso G, Burdach S, Jürgens H et al. (1999) A multivariate and matched pair analysis on high-risk Ewing tumor (ET) patients treated by megatherapy (MGT) and stem cell reinfusion (SCR) in Europe. Proc Annu Meet Am Soc Clin Oncol 18:555 (abstract)

Lau L, Supko JG, Blaney S, Hershon L, Seibel N, Krailo M et al. (2005) A phase I and pharmacokinetic study of ecteinascidin-743 (Yondelis) in children with refractory solid tumors. A Children's Oncology Group study. Clin Cancer Res 11:672–677

Lin PP, Brody RI, Hamelin AC, Bradner JE, Healey JH, Ladanyi M (1999) Differential transactivation by alternative EWS-FLI1 fusion proteins correlates with clinical heterogeneity in Ewing's sarcoma. Cancer Res 59:1428–1432

Mackall C, Berzofsky J, Helman LJ (2000) Targeting tumor specific translocations in sarcomas in pediatric patients for immunotherapy. Clin Orthop 373:25–31

Maksimenko A, Lambert G, Bertrand JR, Fattal E, Couvreur P, Malvy C (2003) Therapeutic potentialities of EWS-Fli-1 mRNA-targeted vectorized antisense oligonucleotides. Ann NY Acad Sci 1002:72–77

Marina NM, Pappo AS, Parham DM et al. (1999) Chemotherapy dose-intensification for pediatric patients with Ewing's family of tumors and desmoplastic small round cell tumor: A feasibility study at St. Jude Children's Research Hospital. J Clin Oncol 17:180–190

Mateo-Lozano S, Tirado OM, Notario V (2003) Rapamycin induces the fusion-type independent downregulation of the EWS/FLI-1 proteins and inhibits Ewing's sarcoma cell proliferation. Oncogene 22:9282–9287

Matsumoto Y, Tanaka K, Nakatani F, Matsunobu T, Matsuda S, Iwamoto Y (2001) Down-regulation and forced expression of EWS-Fli1 fusion gene results in changes in the expression of G(1) regulatory genes. Br J Cancer 84:768–775

Matsunobu T, Tanaka K, Matsumoto Y, Nakatani F, Sakimura R, Hanada M (2004) The prognostic and therapeutic relevance of p27-kip1 in Ewing's family tumors. Clin Cancer Res 10:1003–1012

May WA, Gishizky ML, Lessnick SL et al. (1993a) Ewing sarcoma 11;22 translocation produces a chimeric transcription factor that requires the DNA-binding domain encoded by FLI1 for transformation. Proc Natl Acad Sci USA 90:5752–5756

May WA, Lessnick SL, Braun BS et al. (1993b) The Ewing's sarcoma EWS/FLI-1 fusion gene encodes a more potent transcriptional activator and is a more powerful transforming gene than FLI-1. Mol Cell Biol 13:7393–7398

May W, Arvand A, Thompson A, Braun BS, Wright M, Denny CT (1997) EWS/FLI1-induced manic fringe renders NIH 3t3 cells tumorigenic. Nat Genet 17:495–497

Merchant TE, Kushner BH, Sheldon JM, LaQuaglia M, Healey JH (1999) Effect of low-dose radiation therapy when combined with surgical resection for Ewing sarcoma. Med Pediatr Oncol 33:65–70

Meyer WH, Kun L, Marina N (1992) Ifosfamide plus etoposide in newly diagnosed Ewing's sarcoma of bone. J Clin Oncol 10:1737–1742

Meyers PA, Krailo MD, Ladanyi M, Chan K-W, Sailer SL, Dickman PS et al. (2001) High-dose melphalan, etoposide, total-body irradiation, and autologous stem-cell reconstitution as consolidation therapy for high-risk Ewing's sarcoma does not improve prognosis. J Clin Oncol 19:2812–2820

Miller SL, Hoffer FA, Reddick WE, Wu S, Glass JO, Gronemeyer SA et al. (2001) Tumor volume or dynamic contrast-enhanced MRI for prediction of clinical outcome of Ewing sarcoma family of tumors. Pediatr Radiol 31:518–523

Miser JS, Kinsella TJ, Triche TJ, Tsokos M, Jarosinski P, Forquer R et al. (1987) Ifosfamide with mesna uroprotection and etoposide: An effective regimen in the treatment of recurrent sarcomas and other tumors of children and young adults. J Clin Oncol 5:1191–1198

Miser JS, Krailo M, Meyers P, Rausen A, Link M, Tarbell N et al. (1996) Metastatic Ewing's sarcoma (ES) and primitive neuroectodermal tumor (PNET) of bone: Failure of new regimens to improve outcome. Proc Annu Meet Am Soc Clin Oncol 15:467 (abstract)

Miser JS, Krailo MD, Tarbell NJ, Link MP, Fryer CJH, Pritchard DJ et al. (2004) Treatment of metastatic Ewing's sarcoma or primitive neuroectodermal tumor of bone: evaluation of combination ifosfamide and etoposide – A Children's Cancer Group and Pediatric Oncology Group study. J Clin Oncol 22:2873–2876

Mitsiades N, Poulaki V, Mitsiades C, Tsokos M (2001) Ewing's sarcoma family of tumors are sensitive to tumor necrosis factor-related apoptosis-inducing ligand and express death receptor 4 and death receptor 5. Cancer Res 61:2704–2712

Nesbit ME, Gehan EA, Burgert EO, Vietti TJ, Cangir A, Tefft M et al. (1990) Multimodal therapy for the management of primary, nonmetastatic Ewing's sarcoma of bone: A long-term follow-up of the first intergroup study. J Clin Oncol 8:1664–1674

Nishimori H, Sasaki Y, Yoshida K et al. (2002) The Id2 gene is a novel target of transcriptional activation by EWS-ETS fusion proteins in Ewing family tumors. Oncogene 21:8302–8309

Nitsch R, Bechmann I, Deisz RA, Haas D, Lehmann TN, Wending U et al. (2000) Human brain-cell death induced by tumour-necrosis factor-related apoptosis-inducing ligand (TRAIL). Lancet 356:827–828

Oberlin O, Le Deley MC, N'Guyen Bui B, Gentet JC, Philip T, Terrier P et al. (2001) Prognostic factors in localized Ewing's tumours and peripheral neuroectodermal tumours: The third study of the French Society of Paediatric Oncology (EW88 study). Br J Cancer 85:1646–1654

Ozaki T, Paulussen M, Poremba C et al. (2001) Genetic imbalances revealed by comparative genomic hybridization in Ewing tumors. Genes Chromosomes Cancer 32:164–171

Pagano M, Tam SW, Theodoras AM, Beer-Romero P, Del Sal G, Chau V et al. (1995) Role of the ubiquitin-proteasome pathway in regulating abundance of the cyclin-dependent kinase inhibitor p27. Science 269:682–685

Parham DM, Roloson GJ, Feely M, Green DM, Bridge JA, Beckwith JB (2001) Primary malignant neuroepithelial tumors of the kidney. A clinicopathologic analysis of 146 adult and pediatric cases from the National Wilms' Tumor Study Group Pathology Center. Am J Surg Pathol 25:133–146

Parkin DM, Stiller CA, Nectoux J (1993) International variations in the incidence of childhood bone tumours. Int J Cancer 53:371–376

Paulussen M, Ahrens S, Craft AW, Dunst J, Frölich B, Jabar S et al. (1998a) Ewing's tumors with primary lung metastases: Survival analysis of 114 (European Intergroup) Cooperative Ewing's Sarcoma Studies patients. J Clin Oncol 16: 3044–3052

Paulussen M, Ahrens S, Burdach S, Craft A, Dockhorn-Dworniczak B, Dunst J et al. (1998b) Primary metastatic (stage IV) Ewing tumor: Survival analysis of 171 patients from the EICESS studies. Ann Oncol 9:275–281

Paulussen M, Ahrens S, Dunst J, Winkelmann W, Exner GU, Kotz R et al. (2001a) Localized Ewing tumor of bone: Final results of the Cooperative Ewing's Sarcoma Study CESS-86. J Clin Oncol 19:1818–1829

Paulussen M, Ahrens S, Lehnert M, Taeger D, Hense HW, Wagner A et al. (2001b) Second malignancies after Ewing tumor treatment in 690 patients from a cooperative German/Austrian/Dutch study. Ann Oncol 12:1619–1630

Peart MJ, Tainton KM, Ruefli AA, Dear AE, Sedelies KA, O'Reilly LA et al. (2003) Novel mechanisms of apoptosis induced by histone deacetylase inhibitors. Cancer Res 63:4460–4471

Pedersen-Bjergaard J, Sigsgaard TC, Nielsen D et al. (1992) Acute monocytic or myelomonocytic leukemia with balanced chromosome translocations to band 11q23 after therapy with 4-epi-doxorubicin and cisplatin or cyclophosphamide for breast cancer. J Clin Oncol 10:1444–1451

Pedersen-Bjergaard J, Philip P, Larsen SO et al. (1993) Therapy-related myelodysplasia and acute myeloid leukemia. Cytogenetic characteristics of 115 consecutive cases and risk in seven cohorts of patients treated intensively for malignant diseases in the Copenhagen series. Leukemia 7:1975–1986

Perlman EJ, Dickman PS, Askin FB, Grier HE, Miser JS, Link MP (1994) Ewing's sarcoma – routine diagnostic utilization of MIC2 analysis: a Pediatric Oncology Group/Children's Cancer Group Intergroup Study. Hum Pathol 25:304–307

Picci P, Bohling T, Bacci G, Ferrari S, Sangiorgi L, Mercuri M et al. (1997) Chemotherapy-induced tumor necrosis as a prognostic factor in localized Ewing's sarcoma of the extremities. J Clin Oncol 15:1553–1559

Prieur A, Tirode F, Cohen P, Delattre O (2004) EWS/FLI-1 silencing and gene profiling of Ewing cells reveal downstream oncogenic pathways and a crucial role for repression of insulin-like growth factor binding protein 3. Mol Cell Biol 24:7275–7283

Raney RB, Asmar L, Newton WA, Bagwell C, Breneman JC, Crist W et al. (1997) Ewing's sarcoma of soft tissues in childhood: a report from the Intergroup Rhabdomyosarcoma Study, 1972–1991. J Clin Oncol 15:574–582

Razek A, Perez CA, Tefft M, Nesbit M, Vietti T, Burgert EO et al. (1980) Intergroup Ewing's Sarcoma Study: Local control related to radiation dose, volume, and site of primary lesion in Ewing's sarcoma. Cancer 46:516–521

Rill DR, Santana VM, Roberts WM, Nilson T, Bowman LC, Krance RA et al. (1994) Direct demonstration that autologous bone marrow transplantation for solid tumors can return a multiplicity of tumorigenic cells. Blood 84:380–383

Rodriguez-Galindo C (2004) Pharmacological management of Ewing sarcoma family of tumours. Expert Opin Pharmacother 5:1257–1270

Rodriguez-Galindo C, Poquette CA, Marina NM, Head DR, Cain A, Meyer WH et al. (2000a) Hematologic abnormalities and acute myeloid leukemia in children and adolescents administered intensified chemotherapy for the Ewing sarcoma family of tumors. J Pediatr Hematol Oncol 22:321–329

Rodriguez-Galindo C, Radomski KM, Stewart CF, Furman W, Santana VM, Houghton PJ (2000b) Clinical use of topoisomerase I inhibitors in anticancer treatment. Med Pediatr Oncol 35:385–402

Rodriguez-Galindo C, Billups CA, Kun LE, Rao BN, Pratt CB, Merchant TE et al. (2002) Survival after recurrence of Ewing tumors: The St Jude Children's Research Hospital Experience, 1979–1999. Cancer 94:561–569

Rodriguez-Galindo C, Spunt SL, Pappo AS (2003) Treatment of Ewing sarcoma family of tumors: current status and outlook for the future. Med Pediatr Oncol 40:276–287

Rosito P, Mancini A, Rondelli R, Abate ME, Pession A, Bedei L et al. (1999) Italian cooperative study for the treatment of children and young adults with localized Ewing sarcoma of bone. A preliminary report of 6 years of experience. Cancer 86:421–428

Sanceau J, Poupon M-F, Delattre O, Sastre Garau X, Wietzerbin J (2002) Strong inhibition of Ewing tumor xenograft growth by combination of human interferon-alpha or interferon-beta with ifosfamide. Oncogene 21:7700–7709

Sandoval C, Pui C-H, Bowman LC et al. (1993) Secondary acute myeloid leukemia in children previously treated with alkylating agents, intercalating topoisomerase-II inhibitors, and irradiation. J Clin Oncol 11:1039–1045

Sandoval C, Meyer WH, Parham DM, Kun LE, Hustu HO, Luo X et al. (1996) Outcome in 43 children presenting with metastatic Ewing sarcoma: The St Jude Children's Research Hospital Experience, 1962 to 1992. Med Pediatr Oncol 26: 180–185

Saylors RL, Stine KC, Sullivan J, Kepner JLBM, Wall DA, Bernstein ML et al. (2001) Cyclophosphamide plus topotecan in children with recurrent or refractory solid tumors: a pediatric oncology group (POG) phase II study. J Clin Oncol 19:3463–3469

Schiffman KS, Bensinger WI, Appelbaum FR, Rowley S, Lilleby K, Clift RA et al. (1996) Phase II study of high-dose busulfan, melphalan and thiotepa with autologous peripheral blood stem cell support in patients with malignant disease. Bone Marrow Transplant 17:943–950

Schleiermacher G, Peter M, Oberlin O, Philip T, Rubie H, Mechinaud F et al. (2003) Increased risk of systemic relapses associated with bone marrow micrometastasis and circulating tumor cells in localized Ewing tumor. J Clin Oncol 21:85–91

Schuck A, Ahrens S, Paulussen M, Kuhlen M, Könemann S, Rübe C et al. (2003) Local therapy in localized Ewing tumors: Results of 1058 patients treated in the CESS 81, CESS 86, and EICESS 92 trials. Int J Radiat Oncol Biol Phys 55:168–177

Scotlandi K, Benini S, Sarti M et al. (1996) Insulin-like growth factor I receptor-mediated circuit in Ewing's sarcoma/peripheral neuroectodermal tumor: a possible therapeutic target. Cancer Res 56:4570–4574

Scotlandi K, Avnet S, Benini S et al. (2002) Expression of an IGF-I receptor dominant negative mutant induces apoptosis, inhibits tumorigenesis and enhances chemosensitivity in Ewing's sarcoma cells. Int J Cancer 101:11–16

Scotlandi K, Manara MC, Strammiello R, Landuzzi L, Benini S, Perdichizzi S et al. (2003) *c-kit* receptor expression in Ewing's sarcoma: Lack of prognostic value but therapeutic targeting opportunities in appropriate conditions. J Clin Oncol 21:1952–1960

Shamberger RC, LaQuaglia MP, Gebhardt MC, Neff JR, Tarbell NJ, Marcus KC et al. (2003) Ewing sarcoma/primitive neuroectodermal tumor of the chest wall. Impact of initial versus delayed resection on tumor margins, survival, and use of radiation therapy. Ann Surg 238:563–568

Shankar AG, Pinkerton CR, Atra A, Ashley S, Lewis I, Spooner D et al. (1999) Local therapy and other factors influencing site of relapse in patients with localised Ewing's sarcoma. Eur J Cancer 35:1698–1704

Shankar AG, Ashley S, Craft AW, Pinkerton CR (2003) Outcome after relapse in an unselected cohort of children and adolescents with Ewing sarcoma. Med Pediatr Oncol 40:141–147

Shek TWH, Chan GCF, Khong PL, Chung LP, Cheung ANY (2001) Ewing sarcoma of the small intestine. J Pediatr Hematol Oncol 23:530–532

Silvany RE, Eliazer S, Wolff NC, Ilaria RL (2000) Interference with the constitutive activation of REK1 and ERK2 impairs EWS/FLI-1-dependent transformation. Oncogene 19:4523–4530

Smithey BE, Pappo AS, Hill DA (2002) c-kit expression in pediatric solid tumors. Am J Surg Pathol 26:486–492

Spunt SL, McCarville MB, Kun LE, Poquette CA, Cain AM, Brandao L et al. (2001) Selective use of whole-lung irradiation for patients with Ewing sarcoma family tumors and pulmonary metastases at the time of diagnosis. J Pediatr Hematol Oncol 23:93–98

Spunt S, Harper J, Krasin M, Billups C, Rodriguez-Galindo C (2004) Ewing sarcoma family of tumors (ESFT) as a second malignant neoplasm (SMN) following treatment of a primary malignant neoplasm (PMN) during childhood. Proc Annu Meet Am Soc Clin Oncol 22:808 (abstract)

Strauss SJ, McTiernan A, Driver D, Hall-Craggs M, Sandison A, Cassoni AM et al. (2003) Single center experience of a new intensive induction therapy for Ewing's family of tumors: Feasibility, toxicity, and stem cell mobilization properties. J Clin Oncol 21:2974–2981

Sturla LM, Westwood G, Selby PJ, Lewis IJ, Burchill SA (2000) Induction of cell death by basic fibroblast growth factor in Ewing's sarcoma. Cancer Res 60:6160–6170

Tanaka K, Iwakuma T, Harimaya K, Sato H, Iwamoto Y (1997) EWS-Fli1 antisense oligodeoxynucleotide inhibits proliferation of human Ewing's sarcoma and primitive neuroectodermal tumor cells. J Clin Invest 99:239–247

Terrier Ph, Henry-Amar M, Triche TJ, Horowitz ME, Terrier-Lacombe MJ, Miser JS et al. (1995) Is neuroectodermal differentiation of Ewing's sarcoma of bone associated with an unfavourable prognosis? Eur J Cancer 31A:307–314

Thompson AD, Braun BS, Arvand A et al. (1996) EAT-2 is a novel SH2 domain containing protein that is upregulated by Ewing's sarcoma EWS/FLI1 fusion gene. Oncogene 13: 2649–2658

Torchia EC, Jaishankar S, Baker SJ (2003) Ewing tumor fusion proteins block the differentiation of pluripotent marrow stromal cells. Cancer Res 63:3464–3468

Toretsky JA, Kalebic T, Blakesley V, LeRoith D, Helman LJ (1997) The insulin-like growth factor-I receptor is required for EWS/FLI-1 transformation of fibroblasts. J Biol Chem 272:30822–30827

Toretsky JA, Thakar M, Eskenazi AE, Frantz CN (1999) Phosphoinositide 3-hydroxide kinase blockade enhances apoptosis in the Ewing's sarcoma family of tumors. Cancer Res 59:5745–5750

Tsuchiya T, Sekine K, Hinohara S, Namiki T, Nobori T, Kaneko Y (2000) Analysis of the p16INK4, p14ARF, p15, TP53, and MDM2 genes and their prognostic implications in osteosarcoma and Ewing sarcoma. Cancer Genet Cytogenet 120:91–98

Tucker MA, D'Angio GJ, Boice JD, Strong LC, Li FP, Stovall M et al. (1987a) Bone sarcomas linked to radiotherapy and chemotherapy in children. N Engl J Med 317:588–593

Tucker MA, Meadows AT, Boice JD et al. (1987b) Leukemia after therapy with alkylating agents for childhood cancer. J Natl Cancer Inst 78:459–464

Uren A, Merchant MS, Sun CJ et al. (2003) Beta-platelet-derived growth factor receptor mediates motility and growth of Ewing's sarcoma cells. Oncogene 22:2334–2342

van Valen F, Fulda S, Schafer K-L, Truckenbord B, Hotfilder M, Poremba C et al. (2003) Selective and nonselective toxicity of TRAIL/Apo2L combined with chemotherapy in human bone tumour cells vs. normal human cells. Int J Cancer 107:929–940

Wagner LM, Crews KR, Iacono LC, Houghton PJ, Fuller CE, McCarville MB et al. (2004) Phase I trial of temozolomide and protracted irinotecan in pediatric patients with refractory solid tumors. Clin Cancer Res 10:840–848

Walczak H, Miller RE, Ariail K, Gliniak B, Griffith TS, Kubin M et al. (1999) Tumoricidal activity of tumor necrosis factor-related apoptosis-inducing ligand *in vivo*. Nat Med 5:157–163

West DC, Grier HE, Swallow MM, Demetri GD, Granowetter L, Sklar J (1997) Detection of circulating tumor cells in patients with Ewing's sarcoma and peripheral primitive neuroectodermal tumor. J Clin Oncol 15:583–588

Wingett D, Forcier K, Nielson CP (1999) A role for CD99 in T cell activation. Cell Immunol 193:17–23

Womer RB, Daller RT, Fenton JG, Miser JS (2000) Granulocyte colony stimulating factor permits dose intensification by interval compression in the treatment of Ewing's sarcomas and soft tissue sarcomas in children. Eur J Cancer 36:87–94

Yovine A, Riofrio M, Blay JY, Brain E, Alexandre J, Kahatt C et al. (2004) Phase II study of ecteinascidin-743 in advanced pretreated soft tissue sarcoma patients. J Clin Oncol 22:890–899

Zoubek A, Pfleiderer C, Salzer-Kuntschik M et al. (1994) Variability of EWS chimaeric transcripts in Ewing tumours: a comparison of clinical and molecular data. Br J Cancer 70:908–913

Zoubek A, Dockhorn-Dworniczak B, Delattre O, Christiansen H, Niggli F, Gatterer-Menz I et al. (1996) Does expression of different EWS chimeric transcripts define clinically distinct risk groups of Ewing tumor patients? J Clin Oncol 14:1245–1251

Zoubek A, Ladenstein R, Windhager R, Amann G, Fischmeister G, Kager L et al. (1998) Predictive potential of testing for bone marrow involvement in Ewing tumor patients by RT-PCR: A preliminary evaluation. Int J Cancer 79:56–60

Zucman J, Melot T, Desmaze C et al. (1993) Combinatorial generation of variable fusion proteins in the Ewing family of tumours. EMBO J 12:4481–4487

Zwerner JP, May WA (2001) PDGF-C is an EWS/FLI induced transforming growth factor in Ewing family tumors. Oncogene 20:626–633

Zwerner JP, May WA (2002) Dominant negative PDGF-C inhibits growth of Ewing family tumor cell lines. Oncogene 21:3847–3854

Osteosarcoma

Paul A. Meyers

Contents

10.1 Incidence

Primary malignant tumors of bone are rare, with an estimated incidence of 8.7 per million in children and young adults under the age of 20 (Gurney and Bulterys 1999). Osteosarcoma is the most common primary malignant bone tumor, and there are roughly 400 new cases diagnosed each year in the United States (Dorfman and Czerniak 1995; Huvos 1991). Osteosarcoma has a bimodal age distribution with a peak during adolescence and a second peak in older adults. When osteosarcoma occurs in older patients it is more likely to represent a secondary malignancy, frequently following Paget's disease. Osteosarcoma in adolescents and young adults occurs slightly more frequently in males, and the peak age of incidence is slightly older in males (18 years) than in females (16 years) (Dahlin and Unni 1986; Dorfman and Czerniak 1995; Gurney and Bulterys 1999; Huvos 1991).

10.2 Etiology/Pathogenesis

The etiology and pathogenesis for most cases of osteosarcoma is unknown. The peak onset during adolescence coincides with the adolescent growth spurt, suggesting that a period of rapid bone growth plays a role in the evolution of this tumor. The earlier peak in girls than in boys corresponds to the earlier growth spurt in girls (Price 1958). It has long been recognized that osteosarcoma is much more common in large than in small dogs (Tjalma 1966). A study of a single breed of large dogs failed to demonstrate a correlation between height and the occurrence of osteosarcoma (Cooley et al. 2002). A large epidemiologic study of humans with bone tumors demonstrated that osteosarcoma is more common in tall individuals (Cotterill et al. 2004). Osteosarcoma is a well documented secondary malignancy arising following radiation, both therapeutic and inadvertent. The interval between irradiation and the appearance of osteosarcoma has ranged from 4 to more than 40 years (median, 12–16 years), and bone sarcoma has occurred after irradiation for benign as well as malignant conditions (Huvos 1991; Sim et al. 1972). Osteosarcoma occurs following the use of bone-seeking radioisotopes (Loutit 1970), such as intravenous radium-224 for the treatment of ankylosing spondylitis and tuberculosis, and Thorotrast used as a diagnostic radiocontrast agent (Loutit 1970; Spiess and Mays 1970; Harrist et al. 1979). Osteosarcoma has been reported in patients with Paget's disease, and cases of osteosarcoma in patients older than 40 years are almost exclusively associated with this premalignant condition (Huvos 1991). Approximately 2% of patients with Paget's disease develop osteosarcoma, and the occurrence of osteosarcoma is not necessarily related to the extent of involvement of the skeleton by Paget's disease (Huvos 1991). Histologically, osteosarcomas in patients with Paget's disease are indistinguishable from conventional osteosarcoma, although multiple bone involvement is frequent and the prognosis for such patients is poor (Dahlin and Unni 1977). Certain genetic alterations predispose patients to the development of osteosarcoma. Children and young adults who are survivors of retinoblastoma have a dramatically increased risk to develop osteosarcoma (Abramson et al. 1984; Draper et al. 1986; Meadows et al. 1980; Smith et al. 1989). The Li-Fraumeni syndrome features sarcomas in young patients and pre-menopausal breast cancer in the mothers of the young patients (Li and Fraumeni 1969a, b). The syndrome has been shown to be the result of a germ-line deletion of one copy of the p53 gene and is associated with a high risk to develop osteosarcoma (Friend et al. 1986). The Rothmund-Thomson syndrome is a rare genodermatosis that features a progressive, early-onset poikiloderma, a high incidence of juvenile cataracts, stunted growth, and a wide range of skeletal abnormalities. The genetic abnormality has been shown to be a mutation in the RECQ4 gene, suggesting a role for this gene in the pathogenesis of osteosarcoma (Balraj et al. 2002; Drouin et al. 1993; Wang et al. 2003).

10.3 Molecular Biology

Osteosarcomas exhibit complex unbalanced karyotypes with alterations of both the p53 and retinoblastoma (Rb) pathways (Borden et al. 2003). Despite the apparently random alterations in the karyotype, recurring abnormalities are present. The majority of osteosarcomas are clonal, although they do exhibit heterogeneity, even in tumors from an individual patient (Bridge et al. 1997). The majority of karyotypes reported from osteosarcoma tumor samples display a marker chromosome. Ring chromosomes, and multiple structural and numerical abnormalities, are common (Bridge et al. 1997; Sandberg and Bridge 2003). Some of the recurring cytogenetic abnormalities which have been described include: gains of chromosome 1, loss of chromosomes 9, 10, 13, and 17, and abnormalities of the long arm of chromosome 6 (Diller et al. 1990; Harris 1986; Huang et al. 1988; Lane 1992). Recurring structural abnormalities have been described in chromosomes 11, 19, and 20 (Bayani et al. 2003; Bridge et al. 1997; Sandberg and Bridge 2003).

The pathogenesis of osteosarcoma requires mutations in both the p53 and Rb pathways. The p53 gene codes for a protein which increases in response to DNA damage and is thought to arrest progression through the cell cycle or cause programmed cell death (apoptosis) (Diller et al. 1990; Lane 1992). The Rb gene controls a critical check point in the progression through the cell cycle (Harris 1986; Huang et al. 1988; Murphree and Benedict 1984). Most osteosarcoma tumor specimens exhibit inactivation of these tumor suppressor pathways, and a small percentage of patients with osteosarcoma have a germline mutation in the p53 gene (Miller et al. 1990; Toguchida et al. 1992). Loss of heterozygosity is reported in osteosarcoma in regions of chromosomes 3q, 13q, 17p, and 18q which include the loci for p53 and Rb (Kruzelock and Hansen 1995; Kruzelock et al.

1997). The occurrence of osteosarcoma is much higher in survivors of retinoblastoma who have a positive family history or present with bilateral disease. This finding supports a role for a germ-line mutation of the Rb gene (Abramson et al. 1984; Draper et al. 1986). Mutations in other cell cycle regulatory genes have been described in osteosarcoma, including amplification of the product of the murine double minute 2 (mdm2) gene and cyclin dependent kinase 4 (CDK4) (Ladanyi et al. 1993; Wei et al. 1999).

Many authors have sought to identify a possible link between viral infection and the occurrence of osteosarcoma. In animals, there are clear links between viruses and bone sarcomas (Finkel et al. 1966; Friedlaender and Mitchell 1976). A cell free extract obtained from human osteosarcoma can cause osteosarcoma in hamsters (Finkel et al. 1968). SV40 is a DNA polyomavirus which interacts with both the p53 and Rb genes and promotes cellular proliferation. A majority of osteosarcoma samples exhibit evidence of incorporation of SV40 DNA into their genome (Carbone et al. 1996; Lednicky et al. 1997). There was no correlation between the presence of SV40 DNA and the mutation status of p53 and Rb, and there is still no convincing evidence that viruses play a major etiologic role in human osteosarcoma (Mendoza et al. 1998).

10.4 Pathology

Osteosarcoma has many different histologic subtypes. The hallmark of osteosarcoma is a proliferation of malignant mesenchymal cells associated with production of extracellular matrix osteoid which may be ossified (Huvos 1991; Dorfman and Czerniak 1995). The amount of osteoid and the extent of ossification varies from patient to patient and within large tumors. Small biopsies may not obtain representative tissue. It is not uncommon for a biopsy to demonstrate unequivocal malignant mesenchymal cells, but in the absence of unequivocal osteoid, the diagnosis of osteosarcoma cannot be confirmed. Subsequent resection allows careful pathologic evaluation of the entire tumor and identification of osteoid confirms the diagnosis of osteosarcoma.

Dahlin described three categories of conventional osteosarcoma, based on the predominant differentiation of the tumor cells (Dahlin and Unni 1986, 1977; Dahlin and Coventry 1967). Roughly half of the cases exhibit abundant osteoid production and are called osteoblastic osteosarcoma. Roughly one-quarter exhibit extensive cartilaginous differentiation and are classified as chondroblastic. Another quarter have a predominantly spindle cell stroma and are characterized as fibroblastic. All osteosarcomas exhibit significant heterogeneity, and small biopsies may not be representative of the overall histology of a tumor. Furthermore, no consistent correlation has been shown between histologic subtype and outcome, although some series report a lower rate of favorable necrosis following chemotherapy for chondroblastic osteosarcoma (Bacci et al. 1998a, 2003, 2000).

Several variants of osteosarcoma are distinguished from classic osteosarcoma because of differences in biologic behavior. Primary osteosarcoma of the jaw occurs most often in older patients, most commonly exhibits chondroid differentiation, and is associated with a more indolent course, with a tendency for local recurrence rather than distant metastases, especially if the tumors are low grade (Bertoni et al. 1991; Clark et al. 1983; Gadwal et al. 2001). A meta-analysis of published series of osteosarcoma of the head and face suggests that these patients benefit from the addition of systemic chemotherapy (Smeele et al. 1997) although. It is difficult to dissect the relative contribution of chemotherapy to the outcome (Patel et al. 2002). By contrast, osteosarcoma occurring in patients with Paget's disease has a typically aggressive clinical course with few survivors (Dahlin and Unni 1977). Extraosseous osteosarcoma is an uncommon variant that arises outside of bone and occurs most frequently in the soft tissues of the lower extremity in middle-aged adults (Bane et al. 1990; Patel and Benjamin 1995; Wurlitzer et al. 1972). Local recurrences and distant metastases invariably follow limited surgery (Bane et al. 1990; Wurlitzer et al. 1972). Multifocal osteosarcoma is a rare entity in which multiple synchronous skeletal tumors are present at diagnosis and each lesion resembles a primary tumor radiographically, suggesting a multicentric origin of the sarcoma. It is not clear whether such sarcomas arise in multiple sites or whether one of the lesions is the true primary that has spread rapidly to other skeletal sites in the absence of lung metastases (Fitzgerald et al. 1973; Hopper et al. 1993). Interestingly, a study of four patients with multifocal osteosarcoma revealed germline mutations of the p53 gene in two of the cases (Iavarone et al. 1992).

10.5 Clinical Presentation and Natural History

The most common presentation for osteosarcoma is pain at the site of the primary tumor. Pain is usually episodic at first, then becomes more intense and persistent. Pain can precede diagnosis by many months (Bielack et al. 2002; Pollock et al. 1991). Osteosarcoma can arise in any bone of the body, but it is most common in the metaphyses of the long bones, especially in children and young adults. In every series, the single most common site of primary tumor is the distal femur (Dahlin and Unni 1977; Dahlin and Coventry 1967; Huvos 1991; Weinfeld and Dudley 1962). The next two most common sites are the proximal tibia and the proximal humerus. At least half of osteosarcomas arise around the knee joint. Approximately 15–20% of patients with osteosarcoma have clinically detectable metastatic disease at initial presentation (Bielack et al. 2002; Kaste et al. 1999). By far the most common site for metastatic disease is the lungs, but metastases have been described in bones, soft tissues, and lymph nodes. The presence of multiple bone lesions may represent multifocal osteosarcoma, which has been uniformly fatal (Fitzgerald et al. 1973; Hopper et al. 1993).

10.6 Diagnostic Evaluation

The initial evaluation of the child or young adult with a primary bone lesion requires a complete history, physical examination and plain radiographs of the affected bone. Three dimensional imaging studies of the primary tumor site are essential to define the nature and extent of the tumor. Both MRI and CT scans have been employed and provide different and valuable information about soft tissue spread and joint involvement.

Detailed examination of the lungs and bones is required to determine the presence of clinically detectable metastatic disease. CT of the chest is more sensitive in detecting pulmonary metastases than conventional chest radiograph. CT scan is the choice for screening patients with osteosarcoma for metastatic disease, although false positive results can be a problem with this technique (Kesselring and Penn 1982; Muhm et al. 1978; Neifeld et al. 1977; Schaner et al. 1978; Vanel et al. 1984). If there is any doubt that a lesion on CT scan represents metastatic disease, histologic confirmation is indicated, especially if the lesion does not appear on plain radiographs. Metastases to other bones of the skeleton are seen in approximately 10% of patients with osteosarcoma and a radionuclide bone scan is indicated in screening for metastatic disease. Scanning with methylene diphosphonate labeled with technetium-99m is a very sensitive technique for the detection of metastatic bony sites, and is more sensitive than plain radiographs (McKillop et al. 1981; Kirchner and Simon 1981). Additional baseline studies are being performed to serve as reference for subsequent follow-up which can help to evaluate tumor response to initial treatment. These include dynamic MRI, PET scan, and thallium scanning.

Successful treatment of osteosarcoma requires a combination of systemic chemotherapy and surgical resection of all sites of clinically detectable metastatic disease. Evaluations prior to chemotherapy include a complete blood count with platelet count and differential, tests of renal function, including serum BUN and creatinine and creatinine clearance determination, evaluation of liver function including transaminases and bilirubin, coagulation profile, hepatitis and HIV testing. Both alkaline phosphatase and lactic dehydrogenase (LDH) levels correlate with prognosis, and decrease in elevated alkaline phosphatase and LDH have been associated with favorable response to treatment (Bacci et al. 1993, 1994; Meyers et al. 1992). Almost all chemotherapy regimens for the treatment of osteosarcoma include doxorubicin and cisplatin, so baseline evaluation of cardiac and auditory function are required. Both radionuclide cardiac angiography and echocardiogram have been used to follow cardiac function. Formal audiometric testing is performed at baseline and during treatment.

The degree of necrosis in the primary tumor following induction chemotherapy correlates well with the subsequent probability for event-free survival (Bielack et al. 2002; Meyers et al. 1992). Knowledge of the degree of necrosis prior to surgery can assist the surgeon in planning resection of the primary tumor. Several non-invasive techniques are being investigated for their ability to predict the degree of necrosis in the primary tumor specimen. It is important to note that none of them has yet been shown to predict ultimate event free survival, for which necrosis is only a surrogate.

The follow-up evaluation of the patient with osteosarcoma includes imaging of the lungs frequently during the first 2 years following completion of therapy and less frequently thereafter. Imaging of the lungs is necessary because pulmonary recurrence will be asymptomatic until metastatic lesions are very large, and salvage following pulmonary recurrence is more likely if detected at an early stage. There is no consensus among investigators about the frequency of evaluation or whether plain radiographs or CT scans are preferable. CT scan will identify lesions at a smaller size than plain radiographs, but there is no evidence that the detection of lesion which is only a few millimeters smaller provides a survival advantage to the patient following recurrence.

10.7 Biopsy

Even though the physical findings and plain radiograph often appear pathognomonic for osteosarcoma, a biopsy is still mandatory. Since most biopsies in children are performed with general anesthesia, the chest CT scan of the chest should be performed prior to the biopsy to avoid the possibility that postoperative atelectasis will be confused with pulmonary metastasis. The biopsy should be performed or directed by an orthopedic surgeon familiar with the management of malignant bone tumors and experienced in the required techniques (Mankin et al. 1982, 1996; Springfield and Rosenberg 1996), and preferably by the surgeon who will ultimately perform the definitive surgical procedure (Springfield and Rosenberg 1996; Mankin et al. 1996).

The surgeon should plan the biopsy carefully, with consideration of subsequent definitive surgery (or radiotherapy), because a poorly conceived and poorly placed biopsy may jeopardize the subsequent treatment, especially a limb-salvage procedure (Mankin et al. 1996; Peabody and Simon 1996).

10.8 Staging

Standard staging systems do not work well for osteosarcoma. The first successful staging system was devised by Enneking et al. for the Musculoskeletal Tumor Society (MSTS) (Enneking et al. 1980). Stage I refers to low-grade tumors, Stage II to high grade tumors, and Stage III to tumors with clinically detectable metastasis. A suffix is added to the stage which describes the extent of the primary tumor. Intracompartmental tumors are labeled A and extracompartmental tumors are labeled B. Almost all conventional osteosarcomas are Stage IIB in the MSTS classification. An effort has been made to adapt the TNM staging of the UICC to bone sarcomas (Sobin and Wittekind 2002). Tumors less than or equal to 8 cm are classified as T1; tumors larger than 8 cm are classified as T2; and tumors associated with skip metastases are classified as T3. Clinically detectable metastases in the lung are graded as M1a; metastases in any other site are graded as M1b.

10.9 Prognostic Factors

Several clinical characteristics are thought to be of prognostic significance for patients with osteosarcoma, independent of therapy (Bielack et al. 2002). They may become less important as the outcome for patients with osteosarcoma continues to improve. The single most important predictor of outcome is the presence of clinically detectable metastatic disease at diagnosis. Patients with overt metastatic disease have an unfavorable outcome. Although aggressive approaches to patients presenting with metastases have improved their prognosis somewhat, the majority of such patients ultimately die of their disease.

The primary site of disease is an important variable. Several series (Bielack et al. 2002; Lockshin and Higgins 1968; Simon 1978) report that patients with axial skeleton primaries have a poor prognosis (Bielack et al. 2002; Lockshin and Higgins 1968; Simon 1978). Surgical excision with clean margins is a prerequisite for long-term disease control, and tumors arising in certain axial skeleton sites (e.g., skull, vertebrae) are not amenable to curative surgery. Incomplete resection of the primary tumor (regardless of the primary site) is associated with a poor outcome (Bielack et al. 2002; Jaffe et al. 2002). In general, more distal primaries have been associated with a more favorable prognosis, and tumors of the proximal femur and humerus with a less favorable outcome (Bielack et al. 2002).

Tumor size correlates with prognosis: smaller tumors are associated with a higher probability of event free survival than larger tumors (Bielack et al. 2002). Additional patient characteristics reported to be associated with a favorable outcome are older age, female sex, and lower levels of alkaline phosphatase and LDH (Bielack et al. 2002; Meyers et al. 1992).

Several studies have attempted to identify molecular markers of prognosis. A study of a small number of patients with osteosarcoma examined LOH at the RB gene locus and found that patients whose tumors demonstrated no LOH at RB were less likely to present with metastatic disease, and all such patients were projected to survive without recurrence at 5 years (Feugeas et al. 1996). In patients with osteosarcoma, overexpression of the human epidermal growth factor receptor 2 (HER2/erbB-2) has been associated with an inferior outcome in some studies (Gorlick et al. 1999; Onda et al. 1996). Ezrin is a membrane-cytoskeleton linkage protein. High ezrin expression in dog tumors was associated with early development of metastases. A significant association between high ezrin expression and poor outcome in pediatric osteosarcoma patients has been reported (Khanna et al. 2004). The role of telomeres has also been investigated. One study has demonstrated that the absence of both telomerase activation and activation of alternative lengthening of telomeres was more strongly associated with improved survival than was stage (Ulaner et al. 2003). The Wingless-type (Wnt) family of proteins and its coreceptor LRP5 have been studied in osteosarcoma. The presence of LRP5 correlated significantly with tumor metastasis and the chondroblastic subtype of OS (Hoang et al. 2004). Caution must be exercised in the interpretation of all of the studies of novel prognostic factors. Prognostic factors are typically identified (as in the case of most of the factors included here) through retrospective analysis. Demonstration that a candidate factor is a robust predictor of outcome requires validation in a prospective evaluation (Meyers 2002). None of the biological factors that have been reported to have prognostic value in osteosarcoma are currently sufficiently robust to justify treatment stratification. Further studies to confirm or refute the value of these biological markers are clearly indicated.

The amount of necrosis observed in the resected primary tumor specimen following induction chemotherapy correlates well with subsequent outcome (Bielack et al. 2002; Meyers et al. 1992, 1998). Necrosis is not a true prognostic factor, since it cannot be assessed prior to the initiation of therapy. Several classification schemes have been developed, but in general patients who demonstrate fewer than 2% residual viable tumor cells in the resection specimen have a better prognosis than those patients with higher proportions of viable tumor cells remaining. In theory, more aggressive therapy can be administered to those with a poor histologic response; however, to date no studies have demonstrated the efficacy of this approach.

Resistance to chemotherapy is probably responsible for poor outcome in some patients with osteosarcoma. The MDR-1 gene encodes the p-glycoprotein, an active pump mechanism which excludes certain classes of drugs from the cells, including some chemotherapeutic agents. Some studies have shown that the overexpression of p-glycoprotein is associated with unfavorable necrosis in the primary tumor following chemotherapy and an unfavorable outcome in patients with osteosarcoma treated with multiagent chemotherapy (Baldini et al. 1995; Chan et al. 1997). The method for assessing expression of p-glycoprotein may be important. Studies have failed to show a correlation between MDR1 expression as assessed by RT-PCR and immunohistochemistry for p-glycoprotein (Wunder et al. 2000). One evaluation of diagnostic specimens from patients with osteosarcoma failed to show any correlation among p-glycoprotein immunohistochemistry, MDR expression assessed by measurement of MDR mRNA, MDR expression assessed by in vivo imaging with sestamibi, and histologic response (Gorlick et al. 2001). Studies have also been performed to investigate mechanisms by which osteosarcoma may develop resistance to methotrexate. Mutations within the reduced folate carrier gene are common in osteosarcoma, resulting in loss of activity of the carrier, and this translates into a lower probability of favorable histologic response in the primary tumor after treatment with multiagent chemotherapy which includes high-dose methotrexate (Guo et al. 1999; Yang et al. 2003).

10.10 Treatment

Successful treatment of osteosarcoma requires effective systemic chemotherapy and complete surgical resection, preferably with wide margins, of all clinically detectable disease, including sites of metastasis (Bielack et al. 2002; Meyers et al. 1992, 1993). Prior to the introduction of systemic chemotherapy, 2-year survival following the diagnosis of osteosarcoma ranged from 10% to 20% (Dahlin and Coventry 1967; Friedman and Carter 1972; Marcove et al. 1970; Weinfeld and Dudley 1962). Chemotherapy trials in patients with measurable disease have demonstrated activity for cisplatin (Baum et al. 1981; Gasparini et al. 1985; Ochs et al. 1978), doxorubicin (Cortes et al. 1974; Pratt and Shanks 1974), high-dose methotrexate with leucovorin rescue (Cortes et al. 1974; Pratt and Shanks 1974), ifosfamide (Harris et al. 1995), and ifosfamide with etoposide (Goorin et al. 2002). Several early series of multiagent adjuvant chemotherapy following surgical extirpation of the primary tumor concluded that chemotherapy significantly reduced the incidence of recurrence compared to historical controls (Goorin et al. 1981; Pratt et al. 1977, 1978; Sutow et al. 1978; Sutow et al. 1975). Other investigators were concerned that the apparent benefit of adjuvant chemotherapy was due to improved detection of metastatic disease with modern CT scans, improved surgery, or patient selection (Carter 1984; Taylor et al. 1985). Two prospective trials randomly assigned young patients with osteosarcoma to observation or adjuvant chemotherapy following surgery and clearly demonstrated the benefit of chemotherapy (Eilber et al. 1987; Link et al. 1986). In both studies, patients who did not receive adjuvant chemotherapy experienced a high rate of recurrence, confirming that the natural history of the disease had not changed.

The group at the Memorial Sloan-Kettering Cancer Center introduced the concept of an initial period of chemotherapy prior to definitive surgical resection of the primary tumor (Rosen et al. 1976, 1979). The impetus for this approach was the contemporaneous development of techniques to resect the primary tumor and preserve an anatomic and functional extremity. In that era, all endoprosthetic replacements were custom made, and chemotherapy was used to control the disease until the prosthesis was ready for insertion. The investigators noted that tumors frequently decreased in size in response to this initial period of chemotherapy variously referred to as preoperative, neoadjuvant, or induction chemotherapy. The strategy of primary definitive surgery followed by adjuvant chemotherapy has been compared to the strategy of induction chemotherapy followed by definitive surgery followed by maintenance chemotherapy in a randomized prospective trial (Goorin et al. 2003). The outcome was the same for both strategies. Most orthopedic oncologists who treat osteosarcoma believe that induction chemotherapy improves the chances for and quality of limb preservation surgery, and most patients with osteosarcoma currently receive induction chemotherapy prior to definitive surgical resection.

The administration of induction chemotherapy prior to definitive surgical resection allows the pathologist to assess necrosis in the primary tumor following initial treatment. The degree of necrosis correlates well with the probability for subsequent event-free survival. Early reports suggested that alteration in maintenance chemotherapy for patients with inferior necrosis following induction chemotherapy could improve the prognosis for this unfavorable group (Rosen et al. 1982). With longer follow-up, the apparent benefit was no longer seen, and other investigators have not been able to confirm the value of changing chemotherapy (Meyers et al. 1992; Provisor et al. 1997; Winkler et al. 1988). Intensification of induction chemotherapy can modestly increase the fraction of patients with favorable necrosis at definitive surgery, but does not result in enhanced event-free survival (Meyers et al. 1998).

Many trials have been performed in an effort to identify the optimal treatment for osteosarcoma. Most of these trials have been conducted by cooperative groups because very few institutions see enough patients with osteosarcoma to perform trials with adequate power. German and Austrian centers have conducted trials under the auspices of the Cooperative Osteosarcoma Study Group (COSS). Concerned about significant toxicity from cisplatin and doxorubicin, COSS investigators carried out a trial (COSS 82) in which cisplatin and doxorubicin were administered only to patients with unfavorable necrosis following induction chemotherapy (Winkler et al. 1988). This strategy proved unsuccessful, since only 44% of patients with unfavorable necrosis achieved event-free survival after salvage chemotherapy with doxorubicin and cisplatin, and the authors concluded that cisplatin and doxorubicin are an important component of therapy for osteosarcoma. More recent COSS trials have incorporated high-dose methotrexate, doxorubicin, and cisplatin, and report a 10-year survival of 71% for patients who presented without clinically detectable metastatic disease (Fuchs et al. 1998). Several investigators have favored the administration of intra-arterial cisplatin, and report very high rates of favorable necrosis in the resected primary tumor (Jaffe et al. 1985, 1983; Wilkins et al. 2003). The strategy relies on enhanced local drug delivery to the primary tumor, which does nothing to enhance drug delivery to the microscopic metastatic disease in the lung or other tissues. COSS experience has shown that intra-arterial administration of cisplatin did not increase the probability of event-free survival compared to intravenous administration in the context of multiagent chemotherapy (Winkler et al. 1990).

Investigators in the United Kingdom and Europe have performed a series of trials under the auspices of the European Osteosarcoma Intergroup (EOI). The EOI performed a trial in which patients were randomly assigned to receive cisplatin and doxorubicin or these two agents in combination with high-dose methotrexate (Bramwell et al. 1992; Souhami et al. 1997). They saw no difference between the two regimens, but event-free survival at 3 years for both arms was less than 50%, considerably lower than achieved with contemporaneous trials in COSS and the Children's Oncology Group (COG). They concluded that high-dose methotrexate did not add benefit to cisplatin and doxorubicin, although all other cooperative groups do feel that this agent provides benefit, and have retained it as part of the overall strategy for the treatment of osteosarcoma. An EOI trial randomized patients between cisplatin and doxorubicin administered every 3 weeks and the same drugs and doses given every 2 weeks and saw no difference in outcome (Lewis et al. 2003).

The COG performed a randomized prospective trial in newly diagnosed patients with osteosarcoma (Meyers et al. 2005). All patients received identical cumulative doses of cisplatin, doxorubicin, and high-dose methotrexate. Patients were randomly assigned to receive or not to receive ifosfamide in addition to the three chemotherapy drugs. In a second randomization, patients were randomly assigned to receive or not to receive the biological agent muramyl tripeptide phosphatidyl ethanolamine encapsulated in liposomes (MTP) following definitive surgical resection. MTP is a derivative of the cell wall of bacille Calmette-Guérin and stimulates macrophages to become tumoricidal in the autologous setting (Kleinerman et al. 1993). The addition of ifosfamide to the other three chemotherapy agents did not enhance outcome. The addition of MTP to the three drug chemotherapy regimen did not enhance outcome. The addition of both ifosfamide and MTP to the three drug chemotherapy regimen appeared to improve the probability for event-free survival. The 3-year event-free survival for this regimen was 78%, one of the best results reported for a multi-institutional cooperative group trial. The mechanism of interaction between the alkylating agent ifosfamide and the biological agent MTP will require further investigation.

Further progress in the improvement of outcome for osteosarcoma will require international cooperation to acquire the large numbers of patients to address clinical questions in a reasonable period of time. The COG, COSS, EOI, and Scandinavian investigators have come together in an ambitious consortium to carry out a cooperative trial. The ad hoc cooperative group, called EURAMOS (for European-American osteosarcoma), will open a prospective randomized trial. Patients will receive a common induction with cisplatin, doxorubicin, and high-dose methotrexate. Patients will undergo definitive resection of the primary tumor. Patients with a favorable response to induction chemotherapy will continue the chemotherapy without modification, but will undergo randomization to receive or not to receive interferon. Scandinavian investigators have studied adjuvant interferon in osteosarcoma for many years, and have reported benefit (Strander et al. 1995). Patients with unfavorable necrosis following induction will be randomized to receive or not to receive ifosfamide and etoposide in addition to the three drugs employed in induction. The dose of ifosfamide will be higher than the dose employed in the COG trial, which failed to demonstrate benefit when added to the other three drugs and the ifosfamide will be given in conjunction with etoposide.

10.11 Surgery

Osteosarcoma is conventionally considered to be unresponsive to radiotherapy, so surgery is considered the mainstay of local control. Removal of all gross and microscopic tumor with a cuff of normal tissue completely surrounding the tumor is required to prevent local recurrence. Primary surgical procedures fall into two major categories; amputation and limb-salvage procedures. Both approaches incorporate the basic principle of en bloc excision of the tumor and biopsy site through normal tissue planes. The great majority of patients with osteosarcoma currently receive induction chemotherapy prior to definitive surgical resection. The choice of operation requires consideration of the location and size of the primary tumor, relationship to adjacent neurovascular structures, the age and skeletal maturity of the patient, the need for and possibility of reconstruction, and an estimate of the necrosis in the primary tumor following induction chemotherapy. Although no randomized studies have been performed, there does not appear to be a survival disadvantage for carefully selected patients treated by experienced surgeons with limb preserving operations (Gherlinzoni et al. 1992; Lindner et al. 1999; Simon 1988; Rosen et al. 1976; Rougraff et al. 1994). One center has shown that patients with a less than wide margin and poor histologic response to presurgical chemotherapy have a higher risk of local recurrence than those with a wide margin and a good histological response (Bacci et al. 1998b; Picci et al. 1994; Scully et al. 1996). If there is doubt that complete excision can be accomplished or if margins of resection are positive, amputation must be performed; local recurrence is intolerable, because metastatic spread of tumor invariably follows (Picci et al. 1994; Scully et al. 1996). The administration of chemotherapy cannot be relied on to compensate for inadequate surgery (Jaffe et al. 2002). Patients with osteosarcoma of the axial skeleton present a difficult problem since it is seldom possible to achieve wide margins of resection (Fahey et al. 1992; Ozaki et al. 2002, 2003). As with patients who have osteosarcoma of the extremity, success depends on the ability to achieve a complete resection (Bielack et al. 2002). More recent analysis demonstrates that patients who do achieve complete resection of axial primaries have a probability for event-free survival comparable to that for patients with extremity primary tumors (Bielack et al. 1995; Ozaki et al. 2003).

10.12 Radiation Therapy

Traditionally, osteosarcoma is thought of as a tumor not sensitive to radiation. For this reason, the standard treatment of osteosarcoma has been the combination of systemic chemotherapy and surgery. Optimal surgery requires obtaining wide margins of resection. This is difficult or impossible for tumors of the axial skeleton. Recent studies suggest that for tumors with positive margins of resection, adjuvant radiation therapy can reduce the risk of local recurrence, and enhance the probability of event-free survival (Machak et al. 2003; Ozaki et al. 2002, 2003). Osteosarcoma is distinguished by the formation of extracellular matrix osteoid and the ossification of that matrix. Bone seeking isotopes simulate the distribution of technetium and target sites of ossification. High-dose radioactive samarium has been used to achieve extremely high dosimetry to bony metastases of osteosarcoma, with clinical benefit (Anderson et al. 2002; Franzius et al. 2001). This technique is currently limited to palliative therapy, because the dose to bone results in an "innocent bystander" effect on the bone marrow, resulting in complete myeloablation, and requiring autologous stem cell reconstitution.

10.13 Recurrent Disease

The prognosis for patients with osteosarcoma who present without clinically metastatic disease has improved. In most large series, 65–75% of patients will achieve long-term event-free survival. This means that one-quarter to one-third of newly diagnosed patients will develop recurrent disease, and this proportion is significantly higher for patients who have clinically detectable metastatic disease at initial presentation. There is no universally accepted strategy to deal with recurrent osteosarcoma. All reports stress the necessity for complete surgical resection of all sites of clinically detectable disease, including lung and bone (Ferrari et al. 2003; Meyer et al. 1987; Saeter et al. 1995; Tabone et al. 1994). The use of adjuvant chemotherapy following resection of recurrent disease is controversial. One group has advocated observation following resection, reserving systemic chemotherapy for subsequent resection (Hawkins et al. 2003).

10.14 Future Directions

The most dramatic improvement in the outlook for patients with osteosarcoma came with the introduction of effective systemic chemotherapy. Unfortunately, there has been no significant improvement in the prognosis for patients with osteosarcoma in the last 15 years. Treatment with multiagent chemotherapy and surgery has achieved a plateau. New directions for treatment are required. Monoclonal antibodies against antigens expressed on the surface of tumor cells have demonstrated benefit in a number of other tumor systems. The human epidermal growth factor HER2 is expressed on the surface of some osteosarcoma tumors, and its expression is associated with increased risk for recurrence (Gorlick et al. 1999). Trastuzumab is a humanized monoclonal antibody against HER2. The COG is conducting a study to determine if the addition of trastuzumab to multiagent chemotherapy will enhance the prognosis of patients who present with the very highest risk metastatic osteosarcoma. The glycolipid antigen GD2 is expressed on the surface of osteosarcoma tumors. Monoclonal antibody against this antigen has been an effective addition to therapy against the developmental tumor, neuroblastoma. This approach could be extended to osteosarcoma. New agents under consideration for the treatment of osteosarcoma include novel antifolate compounds and gemcitabine (Merimsky et al. 2000).

References

Abramson DH, Ellsworth RM, Kitchin FD et al. (1984) Second nonocular tumors in retinoblastoma survivors. Are they radiation-induced? Ophthalmology 91:1351–1355

Anderson PM, Wiseman GA, Dispenzieri A et al. (2002) High-dose samarium-153 ethylene diamine tetramethylene phosphonate: low toxicity of skeletal irradiation in patients with osteosarcoma and bone metastases. J Clin Oncol 20:189–196

Bacci G, Picci P, Ferrari S et al. (1993) Prognostic significance of serum alkaline phosphatase measurements in patients with osteosarcoma treated with adjuvant or neoadjuvant chemotherapy. Cancer 71:1224–1230

Bacci G, Ferrari S, Sangiorgi L et al. (1994) Prognostic significance of serum lactate dehydrogenase in patients with osteosarcoma of the extremities. J Chemother 6:204–210

Bacci G, Ferrari S, Delepine N et al. (1998a) Predictive factors of histologic response to primary chemotherapy in osteosarcoma of the extremity: study of 272 patients preoperatively treated with high-dose methotrexate, doxorubicin, and cisplatin. J Clin Oncol 16:658–663

Bacci G, Ferrari S, Mercuri M et al. (1998b) Predictive factors for local recurrence in osteosarcoma: 540 patients with extremity tumors followed for minimum 2.5 years after neoadjuvant chemotherapy. Acta Orthop Scand 69:230–236

Bacci G, Ferrari S, Bertoni F et al. (2000) Long-term outcome for patients with nonmetastatic osteosarcoma of the extremity treated at the Istituto Ortopedico Rizzoli according to the Istituto Ortopedico Rizzoli/Osteosarcoma-2 Protocol: an updated report. J Clin Oncol 18:4016–4027

Bacci G, Bertoni F, Longhi A et al. (2003) Neoadjuvant chemotherapy for high-grade central osteosarcoma of the extremity. Histologic response to preoperative chemotherapy correlates with histologic subtype of the tumor. Cancer 97:3068–3075

Baldini N, Scotlandi K, Barbanti-Brodano G et al. (1995) Expression of P-glycoprotein in high-grade osteosarcomas in relation to clinical outcome. N Engl J Med 333:1380–1385

Balraj P, Concannon P, Jamal R et al. (2002) An unusual mutation in RECQ4 gene leading to Rothmund-Thomson syndrome. Mutat Res 508:99–105

Bane BL, Evans HL, Ro JY et al. (1990) Extraskeletal osteosarcoma. A clinicopathologic review of 26 cases. Cancer 65:2762–2770

Baum ES, Gaynon P, Greenberg L et al. (1981) Phase II trial cisplatin in refractory childhood cancer: Children's Cancer Study Group Report. Cancer Treat Rep 65:815–822

Bayani J, Zielenska M, Pandita A et al. (2003) Spectral karyotyping identifies recurrent complex rearrangements of chromosomes 8, 17, and 20 in osteosarcomas. Genes Chromosomes Cancer 36:7–16

Bertoni F, Dallera P, Bacchini P et al. (1991) The Istituto Rizzoli-Beretta experience with osteosarcoma of the jaw. Cancer 68:1555–1563

Bielack SS, Wulff B, Delling G et al. (1995) Osteosarcoma of the trunk treated by multimodal therapy: experience of the Cooperative Osteosarcoma Study Group (COSS). Med Pediatr Oncol 24:6–12

Bielack SS, Kempf-Bielack B, Delling G et al. (2002) Prognostic factors in high-grade osteosarcoma of the extremities or trunk: an analysis of 1,702 patients treated on neoadjuvant Cooperative Osteosarcoma Study Group Protocols. J Clin Oncol 20:776–790

Borden EC, Baker LH, Bell RS et al. (2003) Soft tissue sarcomas of adults: state of the translational science. Clin Cancer Res 9:1941–1956

Bramwell VH, Burgers M, Sneath R et al. (1992) A comparison of two short intensive adjuvant chemotherapy regimens in operable osteosarcoma of limbs in children and young adults: the first study of the European Osteosarcoma Intergroup. J Clin Oncol 10:1579–1591

Bridge JA, Nelson M, McComb E et al. (1997) Cytogenetic findings in 73 osteosarcoma specimens and a review of the literature. Cancer Genet Cytogenet 95:74–87

Carbone M, Rizzo P, Procopio A et al. (1996) SV40-like sequences in human bone tumors. Oncogene 13:527–535

Carter SK (1984) Adjuvant chemotherapy in osteogenic sarcoma: the triumph that isn't? J Clin Oncol 2:147–148

Chan HS, Grogan TM, Haddad G et al. (1997) P-glycoprotein expression: critical determinant in the response to osteosarcoma chemotherapy. J Natl Cancer Inst 89:1706–1715

Clark JL, Unni KK, Dahlin DC et al. (1983) Osteosarcoma of the jaw. Cancer 51:2311–2316

Cooley DM, Beranek BC, Schlittler DL et al. (2002) Endogenous gonadal hormone exposure and bone sarcoma risk. Cancer Epidemiol Biomarkers Prev 11:1434–1440

Cortes EP, Holland JF, Wang JJ et al. (1974) Amputation and adriamycin in primary osteosarcoma. N Engl J Med 291: 998–1000

Cotterill SJ, Wright CM, Pearce MS et al. (2004) Stature of young people with malignant bone tumors. Pediatr Blood Cancer 42:59–63

Dahlin DC, Coventry MB (1967) Osteogenic sarcoma. A study of six hundred cases. J Bone Joint Surg Am 49:101–110

Dahlin DC, Unni KK (1977) Osteosarcoma of bone and its important recognizable varieties. Am J Surg Pathol 1:61–72

Dahlin DC, Unni KK (1986) Osteosarcoma. In: Dahlin DC, Unni KK (eds) Bone tumors: general aspects and data on 8542 cases, 4th edn. Charles C. Thomas, Springfield, IL, pp 269–307

Diller L, Kassel J, Nelson CE et al. (1990) p53 functions as a cell cycle control protein in osteosarcomas. Mol Cell Biol 10:5772–5781

Dorfman HD, Czerniak B (1995) Bone cancers. Cancer 75: 203–210

Draper GJ, Sanders BM, Kingston JE (1986) Second primary neoplasms in patients with retinoblastoma. Br J Cancer 53:661–671

Drouin CA, Mongrain E, Sasseville D et al. (1993) Rothmund-Thomson syndrome with osteosarcoma. J Am Acad Dermatol 28:301–305

Eilber F, Giuliano A, Eckardt J et al. (1987) Adjuvant chemotherapy for osteosarcoma: a randomized prospective trial. J Clin Oncol 5:21–26

Enneking WF, Spanier SS, Goodman MA (1980) A system for the surgical staging of musculoskeletal sarcoma. Clin Orthop:106–120

Fahey M, Spanier SS, Vander Griend RA (1992) Osteosarcoma of the pelvis. A clinical and histopathological study of twenty-five patients. J Bone Joint Surg Am 74:321–330

Ferrari S, Briccoli A, Mercuri M et al. (2003) Postrelapse survival in osteosarcoma of the extremities: prognostic factors for long-term survival. J Clin Oncol 21:710–715

Feugeas O, Guriec N, Babin-Boilletot A et al. (1996) Loss of heterozygosity of the RB gene is a poor prognostic factor in patients with osteosarcoma. J Clin Oncol 14:467–472

Finkel MP, Biskis BO, Jinkins PB (1966) Virus induction of osteosarcomas in mice. Science 151:698–701

Finkel MP, Biskis BO, Farrell C (1968) Osteosarcomas appearing in Syrian hamsters after treatment with extracts of human osteosarcomas. Proc Natl Acad Sci USA 60:1223–1230

Fitzgerald RH Jr, Dahlin DC, Sim FH (1973) Multiple metachronous osteogenic sarcoma. Report of twelve cases with two long-term survivors. J Bone Joint Surg Am 55:595–605

Franzius C, Bielack S, Flege S et al. (2001) High-activity samarium-153-EDTMP therapy followed by autologous peripheral blood stem cell support in unresectable osteosarcoma. Nuklearmedizin 40:215–220

Friedlaender GE, Mitchell MS (1976) A virally induced osteosarcoma in rats. A model for immunological studies of human osteosarcoma. J Bone Joint Surg Am 58:295–302

Friedman MA, Carter SK (1972) The therapy of osteogenic sarcoma: current status and thoughts for the future. J Surg Oncol 4:482–510

Friend SH, Bernards R, Rogelj S et al. (1986) A human DNA segment with properties of the gene that predisposes to retinoblastoma and osteosarcoma. Nature 323:643–646

Fuchs N, Bielack SS, Epler D et al. (1998) Long-term results of the co-operative German-Austrian-Swiss Osteosarcoma Study Group's protocol COSS-86 of intensive multidrug chemotherapy and surgery for osteosarcoma of the limbs. Ann Oncol 9:893–899

Gadwal SR, Gannon FH, Fanburg-Smith JC et al. (2001) Primary osteosarcoma of the head and neck in pediatric patients: a clinicopathologic study of 22 cases with a review of the literature. Cancer 91:598–605

Gasparini M, Rouesse J, van Oosterom A et al. (1985) Phase II study of cisplatin in advanced osteogenic sarcoma. European Organization for Research on Treatment of Cancer Soft Tissue and Bone Sarcoma Group. Cancer Treat Rep 69:211–213

Gherlinzoni F, Picci P, Bacci G et al. (1992) Limb sparing versus amputation in osteosarcoma. Correlation between local control, surgical margins and tumor necrosis: Istituto Rizzoli experience. Ann Oncol 3 Suppl 2:S23–27

Goorin AM, Frei E 3rd, Abelson HT (1981) Adjuvant chemotherapy for osteosarcoma: a decade of experience. Surg Clin North Am 61:1379–1389

Goorin AM, Harris MB, Bernstein M et al. (2002) Phase II/III trial of etoposide and high-dose ifosfamide in newly diagnosed metastatic osteosarcoma: a pediatric oncology group trial. J Clin Oncol 20:426–433

Goorin AM, Schwartzentruber DJ, Devidas M et al. (2003) Presurgical chemotherapy compared with immediate surgery and adjuvant chemotherapy for nonmetastatic osteosarcoma: Pediatric Oncology Group Study POG-8651. J Clin Oncol 21:1574–1580

Gorlick R, Huvos AG, Heller G et al. (1999) Expression of HER2/erbB-2 correlates with survival in osteosarcoma. J Clin Oncol 17:2781–2788

Gorlick R, Liao AC, Antonescu C et al. (2001) Lack of correlation of functional scintigraphy with (99m)technetium-methoxyisobutylisonitrile with histological necrosis following induction chemotherapy or measures of P-glycoprotein expression in high-grade osteosarcoma. Clin Cancer Res 7:3065–3070

Guo W, Healey JH, Meyers PA et al. (1999) Mechanisms of methotrexate resistance in osteosarcoma. Clin Cancer Res 5:621–627

Gurney JG Swensen AR, Bulterys M (1999) Malignant bone tumors. In: Ries LAG Smith MA, Gurney JG et al. (eds) Cancer incidence and survival among children and adolescents: United States SEER Program 1975–1995. National Cancer Institute SEER Program, Bethesda, MD, pp 99–110

Harris H (1986) Malignant tumours generated by recessive mutations. Nature 323:582–583

Harris MB, Cantor AB, Goorin AM et al. (1995) Treatment of osteosarcoma with ifosfamide: comparison of response in pediatric patients with recurrent disease versus patients previously untreated: a Pediatric Oncology Group study. Med Pediatr Oncol 24:87–92

Harrist TJ, Schiller AL, Trelstad RL et al. (1979) Thorotrast-associated sarcoma of bone: A case report and review of the literature. Cancer 44:2049–2058

Hawkins DS, Arndt CA (2003) Pattern of disease recurrence and prognostic factors in patients with osteosarcoma treated with contemporary chemotherapy. Cancer 98:2447–2456

Hoang BH, Kubo T, Healey JH et al. (2004) Expression of LDL receptor-related protein 5 (LRP5) as a novel marker for disease progression in high-grade osteosarcoma. Int J Cancer 109:106–111

Hopper KD, Eggli KD, Haseman DB et al. (1993) Osteosarcomatosis and metastatic osteosarcoma. Cancer Treat Res 62:163–171

Huang HJ, Yee JK, Shew JY et al. (1988) Suppression of the neoplastic phenotype by replacement of the RB gene in human cancer cells. Science 242:1563–1566

Huvos A (1991) Bone tumors: diagnosis, treatment and prognosis, 2nd edn. WB Saunders, Philadelphia, PA

Iavarone A, Matthay KK, Steinkirchner TM et al. (1992) Germline and somatic p53 gene mutations in multifocal osteogenic sarcoma. Proc Natl Acad Sci USA 89:4207–4209

Jaffe N, Knapp J, Chuang VP et al. (1983) Osteosarcoma: intra-arterial treatment of the primary tumor with *cis*-diammine-dichloroplatinum II (CDP). Angiographic, pathologic, and pharmacologic studies. Cancer 51:402–407

Jaffe N, Robertson R, Ayala A et al. (1985) Comparison of intra-arterial *cis*-diamminedichloroplatinum II with high-dose methotrexate and citrovorum factor rescue in the treatment of primary osteosarcoma. J Clin Oncol 3:1101–1104

Jaffe N, Carrasco H, Raymond K et al. (2002) Can cure in patients with osteosarcoma be achieved exclusively with chemotherapy and abrogation of surgery? Cancer 95:2202–2210

Kaste SC, Pratt CB, Cain AM et al. (1999) Metastases detected at the time of diagnosis of primary pediatric extremity osteosarcoma at diagnosis: imaging features. Cancer 86:1602–1608

Kesselring FO, Penn W (1982) Radiological aspects of 'classic' primary osteosarcoma: value of some radiological investigations: A review. Diagn Imaging 51:78–92

Khanna C, Wan X, Bose S et al. (2004) The membrane-cytoskeleton linker ezrin is necessary for osteosarcoma metastasis. Nat Med 10:182–186

Kirchner PT, Simon MA (1981) Radioisotopic evaluation of skeletal disease. J Bone Joint Surg Am 63:673–681

Kleinerman ES, Maeda M, Jaffe N (1993) Liposome-encapsulated muramyl tripeptide: a new biologic response modifier for the treatment of osteosarcoma. Cancer Treat Res 62:101–107

Kruzelock RP, Hansen MF (1995) Molecular genetics and cytogenetics of sarcomas. Hematol Oncol Clin North Am 9:513–540

Kruzelock RP, Murphy EC, Strong LC et al. (1997) Localization of a novel tumor suppressor locus on human chromosome 3q important in osteosarcoma tumorigenesis. Cancer Res 57:106–109

Ladanyi M, Cha C, Lewis R et al. (1993) MDM2 gene amplification in metastatic osteosarcoma. Cancer Res 53:16–18

Lane DP (1992) Cancer. p53, guardian of the genome. Nature 358:15–16

Lednicky JA, Stewart AR, Jenkins JJ 3rd et al. (1997) SV40 DNA in human osteosarcomas shows sequence variation among T-antigen genes. Int J Cancer 72:791–800

Lewis IJ, Nooij M (2003) Chemotherapy at standard or increased dose intensity in patients with operable osteosarcoma of the extremity: A randomized controlled trial conducted by the European Osteosarcoma Intergroup. American Society of Clinical Oncology, Chicago, IL, p 816

Li FP, Fraumeni JF Jr (1969a) Rhabdomyosarcoma in children: epidemiologic study and identification of a familial cancer syndrome. J Natl Cancer Inst 43:1365–1373

Li FP, Fraumeni JF Jr (1969b) Soft-tissue sarcomas, breast cancer, and other neoplasms. A familial syndrome? Ann Intern Med 71:747–752

Lindner NJ, Ramm O, Hillmann A et al. (1999) Limb salvage and outcome of osteosarcoma. The University of Muenster experience. Clin Orthop 358:120–127

Link MP, Goorin AM, Miser AW et al. (1986) The effect of adjuvant chemotherapy on relapse-free survival in patients with osteosarcoma of the extremity. N Engl J Med 314: 1600–1606

Lockshin MD, Higgins IT (1968) Prognosis in osteogenic sarcoma. Clin Orthop 58:85–103

Loutit J (1970) Malignancy from radium. Br J Cancer 24:195–207

Machak GN, Tkachev SI, Solovyev YN et al. (2003) Neoadjuvant chemotherapy and local radiotherapy for high-grade osteosarcoma of the extremities. Mayo Clin Proc 78:147–155

Mankin HJ, Lange TA, Spanier SS (1982) The hazards of biopsy in patients with malignant primary bone and soft-tissue tumors. J Bone Joint Surg Am 64:1121–1127

Mankin HJ, Mankin CJ, Simon MA (1996) The hazards of the biopsy, revisited. Members of the Musculoskeletal Tumor Society [see comments]. J Bone Joint Surg Am 78:656–663

Marcove RC, Mike V, Hajek JV et al. (1970) Osteogenic sarcoma under the age of twenty-one. A review of one hundred and forty-five operative cases. J Bone Joint Surg Am 52:411–423

McKillop JH, Etcubanas E, Goris ML (1981) The indications for and limitations of bone scintigraphy in osteogenic sarcoma: a review of 55 patients. Cancer 48:1133–1138

Meadows AT, Strong LC, Li FP et al. (1980) Bone sarcoma as a second malignant neoplasm in children: influence of radiation and genetic predisposition for the Late Effects Study Group. Cancer 46:2603–2606

Mendoza SM, Konishi T, Miller CW (1998) Integration of SV40 in human osteosarcoma DNA. Oncogene 17:2457–2462

Merimsky O, Meller I, Flusser G et al. (2000) Gemcitabine in soft tissue or bone sarcoma resistant to standard chemotherapy: a phase II study. Cancer Chemother Pharmacol 45:177–181

Meyer WH, Schell MJ, Kumar AP et al. (1987) Thoracotomy for pulmonary metastatic osteosarcoma. An analysis of prognostic indicators of survival. Cancer 59:374–379

Meyers P (2002) Prognostic factors for sarcomas: Hard and soft. J Clin Oncol 20:627–629

Meyers PA, Heller G, Healey J et al. (1992) Chemotherapy for nonmetastatic osteogenic sarcoma: the Memorial Sloan-Kettering experience. J Clin Oncol 10:5–15

Meyers PA, Heller G, Healey JH et al. (1993) Osteogenic sarcoma with clinically detectable metastasis at initial presentation. J Clin Oncol 11:449–453

Meyers PA, Gorlick R, Heller G et al. (1998) Intensification of preoperative chemotherapy for osteogenic sarcoma: results of the Memorial Sloan-Kettering (T12) protocol. J Clin Oncol 16:2452–2458

Meyers P, Schwartz CL, Krailo M, Kleinerman ES, Betcher D, Bernstein ML, Conrad E, Ferguson W, Gebhardt M, Goorin AM, Harris MB, Healey J, Huvos A, Link M, Montebello J, Nadel H, Nieder M, Sato J, Siegal G, Weiner M, Wells R, Wold L, Womer R, Grier H (2005) Osteosarcoma: A randomized, prospective trial of the addition of ifosfamide and/or muramyl tripeptide to cisplatin, doxorubicin, and high-dose methotrexate. J Clin Oncol 23(9)2004–2011

Miller CW, Aslo A, Tsay C et al. (1990) Frequency and structure of p53 rearrangements in human osteosarcoma. Cancer Res 50:7950–7954

Muhm JR, Brown LR, Crowe JK et al. (1978) Comparison of whole lung tomography and computed tomography for detecting pulmonary nodules. AJR Am J Roentgenol 131:981–984

Murphree AL, Benedict WF (1984) Retinoblastoma: clues to human oncogenesis. Science 223:1028–1033

Neifeld JP, Michaelis LL, Doppman JL (1977) Suspected pulmonary metastases: correlation of chest x-ray, whole lung tomograms, and operative findings. Cancer 39:383–387

Ochs JJ, Freeman AI, Douglass HO Jr. et al. (1978) *cis*-Dichlorodiammineplatinum (II) in advanced osteogenic sarcoma. Cancer Treat Rep 62:239–245

Onda M, Matsuda S, Higaki S et al. (1996) ErbB-2 expression is correlated with poor prognosis for patients with osteosarcoma. Cancer 77:71–78

Ozaki T, Flege S, Liljenqvist U et al. (2002) Osteosarcoma of the spine: experience of the Cooperative Osteosarcoma Study Group. Cancer 94:1069–1077

Ozaki T, Flege S, Kevric M et al. (2003) Osteosarcoma of the pelvis: experience of the Cooperative Osteosarcoma Study Group. J Clin Oncol 21:334–341

Patel SG, Meyers P, Huvos AG et al. (2002) Improved outcomes in patients with osteogenic sarcoma of the head and neck. Cancer 95:1495–1503

Patel SR, Benjamin RS (1995) Primary extraskeletal osteosarcoma – experience with chemotherapy. J Natl Cancer Inst 87:1331–1333

Peabody TD, Simon MA (1996) Making the diagnosis: keys to a successful biopsy in children with bone and soft-tissue tumors. Orthop Clin North Am 27:453–459

Picci P, Sangiorgi L, Rougraff BT et al. (1994) Relationship of chemotherapy-induced necrosis and surgical margins to local recurrence in osteosarcoma. J Clin Oncol 12:2699–2705

Pollock BH, Krischer JP, Vietti TJ (1991) Interval between symptom onset and diagnosis of pediatric solid tumors. J Pediatr 119:725–732

Pratt CB, Shanks EC (1974) Doxorubicin in treatment of malignant solid tumors in children. Am J Dis Child 127: 534–536

Pratt C, Shanks E, Hustu O et al. (1977) Adjuvant multiple drug chemotherapy for osteosarcoma of the extremity. Cancer 39:51–57

Pratt CB, Rivera G, Shanks E et al. (1978) Combination chemotherapy for osteosarcoma. Cancer Treat Rep 62:251–257

Price CH (1958) Primary bone-forming tumours and their relationship to skeletal growth. J Bone Joint Surg Br 36: 1137–1150

Provisor AJ, Ettinger LJ, Nachman JB et al. (1997) Treatment of nonmetastatic osteosarcoma of the extremity with preoperative and postoperative chemotherapy: a report from the Children's Cancer Group. J Clin Oncol 15:76–84

Rosen G, Murphy ML, Huvos AG et al. (1976) Chemotherapy, en bloc resection, and prosthetic bone replacement in the treatment of osteogenic sarcoma. Cancer 37:1–11

Rosen G, Marcove RC, Caparros B et al. (1979) Primary osteogenic sarcoma: the rationale for preoperative chemotherapy and delayed surgery. Cancer 43:2163–2177

Rosen G, Caparros B, Huvos AG et al. (1982) Preoperative chemotherapy for osteogenic sarcoma: selection of postoperative adjuvant chemotherapy based on the response of the primary tumor to preoperative chemotherapy. Cancer 49:1221–1230

Rougraff BT, Simon MA, Kneisl JS et al. (1994) Limb salvage compared with amputation for osteosarcoma of the distal end of the femur. A long-term oncological, functional, and quality-of-life study. J Bone Joint Surg Am 76:649–656

Saeter G, Hoie J, Stenwig AE et al. (1995) Systemic relapse of patients with osteogenic sarcoma. Prognostic factors for long term survival. Cancer 75:1084–1093

Sandberg AA, Bridge JA (2003) Updates on the cytogenetics and molecular genetics of bone and soft tissue tumors: osteosarcoma and related tumors. Cancer Genet Cytogenet 145:1–30

Schaner EG, Chang AE, Doppman JL et al. (1978) Comparison of computed and conventional whole lung tomography in detecting pulmonary nodules: a prospective radiologic-pathologic study. AJR Am J Roentgenol 131:51–54

Scully SP, Temple HT, O'Keefe RJ et al. (1996) The surgical treatment of patients with osteosarcoma who sustain a pathologic fracture. Clin Orthop:227–232

Sim FH, Cupps RE, Dahlin DC et al. (1972) Postradiation sarcoma of bone. J Bone Joint Surg Am 54:1479–1489

Simon MA (1988) Limb salvage for osteosarcoma. J Bone Joint Surg Am 70:307–310

Simon R (1978) Clinical prognostic factors in osteosarcoma. Cancer Treat Rep 62:193–197

Smeele LE, Kostense PJ, van der Waal I et al. (1997) Effect of chemotherapy on survival of craniofacial osteosarcoma: a systematic review of 201 patients. J Clin Oncol 15:363–367

Smith LM, Donaldson SS, Egbert PR et al. (1989) Aggressive management of second primary tumors in survivors of hereditary retinoblastoma. Int J Radiat Oncol Biol Phys 17:499–505

Sobin LH, Wittekind C (2002) UICC TNM classification of malignant tumors, 6th edn. Wiley, New York, NY

Souhami RL, Craft AW, Van der Eijken JW et al. (1997) Randomised trial of two regimens of chemotherapy in operable osteosarcoma: a study of the European Osteosarcoma Intergroup. Lancet 350:911–917

Spiess H, Mays CW (1970) Bone cancers induced by 224 Ra (Th X) in children and adults. Health Phys 19:713–729

Springfield DS, Rosenberg A (1996) Biopsy: complicated and risky. J Bone Joint Surg Am 78:639–643

Strander H, Bauer HC, Brosjo O et al. (1995) Long-term adjuvant interferon treatment of human osteosarcoma. A pilot study. Acta Oncol 34:877–880

Sutow WW, Sullivan MP, Fernbach DJ et al. (1975) Adjuvant chemotherapy in primary treatment of osteogenic sarcoma. A Southwest Oncology Group study. Cancer 36:1598–1602

Sutow WW, Gehan EA, Dyment PG et al. (1978) Multidrug adjuvant chemotherapy for osteosarcoma: interim report of the Southwest Oncology Group Studies. Cancer Treat Rep 62:265–269

Tabone MD, Kalifa C, Rodary C et al. (1994) Osteosarcoma recurrences in pediatric patients previously treated with intensive chemotherapy. J Clin Oncol 12:2614–2620

Taylor WF, Ivins JC, Pritchard DJ et al. (1985) Trends and variability in survival among patients with osteosarcoma: a 7-year update. Mayo Clin Proc 60:91–104

Tjalma RA (1966) Canine bone sarcoma: estimation of relative risk as a function of body size. J Natl Cancer Inst 36:1137–1150

Toguchida J, Yamaguchi T, Dayton SH et al. (1992) Prevalence and spectrum of germline mutations of the p53 gene among patients with sarcoma. N Engl J Med 326:1301–1308

Ulaner GA, Huang HY, Otero J et al. (2003) Absence of a telomere maintenance mechanism as a favorable prognostic factor in patients with osteosarcoma. Cancer Res 63:1759–1763

Vanel D, Henry-Amar M, Lumbroso J et al. (1984) Pulmonary evaluation of patients with osteosarcoma: roles of standard radiography, tomography, CT, scintigraphy, and tomoscintigraphy. AJR Am J Roentgenol 143:519–523

Wang LL, Gannavarapu A, Kozinetz CA et al. (2003) Association between osteosarcoma and deleterious mutations in the RECQL4 gene in Rothmund-Thomson syndrome. J Natl Cancer Inst 95:669–674

Wei G, Lonardo F, Ueda T et al. (1999) CDK4 gene amplification in osteosarcoma: reciprocal relationship with INK4A gene alterations and mapping of 12q13 amplicons. Int J Cancer 80:199–204

Weinfeld MS, Dudley HR Jr (1962) Osteogenic sarcoma. A follow-up study of the ninety-four cases observed at the Massachusetts General Hospital from 1920 to 1960. Am J Orthop 44A:269–276

Wilkins RM, Cullen JW, Odom L et al. (2003) Superior survival in treatment of primary nonmetastatic pediatric osteosarcoma of the extremity. Ann Surg Oncol 10:498–507

Winkler K, Beron G, Delling G et al. (1988) Neoadjuvant chemotherapy of osteosarcoma: results of a randomized cooperative trial (COSS-82) with salvage chemotherapy based on histological tumor response. J Clin Oncol 6:329–337

Winkler K, Bielack S, Delling G et al. (1990) Effect of intraarterial versus intravenous cisplatin in addition to systemic doxorubicin, high-dose methotrexate, and ifosfamide on histologic tumor response in osteosarcoma (study COSS-86). Cancer 66:1703–1710

Wunder JS, Bull SB, Aneliunas V et al. (2000) MDR1 gene expression and outcome in osteosarcoma: a prospective, multicenter study. J Clin Oncol 18:2685–2694

Wurlitzer F, Ayala L, Romsdahl M (1972) Extraosseous osteogenic sarcoma. Arch Surg 105:691–695

Yang R, Sowers R, Mazza B et al. (2003) Sequence alterations in the reduced folate carrier are observed in osteosarcoma tumor samples. Clin Cancer Res 9:837–844

Subject Index

A

B

C

D

E

F

G

N

O

P

Q

R

S

T

U

V

W

X

MIX
Papier aus verantwortungsvollen Quellen
Paper from responsible sources
FSC® C105338

If you have any concerns about our products,
you can contact us on
ProductSafety@springernature.com

In case Publisher is established outside the EU,
the EU authorized representative is:
Springer Nature Customer Service Center GmbH
Europaplatz 3, 69115 Heidelberg, Germany

Printed by Libri Plureos GmbH
in Hamburg, Germany